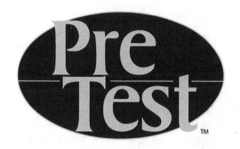

Surgery

PreTest™ Self-Assessment and Review

Notice

Medicine is an ever-changing science. As new research and clinical experience broaden our knowledge, changes in treatment and drug therapy are required. The authors and the publisher of this work have checked with sources believed to be reliable in their efforts to provide information that is complete and generally in accord with the standards accepted at the time of publication. However, in view of the possibility of human error or changes in medical sciences, neither the authors nor the publisher nor any other party who has been involved in the preparation or publication of this work warrants that the information contained herein is in every respect accurate or complete, and they disclaim all responsibility for any errors or omissions or for the results obtained from use of the information contained in this work. Readers are encouraged to confirm the information contained herein with other sources. For example and in particular, readers are advised to check the product information sheet included in the package of each drug they plan to administer to be certain that the information contained in this work is accurate and that changes have not been made in the recommended dose or in the contraindications for administration. This recommendation is of particular importance in connection with new or infrequently used drugs.

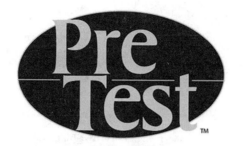

Surgery
PreTest™ Self-Assessment and Review
Twelfth Edition

Lillian S. Kao, MD
Associate Professor
Department of Surgery
University of Texas—Houston Medical School
Houston, Texas

Tammy Lee, MD
Assistant Professor
Department of Surgery
University of Texas—Houston Medical School
Houston, Texas

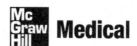

New York Chicago San Francisco Lisbon London Madrid Mexico City
Milan New Delhi San Juan Seoul Singapore Sydney Toronto

The **McGraw·Hill** Companies

Surgery: PreTest™ Self-Assessment and Review, Twelfth Edition

Copyright © 2009, 2006, 2003, 2001, 1998, 1995, 1992, 1989, 1987, 1985, 1982, 1978 by The McGraw-Hill Companies, Inc. All rights reserved. Printed in the United States of America. Except as permitted under the United States Copyright Act of 1976, no part of this publication may be reproduced or distributed in any form or by any means, or stored in a data base or retrieval system, without the prior written permission of the publisher.

PreTest™ is a trademark of The McGraw-Hill Companies, Inc.

2 3 4 5 6 7 8 9 0   DOC/DOC   12 11 10

ISBN 978-0-07-159863-7
MHID 0-07-159863-4

The book was set in Berkeley by International Typesetting and Composition.
The editors were Kirsten Funk and Karen Davis.
The production supervisor was Sherri Souffrance.
Project management was provided by Smita Rajan, International Typesetting and Composition.
The cover designer was Margaret Webster-Shapiro.
RR Donnelley was printer and binder.

This book is printed on acid-free paper.

Library of Congress Cataloging-in-Publication Data

Surgery : PreTest self-assessment and review. — 12th ed. / [edited by]
   Lillian S. Kao, Tammy Lee.
         p. ; cm.
   Includes bibliographical references and index.
   ISBN-13: 978-0-07-159863-7 (pbk.)
   ISBN-10: 0-07-159863-4
   1. Surgery—Examinations, questions, etc.   I. Kao, Lillian S.   II. Lee, Tammy.
   [DNLM: 1. Surgical Procedures, Operative—Examination Questions. WO
   18.2 S961   2009]
   RD37.2.S97   2009
   617.0076—dc22

                                                              2008052735

Student Reviewers

Mary Bonar
Ohio State University College of Osteopathic Medicine
Class of 2008

Edward Gould
SUNY Upstate College of Medicine
Class of 2009

Ranjith Ramasamy, MD
New York Presbyterian Hospital
Weill Medical College at Cornell University
PGY-2

Kevyn To
SUNY Upstate College of Medicine
Class of 2009

Judy Vu
University of Utah School of Medicine
Class of 2010

Contents

Introduction ix

Pre- and Postoperative Care

Questions 1
Answers 18

Critical Care: Anesthesiology, Blood Gases, and Respiratory Care

Questions 37
Answers 55

Skin: Wounds, Infections, and Burns; Hands; Plastic Surgery

Questions 73
Answers 81

Trauma and Shock

Questions 91
Answers 113

Transplants, Immunology, and Oncology

Questions 137
Answers 153

Endocrine Problems and the Breast

Questions 169
Answers 183

Gastrointestinal Tract, Liver, and Pancreas

Questions 197
Answers 226

Cardiothoracic Problems

Questions 253
Answers 268

Peripheral Vascular Problems

Questions 281
Answers 292

Urology

Questions 303
Answers 308

Orthopedics

Questions 315
Answers 321

Neurosurgery

Questions 327
Answers 333

Otolaryngology

Questions 339
Answers 343

Pediatric Surgery

Questions 347
Answers 355

Bibliography 363
Index 365

Introduction

Surgery: PreTest™ Self Assessment and Review, Twelfth Edition, is intended to provide medical students, as well as house officers and physicians, with a convenient tool for assessing and improving their knowledge of medicine. The 500+ questions in this book are similar in format and complexity to those included in Step 2 of the United States Medical Licensing Examination (USMLE). They may also be a useful study tool for Step 3.

For multiple-choice questions, the **one best** response to each question should be selected. For matching sets, a group of questions will be preceded by a list of lettered options. For each question in the matching set, select **one** lettered option that is **most** closely associated with the question. Each question in this book has a corresponding answer, a reference to a text that provides background to the answer, and a short discussion of various issues raised by the question and its answer. A listing of references for the entire book follows the last chapter.

To simulate the time constraints imposed by the qualifying examinations for which this book is intended as a practice guide, the student or physician should allot about 1 minute for each question. After answering all questions in a chapter, as much time as necessary should be spent in reviewing the explanations for each question at the end of the chapter. Attention should be given to all explanations, even if the examinee answered the question correctly. Those seeking more information on a subject should refer to the reference materials listed or to other standard texts in medicine.

Pre- and Postoperative Care

Questions

1. A 48-year-old woman develops constipation postoperatively and self-medicates with Milk of Magnesia. She presents to clinic, at which time her serum electrolytes are checked, and she is noted to have an elevated serum magnesium level. Which of the following represents the earliest clinical indication of hypermagnesemia?

a. Loss of deep tendon reflexes
b. Flaccid paralysis
c. Respiratory arrest
d. Hypotension
e. Stupor

2. Five days after an uneventful cholecystectomy, an asymptomatic middle-aged woman is found to have a serum sodium level of 125 mEq/L. Which of the following is the most appropriate management strategy for this patient?

a. Administration of hypertonic saline solution
b. Restriction of free water
c. Plasma ultrafiltration
d. Hemodialysis
e. Aggressive diuresis with furosemide

3. A 50-year-old patient presents with symptomatic nephrolithiasis. He reports that he underwent a jejunoileal bypass for morbid obesity when he was 39. Which of the following is a complication of jejunoileal bypass?

a. Pseudohyperparathyroidism
b. Hyperuric aciduria
c. Hungry bone syndrome
d. Hyperoxaluria
e. Sporadic unicameral bone cysts

4. Following surgery a patient develops oliguria. You believe the patient is hypovolemic, but you seek corroborative data before increasing intravenous fluids. Which of the following values supports the diagnosis of hypovolemia?

a. Urine sodium of 28 mEq/L
b. Urine chloride of 15 mEq/L
c. Fractional excretion of sodium less than 1
d. Urine/serum creatinine ratio of 20
e. Urine osmolality of 350 mOsm/kg

5. A 45-year-old woman with Crohn disease and a small intestinal fistula develops tetany during the second week of parenteral nutrition. The laboratory findings include:

Na: 135 mEq/L
K: 3.2 mEq/L
Cl: 103 mEq/L
HCO_3: 25 mEq/L
Ca: 8.2 mEq/L
Mg: 1.2 mEq/L
PO_4: 2.4 mEq/L
Albumin: 2.4

An arterial blood gas sample reveals a pH of 7.42, PCO_2 of 38 mm Hg, and PO_2 of 84 mm Hg. Which of the following is the most likely cause of the patient's tetany?

a. Hyperventilation
b. Hypocalcemia
c. Hypomagnesemia
d. Essential fatty acid deficiency
e. Focal seizure

6. A patient with a nonobstructing carcinoma of the sigmoid colon is being prepared for elective resection. Which of the following reduces the risk of postoperative infectious complications?

a. A single preoperative parenteral dose of antibiotic effective against aerobes and anaerobes
b. Avoidance of oral antibiotics to prevent emergence of *Clostridium difficile*
c. Postoperative administration for 48 hours of parenteral antibiotics effective against aerobes and anaerobes
d. Postoperative administration of parenteral antibiotics effective against aerobes and anaerobes until the patient's intravenous lines and all other drains are removed
e. Redosing of antibiotics in the operating room if the case lasts for more than 2 hours

7. A 75-year-old man with a history of myocardial infarction 2 years ago, peripheral vascular disease with symptoms of claudication after half block, hypertension, and diabetes presents with a large ventral hernia. He wishes to have the hernia repaired. Which of the following is the most appropriate next step in his preoperative workup?

a. A normal electrocardiogram (ECG) precludes the need for further cardiac testing.
b. He should undergo an exercise stress test.
c. He should undergo coronary artery bypass prior to operative repair of his ventral hernia.
d. He should undergo a persantine thallium stress test and echocardiography.
e. His history of a myocardial infarction within 3 years is prohibitive for elective surgery. No further testing is necessary.

8. A previously healthy 55-year-old man undergoes elective right hemicolectomy for a Stage I (T2N0M0) cancer of the cecum. His postoperative ileus is somewhat prolonged, and on the fifth postoperative day his nasogastric tube is still in place. Physical examination reveals diminished skin turgor, dry mucous membranes, and orthostatic hypotension. Pertinent laboratory values are as follows:

Arterial blood gases: pH 7.56, P_{CO_2} 50 mm Hg, P_{O_2} 85 mm Hg.
Serum electrolytes (mEq/L): Na^+ 132, K^+ 3.1, Cl^- 80; HCO_3^- 42.
Urine electrolytes (mEq/L): Na^+ 2, K^+ 5, Cl^- 6.

What is the patient's acid–base abnormality?

a. Uncompensated metabolic alkalosis
b. Respiratory acidosis with metabolic compensation
c. Combined metabolic and respiratory alkalosis
d. Metabolic alkalosis with respiratory compensation
e. Mixed respiratory acidosis and respiratory alkalosis

9. A 52-year-old man with gastric outlet obstruction secondary to a duodenal ulcer presents with hypochloremic, hypokalemic metabolic alkalosis. Which of the following is the most appropriate therapy for this patient?

a. Infusion of 0.9% NaCl with supplemental KCl until clinical signs of volume depletion are eliminated
b. Infusion of isotonic (0.15 N) HCl via a central venous catheter
c. Clamping the nasogastric tube to prevent further acid losses
d. Administration of acetazolamide to promote renal excretion of bicarbonate
e. Intubation and controlled hypoventilation on a volume-cycled ventilator to further increase P_{CO_2}

10. A 23-year-old woman is brought to the emergency room from a halfway house, where she apparently swallowed a handful of pills. The patient complains of shortness of breath and tinnitus, but refuses to identify the pills she ingested. Pertinent laboratory values are as follows:

Arterial blood gases: pH 7.45, P_{CO_2} 12 mm Hg, P_{O_2} 126 mm Hg.
Serum electrolytes (mEq/L): Na^+ 138, K^+ 4.8, Cl^- 102, HCO_3^- 8.

An overdose of which of the following drugs would be most likely to cause the acid–base disturbance in this patient?

a. Phenformin
b. Aspirin
c. Barbiturates
d. Methanol
e. Diazepam (Valium)

11. An 18-year-old previously healthy male is placed on intravenous heparin after having a pulmonary embolism (PE) after exploratory laparotomy for a small bowel injury following a motor vehicle collision. Five days later, his platelet count is 90,000/μL and continues to fall over the next several days. The patient's serum is positive for antibodies to the heparin-platelet factor complexes. Which of the following is the most appropriate next management step?

a. Cessation of all anticoagulation therapy
b. Cessation of heparin and immediate institution of high-dose warfarin therapy
c. Cessation of heparin and institution of low-molecular-weight heparin
d. Cessation of heparin and institution of lepirudin
e. Cessation of heparin and transfusion with platelets

12. A 65-year-old man undergoes a technically difficult abdominal–perineal resection for a rectal cancer during which he receives three units of packed red blood cells. Four hours later, in the intensive care unit (ICU), he is bleeding heavily from his perineal wound. Emergency coagulation studies reveal normal prothrombin, partial thromboplastin, and bleeding times. The fibrin degradation products are not elevated, but the serum fibrinogen content is depressed and the platelet count is 70,000/μL. Which of the following is the most likely cause of his bleeding?

a. Delayed blood transfusion reaction
b. Autoimmune fibrinolysis
c. A bleeding blood vessel in the surgical field
d. Factor VIII deficiency
e. Hypothermic coagulopathy

13. A 78-year-old man with a history of coronary artery disease and an asymptomatic reducible inguinal hernia requests an elective hernia repair. Which of the following would be a valid reason for delaying the proposed surgery?

a. Coronary artery bypass surgery 3 months earlier
b. A history of cigarette smoking
c. Jugular venous distension
d. Hypertension
e. Hyperlipidemia

14. A 68-year-old man is admitted to the coronary care unit with an acute myocardial infarction. His postinfarction course is marked by congestive heart failure and intermittent hypotension. On the fourth day in hospital, he develops severe midabdominal pain. On physical examination, blood pressure is 90/60 mm Hg and pulse is 110 beats per minute and regular; the abdomen is soft with mild generalized tenderness and distention. Bowel sounds are hypoactive; stool Hematest is positive. Which of the following is the most appropriate next step in this patient's management?

a. Barium enema
b. Upper gastrointestinal series
c. Angiography
d. Ultrasonography
e. Celiotomy

15. A 30-year-old woman in her last trimester of pregnancy suddenly develops massive swelling of the left lower extremity. Which of the following would be the most appropriate workup and treatment at this time?

a. Venography and heparin
b. Duplex ultrasonography and heparin
c. Duplex ultrasonography, heparin, and vena caval filter
d. Duplex ultrasonography, heparin, warfarin (Coumadin)
e. Impedance plethysmography, warfarin

16. A 20-year-old woman with a family history of von Willebrand disease is found to have an activated partial thromboplastin time (aPTT) of 78/32 (patient/control) on routine testing prior to cholecystectomy. Further investigation reveals a prothrombin time (PT) of 13/12, a platelet count of 350,000/mm^3 and an abnormal bleeding time. Which of the following characteristics of this woman's coagulopathy is true?

a. Infusion of purified factor VIII prior to surgery will correct her coagulopathy.
b. Infusion of cryoprecipitate will not reduce blood loss in the perioperative period.
c. Most of these patients are, or become, seropositive for human immunodeficiency virus (HIV).
d. Epistaxis or menorrhagia is uncommon.
e. Desmopressin (DDAVP) will reduce blood loss in the perioperative period.

17. A 65-year-old man undergoes a low anterior resection for rectal cancer. On the fifth day in hospital, his physical examination shows a temperature of 39°C (102°F), blood pressure of 150/90 mm Hg, pulse of 110 beats per minute and regular, and respiratory rate of 28 breaths per minute. A computed tomography (CT) scan of the abdomen reveals an abscess in the pelvis. Which of the following most accurately describes his present condition?

a. Systemic inflammatory response syndrome (SIRS)
b. Sepsis
c. Severe sepsis
d. Septic shock
e. Severe septic shock

18. A victim of blunt abdominal trauma undergoes a partial hepatectomy. During surgery, he receives twelve units of packed red blood cells. In the recovery room, he is noted to be bleeding from intravenous puncture sites and the surgical incision. Which of the following statements regarding the coagulopathy is most likely true?

a. The patient has an unknown primary bleeding disorder.
b. The coagulopathy is secondary to the partial hepatectomy.
c. The coagulopathy is secondary to dilutional thrombocytopenia and deficiency of clotting factors from the massive blood transfusion.
d. The treatment is oral vitamin K.
e. The treatment is intravenous vitamin K.

19. A 62-year-old woman undergoes a lysis of adhesions and bowel resection for small-bowel obstruction secondary to radiation enteritis after treatment for ovarian cancer. A jejunostomy is placed to facilitate nutritional repletion. Which of the following statements is true regarding postoperative nutrition?

a. Enteral nutrition has no advantages over parenteral nutrition in postoperative patients.
b. Institution of enteral feeding within 24 hours postoperatively is safe.
c. Institution of enteral feeding should be delayed until bowel function returns as evidenced by passage of flatus or a bowel movement.
d. Parenteral nutrition should be instituted immediately postoperatively and continued until enteral feeds have been initiated.
e. Return of gastric motility postoperatively occurs before return of small-bowel motility.

20. A 65-year-old woman has a life-threatening pulmonary embolus 5 days following removal of a uterine malignancy. She is immediately heparinized and maintained in good therapeutic range for the next 3 days, then passes gross blood from her vagina and develops tachycardia, hypotension, and oliguria. Following resuscitation, an abdominal CT scan reveals a major retroperitoneal hematoma. Which of the following is the best next step in management?

a. Immediately reverse heparin by a calculated dose of protamine and place a vena caval filter (eg, a Greenfield filter).
b. Reverse heparin with protamine, explore and evacuate the hematoma, and ligate the vena cava below the renal veins.
c. Switch to low-dose heparin.
d. Stop heparin and observe closely.
e. Stop heparin, give fresh-frozen plasma (FFP), and begin warfarin therapy.

21. A 71-year-old man develops dysphagia for both solids and liquids and weight loss of 60-lb over the past 6 months. He undergoes endoscopy, demonstrating a distal esophageal lesion, and biopsies are consistent with squamous cell carcinoma. He is scheduled for neoadjuvant chemoradiation followed by an esophagectomy and preoperatively is started on total parenteral nutrition, given his severe malnutrition reflected by an albumin of less than 1. Which of the following is most likely to be a concern initially in starting total parenteral nutrition in this patient?

a. Hyperkalemia
b. Hypermagnesemia
c. Hypoglycemia
d. Hypophosphatemia
e. Hypochloremia

22. An elderly diabetic woman with chronic steroid-dependent bronchospasm has an ileocolectomy for a perforated cecum. She is taken to the ICU intubated and is maintained on broad-spectrum antibiotics, renal dose dopamine, and a rapid steroid taper. On postoperative day 2, she develops a fever of 39.2°C (102.5°F), hypotension, lethargy, and laboratory values remarkable for hypoglycemia and hyperkalemia. Which of the following is the most likely explanation for her deterioration?

a. Sepsis
b. Hypovolemia
c. Adrenal insufficiency
d. Acute tubular necrosis
e. Diabetic ketoacidosis

23. A cirrhotic patient with abnormal coagulation studies due to hepatic synthetic dysfunction requires an urgent cholecystectomy. A transfusion of FFP is planned to minimize the risk of bleeding due to surgery. What is the optimal timing of this transfusion?

a. The day before surgery
b. The night before surgery
c. On call to surgery
d. Intraoperatively
e. In the recovery room

24. On postoperative day 5, an otherwise healthy 55-year-old man recovering from a partial hepatectomy is noted to have a fever of 38.6°C (101.5°F). Which of the following is the most common nosocomial infection postoperatively?

a. Wound infection
b. Pneumonia
c. Urinary tract infection
d. Intra-abdominal abscess
e. Intravenous catheter-related infection

25. Ten days after an exploratory laparotomy and lysis of adhesions, a patient, who previously underwent a low anterior resection for rectal cancer followed by postoperative chemoradiation, is noted to have succus draining from the wound. She appears to have adequate source control—she is afebrile with a normal white blood count. The output from the fistula is approximately 150 cc per day. Which of the following factors is most likely to result in failure of the enterocutaneous fistula to close?

a. Previous radiation
b. Previous chemotherapy
c. Recent surgery
d. History of malignancy
e. More than 100 cc output per day

26. A 26-year-old male is resuscitated with packed red blood cells following a motor vehicle collision complicated by a fractured pelvis and resultant hemorrhage. A few hours later the patient becomes hypotensive with a normal central venous pressure (CVP), oliguric, and febrile. Upon examination, the patient is noted to have profuse oozing of blood from his intravenous (IV) sites. Which of the following is the most likely diagnosis?

a. Hypovolemic shock
b. Acute adrenal insufficiency
c. Gram-negative bacteremia
d. Transfusion reaction
e. Ureteral obstruction

27. A 16-year-old male with a history of severe hemophilia A is undergoing an elective inguinal hernia repair. Which of the following is the best option for preventing or treating a bleeding complication in the setting of this disease?

a. Fresh-frozen plasma
b. Combination of desmopressin and fresh-frozen plasma
c. DDAVP
d. Combination of ε-aminocaproic acid and desmopressin
e. Factor IX concentrate

28. A 59-year-old man is planning to undergo a coronary artery bypass. He has osteoarthritis and consumes nonsteroidal anti-inflammatory drugs (NSAIDs) for the pain. Which of the following is the most appropriate treatment prior to surgery to minimize his risk of bleeding from his NSAID use?

a. Begin vitamin K 1 week prior to surgery.
b. Give FFP few hours before surgery.
c. Stop the NSAIDs 1 week prior to surgery.
d. Stop the NSAIDs 3 to 4 days prior to surgery.
e. Stop the NSAIDs the day before surgery.

29. A 63-year-old man undergoes a partial gastrectomy with Billroth II reconstruction for intractable peptic ulcer disease. Which of the following metabolic disturbances is not a potential consequence of this procedure?

a. Megaloblastic anemia
b. Iron-deficiency anemia
c. Osteoporosis
d. Osteitis fibrosa cystica
e. Steatorrhea

30. A 52-year-old woman undergoes a sigmoid resection with primary anastomosis for recurrent diverticulitis. She returns to the emergency room 10 days later with left flank pain and decreased urine output; laboratory examination is significant for a white blood cell (WBC) count of 20,000/mm^3. She undergoes a CT scan that demonstrates new left hydronephrosis, but no evidence of an intra-abdominal abscess. Which of the following is the most appropriate next step in management?

a. Intravenous pyelogram
b. Intravenous antibiotics and repeat CT in 1 week
c. Administration of intravenous methylene blue
d. No further management if urinalysis is negative for hematuria
e. Immediate reexploration

31. A 23-year-old woman undergoes total thyroidectomy for carcinoma of the thyroid gland. On the second postoperative day, she begins to complain of a tingling sensation in her hands. She appears quite anxious and later complains of muscle cramps. Which of the following is the most appropriate initial management strategy?

a. 10 mL of 10% magnesium sulfate intravenously
b. Oral vitamin D
c. 100 μg oral Synthroid
d. Continuous infusion of calcium gluconate
e. Oral calcium gluconate

32. A 42-year-old man sustains a gunshot wound to the abdomen and is in shock. Multiple units of packed red blood cells are transfused in an effort to resuscitate him. He complains of numbness around his mouth and displays carpopedal spasm and a positive Chvostek sign. An electrocardiogram demonstrates a prolonged QT interval. Which of the following is the most appropriate treatment?

a. Intravenous bicarbonate
b. Intravenous potassium
c. Intravenous calcium
d. Intravenous digoxin
e. Intravenous parathyroid hormone

33. A 65-year-old man has an enterocutaneous fistula originating in the jejunum secondary to inflammatory bowel disease. Which of the following would be the most appropriate fluid for replacement of his enteric losses?

a. D5W
b. 3% normal saline
c. Ringer lactate solution
d. 0.9% sodium chloride
e. 6% sodium bicarbonate solution

34. A 62-year-old man is suffering from arrhythmias on the night of his triple coronary bypass. Potassium has been administered. His urine output is 20 to 30 mL/h. Serum potassium level is 6.2. Which of the following medications counteracts the effects of potassium without reducing the serum potassium level?

a. Sodium polystyrene sulfonate (Kayexalate)
b. Sodium bicarbonate
c. 50% dextrose
d. Calcium gluconate
e. Insulin

35. An in-hospital workup of a 78-year-old hypertensive, mildly asthmatic man who is receiving chemotherapy for colon cancer reveals symptomatic gallstones. Preoperative laboratory results are notable for a hematocrit of 24% and urinalysis with 18 to 25 WBCs and gram-negative bacteria. On call to the operating room, the patient receives intravenous penicillin. His abdomen is shaved in the operating room. An open cholecystectomy is performed and, despite a lack of indications, the common bile duct is explored. The wound is closed primarily with a Penrose drain exiting a separate stab wound. On postoperative day 3, the patient develops a wound infection. Which of the following changes in the care of this patient could have decreased the chance of a postoperative wound infection?

a. Increasing the length of the preoperative hospital stay to prophylactically treat the asthma with steroids
b. Treating the urinary infection prior to surgery
c. Shaving the abdomen the night prior to surgery
d. Continuing the prophylactic antibiotics for 3 postoperative days
e. Using a closed drainage system brought out through the operative incision

36. A 72-year-old man undergoes a subtotal colectomy for a cecal perforation due to a sigmoid colon obstruction. He has had a prolonged recovery and has been on total parenteral nutrition (TPN) for 2 weeks postoperatively. After regaining bowel function, he experienced significant diarrhea. Examination of his abdominal wound demonstrates minimal granulation tissue. He complains that he has lost his taste for food. He also has increased hair loss and a new perioral pustular rash. Which of the following deficiencies does he most likely have?

a. Zinc
b. Selenium
c. Molybdenum
d. Chromium
e. Thiamine

37. A 12-year-old boy with a femur fracture after a motor vehicle collision undergoes operative repair. After induction of anesthesia, he develops a fever of 40°C (104°F), shaking rigors, and blood-tinged urine. Which of the following is the best treatment option?

a. Alkalinization of the urine, administration of mannitol, and continuation with the procedure
b. Administration of dantrolene sodium and continuation with the procedure
c. Administration of dantrolene sodium and termination of the procedure
d. Administration of intravenous steroids and an antihistamine agent with continuation of the procedure
e. Administration of intravenous steroids and an antihistamine agent with termination of the procedure

38. A 24-year-old Jehovah's Witness who was in a high-speed motorcycle collision undergoes emergent splenectomy. His estimated blood loss was 1500 mL. Which of the following is most accurate regarding his resuscitation?

a. Vasopressors should be primarily utilized for maintenance of his blood pressure.
b. Synthetic colloids should be administered as the primary resuscitation fluid in a 3:1 ratio to replace the volume of blood lost.
c. Crystalloid solutions should be administered in a 1:1 ratio to replace the volume of blood lost.
d. 0.45% normal saline should be administered in a 3:1 ratio to replace the volume of blood lost.
e. A non-anion-gap acidosis may result from large-volume resuscitation with 0.9% normal saline.

39. A 53-year-old man with no significant medical problems undergoes lysis of adhesions for a small-bowel obstruction. Postoperatively, he is placed on lactated Ringer solution for the first 24 hours. Which of the following is true regarding lactated Ringer?

a. It contains a higher concentration of sodium ions than does plasma.
b. It is most appropriate for replacement of nasogastric tube losses.
c. It is isosmotic with plasma.
d. It has a pH of less than 7.0.
e. It may induce a significant metabolic acidosis.

40. Four days after surgical evacuation of an acute subdural hematoma, a 44-year-old man becomes mildly lethargic and develops asterixis. He has received 2400 mL of 5% dextrose in water intravenously each day since surgery, and he appears well hydrated. Pertinent laboratory values are as follows:

Serum electrolytes (mEq/L): Na^+ 118, K^+ 3.4, Cl^- 82, HCO_3^- 24
Serum osmolality: 242 mOsm/L
Urine sodium: 47 mEq/L
Urine osmolality: 486 mOsm/L

A correct statement about this patient's fluid and electrolyte status is which of the following?

a. His low serum sodium indicates sodium deficiency, which should be treated with 3% saline infusion.
b. He probably has the syndrome of inappropriate secretion of antidiuretic hormone.
c. His blood glucose level should be checked because the hyponatremia may be artifactual.
d. Water restriction is rarely effective in severe cases of hyponatremia.
e. The underlying problem is the inappropriate excretion of sodium (renal sodium wasting).

41. A 43-year-old woman develops acute renal failure following an emergency resection of a leaking abdominal aortic aneurysm. One week after surgery, the following laboratory values are obtained:

Serum electrolytes (mEq/L): Na^+ 127, K^+ 5.9, Cl^- 92, HCO_3^- 15
Blood urea nitrogen: 82 mg/dL
Serum creatinine: 6.7 mg/dL

The patient has gained 4 kg since surgery and is mildly dyspneic at rest. Eight hours after these values are reported, the following electrocardiogram is obtained. Which of the following is the most appropriate initial treatment in the management of this patient?

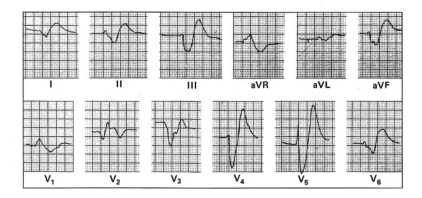

a. 10 mL of 10% calcium gluconate
b. 0.25 mg digoxin every 3 hours for three doses
c. Oral Kayexalate
d. 100 mg lidocaine
e. Emergent hemodialysis

42. A 63-year-old man with a 40-pack per year smoking history undergoes a low anterior resection for rectal cancer and on postoperative day 5 develops a fever, new infiltrate on chest x-ray, and leukocytosis. He is transferred to the ICU for treatment of his pneumonia because of clinical deterioration. Which of the following is a sign of early sepsis?

a. Respiratory acidosis
b. Decreased cardiac output
c. Hypoglycemia
d. Increased arteriovenous oxygen difference
e. Peripheral vasodilation

43. A 60-year-old woman with no previous medical problems undergoes a total colectomy with diverting ileostomy for a cecal perforation secondary to a sigmoid stricture. Postoperatively, she has 2 L of ileostomy output per day. Her heart rate is 110 beats per minute, her respiratory rate is 16 breaths per minute, and her oxygen saturation is 98% on 2 L nasal cannula (NC). Her laboratory values on postoperative day 6 are as follows:

Na^+: 128
K^+: 3.0
Cl^-: 102
HCO_3^-: 20

Which of the following statements is true?

a. Her laboratory abnormalities are most likely secondary to a type IV renal tubular acidosis.
b. Her laboratory abnormalities are most likely compensatory for a primary respiratory problem.
c. She should be treated with fluid replacement and empiric treatment with oral Vancomycin.
d. She should be treated with fluid replacement and stool-bulking agents.
e. She should undergo immediate dialysis.

44. A 39-year-old man is suspected of having had a transfusion reaction during resuscitation for an upper gastrointestinal (GI) bleed. Which of the following is appropriate in the management of this patient?

a. Removal of nonessential foreign body irritants, for example, Foley catheter
b. Fluid restriction
c. 0.1 M HCl infusion
d. Steroids
e. Fluids and mannitol

45. A 45-year-old woman undergoes an uneventful laparoscopic cholecystectomy for which she receives one dose of cephalosporin. One week later, she returns to the emergency room with fever, nausea, and copious diarrhea and is subsequently diagnosed with pseudomembranous colitis. With respect to this disease, which one of the following statements is correct?

a. Surgical intervention is frequently required.
b. After appropriate antibiotic therapy, the relapse rate is less than 5%.
c. Tissue culture assay for *C difficile* toxin B is neither sensitive nor specific; therefore, diagnosis should be based on clinical findings.
d. If surgery is performed, a left hemicolectomy is usually adequate to treat pseudomembranous colitis.
e. Indications for surgical treatment include intractable disease, failure of medical therapy, toxic megacolon, and colonic perforation.

Questions 46 to 49

A patient has a calculated basal energy expenditure of 2000 kcal/day. Match the following clinical situations with the appropriate daily energy requirement. Each lettered option may be used once, more than once, or not at all.

a. 1800 kcal/day
b. 2000 kcal/day
c. 2200 kcal/day
d. 3000 kcal/day
e. 4000 kcal/day

46. Starvation

47. Multiple organ failure

48. Third-degree burns involving 60% of body surface area

49. Postoperative

Pre- and Postoperative Care

Answers

1. The answer is a. *(Brunicardi, p 49.)* The earliest clinical indication of hypermagnesemia is loss of deep tendon reflexes. States of magnesium excess are characterized by generalized neuromuscular depression. Clinically, severe hypermagnesemia is rarely seen except in those patients with advanced renal failure treated with magnesium-containing antacids. However, hypermagnesemia is produced intentionally by obstetricians who use parenteral magnesium sulfate ($MgSO_4$) to treat preeclampsia. $MgSO_4$ is administered until depression of the deep tendon reflexes is observed, a deficit that occurs with modest hypermagnesemia (over 4 mEq/L). Greater elevations of magnesium produce progressive weakness, which culminates in flaccid quadriplegia and in some cases respiratory arrest due to paralysis of the chest bellows mechanism. Hypotension may occur because of the direct arteriolar relaxing effect of magnesium. Changes in mental status occur in the late stages of the syndrome and are characterized by somnolence that progresses to coma.

2. The answer is b. *(Brunicardi, pp 46, 52-54.)* The initial, and often definitive, management of hyponatremia is free-water restriction. Symptomatic hyponatremia, which occurs at serum sodium levels less than or equal to 120 mEq/L, can result in headache, seizures, coma, and signs of increased intracranial pressure and may require infusion of hypertonic saline. Rapid correction should be avoided so as not to cause central pontine myelinolysis, manifested by neurologic symptoms ranging from seizures to brain damage and death. Additionally, a search for the underlying etiology of the hyponatremia should be undertaken. Acute severe hyponatremia sometimes occurs following elective surgical procedures due to a combination of appropriate stimulation of antidiuretic hormone and injudicious administration of excess free water in the first few postoperative days. Other potential etiologies include hyperosmolarity with free-water shifts from the intra- to the extracellular compartment (eg, hyperglycemia), sodium depletion (eg, gastrointestinal or renal losses, insufficient intake), dilution (eg, drug-induced), and the syndrome of inappropriate secretion of antidiuretic hormone (SIADH).

3. The answer is d. (*Greenfield, pp 769-770.*) Any patient who has lost much of the ileum (whether from injury, disease, or elective surgery) is at high risk of developing enteric hyperoxaluria if the colon remains intact. Calcium oxalate stones can subsequently develop due to excessive absorption of oxalate from the colon. Normally, fatty acids are absorbed by the terminal ileum, and calcium and oxalate combine to form an insoluble compound that is not absorbed. In the absence of the terminal ileum, unabsorbed fatty acids reach the colon, where they combine with calcium, leaving free oxalate to be absorbed. Unabsorbed fatty acids and bile acids in the colon also promote oxalate uptake by the colon. Subsequently, the excess oxalate is excreted by the kidneys, promoting calcium oxalate stone formation.

Hungry bone syndrome refers to rapid remineralization of bones leading to hypocalcemia and can be seen postoperatively in patients with secondary or tertiary hyperparathyroidism. Pseudohyperparathyroidism refers to hypercalcemia associated with the production of parathyroid-related peptide. A unicameral bone cyst is a benign lesion found in children.

4. The answer is c. (*Townsend, pp 621-622.*) A fractional excretion of sodium (FENa) of less than 1, which is calculated as (urine sodium × serum creatinine) ÷ (serum sodium × urinary creatinine), supports a prerenal etiology for the patient's oliguria. When oliguria occurs postoperatively, it is important to differentiate between low output caused by the physiologic response to intravascular hypovolemia and that caused by acute tubular necrosis. A FENa of less than 1% in an oliguric setting indicates aggressive sodium reclamation in the tubules. Values above this suggest a tubular injury such that Na cannot be appropriately reclaimed. In the setting of postoperative hypovolemia, all findings would reflect the kidney's efforts to retain volume: the urine sodium would be below 20 mEq/L, the urine chloride would not be helpful except in the metabolically alkalotic patient, the urine osmolality would be over 500 mOsm/kg, the urine/serum creatinine ratio would be above 20, and the blood urea nitrogen (BUN)/creatinine ratio would be above 20.

5. The answer is c. (*Brunicardi, pp 49, 55.*) Magnesium deficiency is common in malnourished patients and patients with large gastrointestinal fluid losses. The neuromuscular effects resemble those of calcium deficiency—

namely, paresthesia, hyperreflexia, muscle spasm, and, ultimately, tetany. The cardiac effects are more like those of hypercalcemia. An electrocardiogram therefore provides a rapid means of differentiating between hypocalcemia (prolonged QT interval, T-wave inversion, heart blocks) and hypomagnesemia (prolonged QT and PR intervals, ST segment depression, flattening or inversion of p waves, torsade de pointes). Hypomagnesemia also causes potassium wasting by the kidney. Many hospital patients with refractory hypocalcemia will be found to be magnesium deficient. Often this deficiency becomes manifest during the response to parenteral nutrition when normal cellular ionic gradients are restored. A normal blood pH and arterial PCO_2 rule out hyperventilation. The serum calcium in this patient is normal when adjusted for the low albumin (add 0.8 mg/dL per 1 g/dL decrease in albumin). Hypomagnesemia causes functional hypoparathyroidism, which can lower serum calcium and thus result in a combined defect.

6. The answer is a. (*Townsend, pp 265-266.*) The appropriate dosing and timing of antibiotic prophylaxis to prevent surgical site infections in an elective procedure is a single dose, no greater than 1 hour prior to the incision. Additionally, most textbooks recommend use of an oral, nonabsorbable antibiotic regimen effective against aerobes and anaerobes in combination with a mechanical bowel preparation before elective colon resections. There is no evidence to support the continuation of antibiotics for more than 12 hours after an elective operation has been completed, and this practice should be avoided to prevent increasing microbial drug resistance. For complex, prolonged procedures, redosing of antibiotics may be appropriate during the procedure based on the drug's half-life. Broad-spectrum antibiotic coverage, including against anaerobic organisms, is required only in cases where such flora are anticipated, such as during colon resections; otherwise, cefazolin is the antibiotic of choice for cases requiring antibiotic prophylaxis.

7. The answer is d. (*Townsend, pp 252-256.*) The patient should undergo persantine thallium stress testing followed by echocardiography to assess his need for coronary angiogram with possible need for angioplasty, stenting, or surgical revascularization prior to repair of his hernia. Although exercise stress testing is an appropriate method for evaluating a patient's cardiac function preoperatively, this patient's functional status is limited by his peripheral vascular disease and therefore a pharmacologic stress test would be the preferred method of cardiac evaluation. An ECG should be performed in this patient with a history of cardiovascular disease, hypertension, and diabetes, but a normal ECG would not preclude further workup. While myocardial infarction (MI) within 6 months of surgery is considered to increase a patient's risk for a cardiac complication after surgery using Goldman's criteria, a remote history of MI is not prohibitive for surgery in and of itself.

8. The answer is d. *(Townsend, pp 81-85.)* The patient has a metabolic alkalosis secondary to gastric losses of HCl, with compensatory hypoventilation as reflected by the elevated arterial pH and P_{CO_2} and supported by the absence of clinical lung disease. The P_{CO_2} would be normal if the metabolic alkalosis was uncompensated. A respiratory acidosis with metabolic compensation would be characterized by decreased pH, increased P_{CO_2} levels, and increased bicarbonate levels. Mixed acid–base abnormalities should be suspected when the pH is normal but the P_{CO_2} and bicarbonate levels are abnormal or if the compensatory responses appear to be excessive or inadequate. The combination of respiratory acidosis and respiratory alkalosis is impossible.

9. The answer is a. *(Townsend, pp 88-89.)* Infusion of 0.9% normal saline (sodium chloride) will correct his hypovolemia and his metabolic alkalosis. The development of a clinically significant metabolic alkalosis is secondary not only to the loss of acid or addition of alkali, but to renal responses that maintain the alkalosis. The normal kidney can tremendously augment its excretion of acid or alkali in response to changes in ingested load. However, in the presence of significant volume depletion and consequent excessive salt and water retention, the tubular maximum for bicarbonate reabsorption is increased. Correction of volume depletion alone is usually sufficient to correct the alkalosis, since the kidney will then excrete the excess bicarbonate. HCl infusion is usually unnecessary. Acetazolamide can be utilized to increase renal excretion of bicarbonate but should be avoided in volume-depleted individuals. Moreover, to the extent that acetazolamide causes natriuresis, it will exacerbate the volume depletion.

10. The answer is b. *(Brunicardi, p 52.)* This patient's history of tinnitus in conjunction with her mixed metabolic acidosis-respiratory alkalosis is pathognomonic of salicylate intoxication. Salicylates directly stimulate the respiratory center and produce respiratory alkalosis. By building up an accumulation of organic acids, salicylates also produce a concomitant metabolic acidosis. The patient is in a state of metabolic acidosis as shown by a markedly increased anion gap of 28 mEq unmeasured anions per liter of plasma.

However, the respiratory response is greater than can be explained by a compensatory response; respiratory compensation alone would not result in an alkalemic pH. The disturbance cannot be pure respiratory alkalosis, since the serum bicarbonate does not drop below 15 mEq/L as a result of renal compensation and the anion gap does not vary by more than 1 to 2 mEq/L from its normal value of 12 in response to a respiratory disturbance. The renal response to hyper-ventilation involves wasting of bicarbonate and compensatory retention of chloride; it does not involve a change in the concentration of unmeasured anions, such as albumin and organic acids.

Phenformin and methanol overdoses also produce high-anion-gap metabolic acidosis, but without the simultaneous respiratory disturbance. Sedatives, such as barbiturates or diazepam, would result in hypoventilation with respiratory acidosis.

11. The answer is d. (*Brunicardi, p 69.*) The patient has heparin-induced thrombocytopenia (HIT), which is a complication of heparin therapy, at both prophylactic and therapeutic doses. HIT is mediated by antibodies to the complexes formed by binding of heparin to platelet factor 4. In a previously unexposed patient, HIT typically manifests after 5 days as a decrease in platelet counts by 50% of the highest preceding value or to a level less than 100,000/mm^3. Complications of HIT are related to venous and/or arterial thromboembolic phenomena. Treatment of HIT consists of cessation of heparin (including low-molecular-weight heparins), institution of a non-heparin anticoagulant such as lepirudin, and conversion to oral warfarin when appropriate. Cessation of heparin alone is inadequate to prevent thromboembolic complications, and warfarin should not be started until the platelet count is above 100,000/mm^3. Platelet transfusion is not indicated, as HIT results in thrombotic rather than hemorrhagic complications.

12. The answer is c. (*Townsend, pp 116-119, 131, 329-330.*) Whenever significant bleeding is noted in the early postoperative period, the presumption should always be that it is due to an error in surgical control of blood vessels in the operative field. Hematologic disorders that are not apparent during the long operation are most unlikely to surface as problems postoperatively. Blood transfusion reactions can cause diffuse loss of clot integrity; the sudden appearance of diffuse bleeding during an operation may be the only evidence of an intraoperative transfusion reaction. In the postoperative period, transfusion reactions usually present as unexplained fever, apprehension, and headache—all symptoms difficult to interpret in the early postoperative period. Factor VIII deficiency (hemophilia) would almost certainly be known by history in a 65-year-old man, but if not, intraoperative bleeding would have been a problem earlier in this long operation. Moreover, factor VIII deficiency causes prolongation of the partial thromboplastin time (PTT), which is normal in this patient. Severely hypothermic patients will not be able to form clots effectively, but clot dissolution does not occur. Care should be taken to prevent the development of hypothermia during long operations through the use of warmed intravenous fluid, gas humidifiers, and insulated skin barriers.

13. The answer is c. (*Townsend, pp 252-256.*) The work of Goldman and others has served to identify risk factors for perioperative myocardial infarction. The highest likelihood is associated with recent myocardial infarction: the more recent the event, the higher the risk up to 6 months. It should be noted, however, that the risk never returns to normal. A non-Q-wave infarction may not have destroyed much myocardium, but it leaves the surrounding area with borderline perfusion, thus the particularly high risk of subsequent perioperative infarction. Evidence of congestive heart failure, such as jugular venous distention, or S_3 gallop also carries a high risk, as does the frequent occurrence of ectopic beats. Old age (age >70 years) and emergency surgery are risk factors independent of these others. Coronary revascularization by coronary artery bypass graft (CABG) tends to protect against myocardial infarction. Smoking, diabetes, hypertension, and hyperlipidemia (all of which predispose to coronary artery disease) are surprisingly not independent risk factors, although they may increase the death rate should an infarct occur. The value of this information and data derived from further testing is that it identifies the patient who needs to be monitored invasively with a systemic arterial catheter and pulmonary arterial catheter. Most perioperative infarcts occur postoperatively when the third-space fluids return to the circulation, which increases the preload and the myocardial oxygen consumption. This generally occurs around the third postoperative day.

14. The answer is c. (*Brunicardi, pp 1047-1049.*) In the absence of peritoneal signs, angiography is the diagnostic test of choice for acute mesenteric ischemia. Patients with peritoneal signs should undergo emergent laparotomy. Acute mesenteric ischemia may be difficult to diagnose. The condition should be suspected in patients with either systemic manifestations of arteriosclerotic vascular disease or low cardiac-output states associated with a sudden development of abdominal pain that is out of proportion to the physical findings. Because of the risk of progression to small-bowel infarction, acute mesenteric ischemia is an emergency, and timely diagnosis is essential. Although patients may have lactic acidosis or leukocytosis, these are late findings. Abdominal films are generally unhelpful and may show a nonspecific ileus pattern. Since the pathology involves the small bowel, a barium enema is not indicated. Upper gastrointestinal series and ultrasonography are also of limited value. CT scanning has a sensitivity of 64% to 82% and is a good initial test, but should still be followed by angiography in a patient with clinically suspected acute mesenteric ischemia, even in the absence of findings on the CT scan. In addition to establishing the diagnosis in this stable patient, angiography may also assist with operative planning and elucidation of the etiology of the acute mesenteric ischemia. The cause may be embolic occlusion or thrombosis of the superior mesenteric artery, primary mesenteric venous occlusion, or nonocclusive mesenteric ischemia secondary to low-cardiac output states. A mortality of 65% to 100% is reported. The majority of affected patients are at high operative risk, but early diagnosis followed by revascularization or resectional surgery or both are the only hope for survival. Celiotomy must be performed once the diagnosis of arterial occlusion or bowel infarction has been made. Initial treatment of nonocclusive mesenteric ischemia includes measures to increase cardiac output and blood pressure. Laparotomy should be performed if peritoneal signs develop.

15. The answer is b. (*Brunicardi, pp 813-821.*) Duplex ultrasound is the diagnostic modality of choice for detection of infrainguinal deep-venous thrombosis (DVT). Although venography is the gold standard, it is no longer routinely used, given the risks of local (thrombosis, pain) and contrast-related (allergic reaction, renal failure) complications. Impedance plethysmography, which measures changes in volume in the lower extremity as related to blood flow, is also used infrequently due to the superiority of duplex scanning in detecting DVTs. In pregnant women, anticoagulation for treatment of DVT is achieved with heparin, which does not cross the placenta, rather than warfarin, which is associated with the risk of spontaneous abortion and birth defects. The vena caval filter is not indicated because there is no contraindication to heparin therapy and no evidence of failure of anticoagulation therapy (pulmonary embolus in the face of adequate anticoagulation).

16. The answer is e. (*Townsend, p 119.*) The patient's elevated aPTT, normal PT, and abnormal bleeding time are consistent with her von Willebrand disease (vWD). von Willebrand factor (vWF) is an important stimulus for platelet aggregation at the site of tissue injury and a major carrier protein for circulating factor VIII. There are three major groups of vWD. Type I, inherited as an autosomal dominant trait, has decreased levels of vWF. Type II is variably inherited and has qualitative defects in vWF. Type III is an autosomal recessive severe bleeding disorder with absent levels of vWF. Patients with vWD present with mucosal bleeding, petechiae, epistaxis, and menorrhagia. vWD produces a depressed ristocetin cofactor assay (which measures the effectiveness of vWF in agglutinating platelets when stimulated with the antibiotic ristocetin). These patients do not generally require treatment unless they need surgery or are severely injured. DDAVP, a synthetic analogue of vasopressin, activates receptors that result in release of vWF from storage sites and causes shortening in the bleeding time in patients with type I vWD and some patients with type II vWD. vWF prevents inactivation of factor VIII; administration of DDAVP results in normalization of factor VIII activities. Transfusion of cryoprecipitate provides vWF, whereas infusions of high-purity concentrates of factor VIII:C are not effective because of the lack of vWF. Because they do not receive frequent transfusions, patients with vWD are not at increased risk for HIV seropositivity.

17. The answer is b. (*Townsend, p 156.*) The correct diagnosis is sepsis. Systemic Inflammatory Response Syndrome (SIRS) involves 2 or more of the following: temperature $> 38°C$ (100°F) or $< 36°C$ (97°F), heart rate > 90 beats per minute, respiratory rate > 20 or $Paco_2$ < 32 mm Hg, WBC count $> 12,000$ or $< 4000/mm^3$ or $> 10\%$ immature neutrophils. Sepsis = SIRS + documented infection. Severe sepsis = sepsis + organ dysfunction or hypoperfusion (lactic acidosis, oliguria, or altered mental status). Septic shock = sepsis + organ dysfunction + hypotension (systolic blood pressure < 90 mm Hg or > 90 mm Hg with vasopressors).

18. The answer is c. (*Brunicardi, pp 77-79.*) The patient has an acquired coagulopathy from the massive blood transfusion. The term massive blood transfusion is defined as a single transfusion greater than 2500 mL or 5000 mL transfused over a period of 24 hours. When large amounts of banked blood are transfused, the recipient develops dilutional thrombocytopenia and deficiencies in factors V and VIII. Treatment involves transfusion of FFP and platelets. Vitamin K will take days to replace the clotting factors. This patient needs to have his coagulopathy corrected immediately to prevent bleeding from his recent surgery. It is unlikely that this patient has an unknown primary clotting disorder.

19. The answer is b. *(Brunicardi, pp 31-32.)* The misconception that the entire bowel does not function in the early postoperative period is still widely held. Intestinal motility and absorption studies have clarified the patterns by which bowel activity resumes. The stomach remains uncoordinated in its muscular activity and does not empty efficiently for about 24 hours after abdominal procedures. The small bowel functions normally within hours of surgery and is able to accept nutrients promptly, either by nasoduodenal or percutaneous jejunal feeding catheters or, after 24 hours, by gastric emptying. The colon is stimulated in large measure by the gastrocolic reflex but ordinarily is relatively inactive for 3 to 4 days. Well-nourished patients who undergo uncomplicated surgical procedures can tolerate up to 10 days without full nutritional support before significant problems with protein breakdown begin to occur. Enteral nutrition is preferred over parenteral nutrition because of decreased risks of nosocomial infections and catheter-related complications.

20. The answer is a. *(Brunicardi 346, 817-818.)* Immediate reversal of heparin anticoagulation is indicated in a heparinized patient with significant life-threatening hemorrhage. Protamine sulfate is a specific antidote to heparin and is given at 1 mg for each 100 U heparin. It is given in cases when hemorrhage begins shortly after a bolus of heparin. For a patient who is undergoing heparin therapy, the dose should be based on the half-life of heparin (90 minutes). Since protamine is also an anticoagulant, only half the calculated circulating heparin should be reversed. The indications for inferior vena cava (IVC) filter placement fall into three categories: a failure or complication of anticoagulation, a known free-floating venous clot, and a prior history of PE. In this critically ill patient, exploration of the retroperitoneal space would be surgically challenging and unnecessary.

21. The answer is d. *(Townsend, pp 168-175.)* Hypophosphatemia is a complication of refeeding syndrome, which occurs in malnourished patients who are administered with intravenous glucose. During periods of starvation, electrolytes are shifted to the extracellular space to maintain adequate serum concentrations. With refeeding, insulin levels rise and electrolytes are shifted back intracellularly, resulting in potential hypokalemia, hypomagnesemia, and hypophosphatemia. Additionally, refeeding results in an increased cellular need for phosphorus for energy production (ATP) and glucose metabolism. Early complications of TPN also include hyperglycemia, hyperchloremic acidosis, and volume overload with resultant heart failure. TPN, particularly in the extremely malnourished patient, should be started slowly; magnesium, potassium, and phosphate levels should be repleted; and dextrose infusions should be limited to prevent complications of refeeding.

22. The answer is c. (*Brunicardi, pp 1463-1465.*) Acute adrenal insufficiency can occur in patients with severe stress, infection, or trauma or as a result of abrupt cessation or too rapid tapering of chronic glucocorticoid therapy, and is classically manifested as changing mental status, increased temperature, cardiovascular collapse, hypoglycemia, and hyperkalemia. The diagnosis can be difficult to make and requires a high index of suspicion. Its clinical presentation is similar to that of sepsis; however, sepsis is generally associated with hyperglycemia and no significant change in potassium. The treatment for adrenal crisis is intravenous steroids, volume resuscitation, and other supportive measures to treat any new or ongoing stress. Dexamethasone is the steroid replacement of choice when empirically treating adrenal insufficiency since hydrocortisone can interfere with confirmatory testing (adrenocorticotropic hormone [ACTH] stimulation test). Steroid treatment can be subsequently converted to oral medication and tapered after treatment of the adrenal crisis.

23. The answer is c. (*Brunicardi, p 78.*) Transfusions with FFP to replenish vitamin K–dependent clotting factors should be administered on call to the operating room. The timing of transfusion is dependent on the quantity of each factor delivered and its half-life. The half-life of the most stable clotting factor, factor VII, is 4 to 6 hours. Thus, transfusion of FFP on call to the operating room ensures that the transfusion is complete prior to the incision, with circulating factors to cover the operative and immediate postoperative period.

24. The answer is c. (*Brunicardi, p 353.*) The most common nosocomial infection is a urinary tract infection. Treatment consists of removal of an indwelling catheter as soon as possible and antibiotic therapy for cultures with greater than 100,000 CFU/mL. Pneumonias, wound infections, intra-abdominal abscesses, and catheter-related bloodstream infections are also all causes of nosocomial infections, and a workup of a postoperative fever should also include careful examination of the patient and other diagnostic tests as appropriate (chest x-ray, blood cultures, abdominal/pelvic CT scan).

25. The answer is a. (*Brunicardi, p 347.*) Factors that predispose to fistula formation and may prevent closure include foreign body, radiation, inflammation, epithelialization of the tract, neoplasm, distal obstruction, and steroids.

Factors that result in unhealthy or abnormal tissue surrounding the enterocutaneous fistula decrease the likelihood of spontaneous resolution. For example, radiation therapy, such as used for treatment of pelvic gynecologic and rectal malignancies, can result in chronic injury to the small intestine characterized by fibrosis and poor wound healing. High-output fistulas, defined as those with more than 500 cc per day output, are usually proximal and unlikely to close. Treatment consists of source control, nutritional supplementation, wound care, and delayed surgical intervention if the fistula fails to close.

26. The answer is d. (*Townsend, p 131.*) Transfusion reactions can be categorized into hemolytic versus allergic nonhemolytic reactions. Hemolytic transfusion reactions are caused by complement-mediated destruction of transfused red blood cells by the recipient's preexisting antibodies. Severe hemolytic transfusion reactions usually involve the transfusion of ABO-incompatible blood, with fatalities occurring in 1 in 600,000 units. Peptides from the complement, released into the blood as the red blood cells are rapidly destroyed, cause hypotension, activate coagulation, and lead to disseminated intravascular coagulation (DIC). Symptoms of a hemolytic transfusion reaction include fever, chills, pain and redness along the infused vein, oozing from IV sites, respiratory distress, anxiety, hypotension, and oliguria. The patient would have a low CVP with hypovolemic shock. Acute adrenal insufficiency, gram-negative bacteremia, and ureteral obstruction would not cause oozing from the IV sites.

27. The answer is d. (*Townsend, pp 118-119.*) Hemophilia A is a coagulation disorder resulting from a deficiency or abnormality of factor VIII. Desmopressin (DDAVP) is a synthetic analogue of antidiuretic hormone that increases levels of factor VIII and von Willebrand factor. DDAVP can be used alone for mild hemophilia A, but is ineffective in severe forms of the disease. For severe hemophilia A, DDAVP is given in combination with an inhibitor of fibrinolysis such as ε-aminocaproic acid (AMICAR). Although FFP contains factor VIII, the levels are too low to prevent or control bleeding in hemophiliacs. Other agents used in treatment of hemophilia A include cryoprecipitate and specific factor VIII concentrates.

28. The answer is d. (*Townsend, p 122.*) NSAIDs block platelet function by causing a reversible defect in the enzyme cyclooxygenase. Unlike aspirin which permanently acetylates cyclooxygenase and leaves affected platelets dysfunctional throughout their 7-day life span, NSAIDs cause a reversible defect that lasts 3 to 4 days. Therefore, the patient's platelets will be functional for surgery if he stops taking the NSAIDs 3 to 4 days prior to the date of surgery. The patient would not benefit from FFP or vitamin K since he does not have problems with his clotting factors.

29. The answer is d. *(Townsend, pp 1252-1253.)* Osteitis cystica fibrosa is a finding in patients with primary hyperparathyroidism and represents subperiosteal resorption, characteristically on the radial aspect of the middle phalanx. This is not a reported complication after partial gastrectomy. Patients who have undergone partial gastrectomy may, however, have osteoporosis secondary to impaired calcium absorption due to the Billroth II reconstruction (since calcium is normally absorbed in the proximal intestine—duodenum and jejunum). Fatty acids may also be malabsorbed due to inadequate mixing of bile salts and lipase with ingested fat, and therefore steatorrhea may result. Either megaloblastic anemia due to vitamin B_{12} deficiency (due to lack of intrinsic factor, which is necessary for B_{12} absorption and is normally produced by the parietal cells of the stomach) or microcytic anemia due to iron deficiency (due to decreased iron intake and impaired absorption in the duodenum) can result after partial gastrectomy.

30. The answer is a. *(Brunicardi, pp 175, 1606.)* The patient should undergo an intravenous pyelogram for a suspected ureteral injury. After gynecologic surgeries, colorectal surgery is the most common cause of iatrogenic ureteral injuries. Intraoperatively, intravenous administration of methylene blue or indigocyanine green may facilitate identification of an injury. However, delay in diagnosis is common, and patients may present with flank pain, fevers, and signs of sepsis, ileus, or decreased urine output. CT scan may demonstrate hydronephrosis or a fluid collection (urinoma). Initial diagnosis and management should include urinalysis, although hematuria may not always be present; percutaneous nephrostomy tube or retrograde ureteral catheterization; percutaneous drainage of fluid collections; and identification of the location of ureteral injury. Surgical management should be delayed if diagnosis is late (10-14 days), and operative strategy is dependent on the location of the injury. Diagnostic imaging such as a pyelogram or nuclear medicine scan may be helpful to identify the site of the injury.

31. The answer is d. *(Brunicardi, p 1448.)* Intravenous calcium infusion is the treatment for severe, symptomatic hypocalcemia, although, typically, oral calcium supplementation (up to 1-2 g every 4 hours) is sufficient in patients with mild symptoms. Since postthyroidectomy hypocalcemia is usually due to transient ischemia of the parathyroid glands and is self-limited, in most cases the problem is resolved in several days. In cases of persistent hypocalcemia, vitamin D preparations may be necessary. There is no role for thyroid hormone replacement or magnesium sulfate in the treatment of hypocalcemia.

32. The answer is c. (*Brunicardi, p 50.*) Hypocalcemia is associated with a prolonged QT interval and may be aggravated by both hypomagnesemia and alkalosis. Additionally, massive transfusion is associated with hypocalcemia secondary to chelation with citrate in banked blood. Severe, symptomatic hypocalcemia, encountered most frequently following parathyroid or thyroid surgery or in patients with acute pancreatitis, should be treated with intravenous calcium gluconate. The myocardium is very sensitive to calcium levels; therefore, calcium is considered a positive inotropic agent. Calcium increases the contractile strength of cardiac muscle as well as the velocity of shortening. In its absence, the efficiency of the myocardium decreases. Hypocalcemia often occurs with hypoproteinemia, even though the ionized serum calcium fraction remains normal.

33. The answer is c. (*Brunicardi, pp 46, 52-53.*) Bile and the fluids found in the duodenum, jejunum, and ileum all have an electrolyte content similar to that of Ringer lactate. Saliva, gastric juice, and right colon fluids have high K^+ and low Na^+ content. Pancreatic secretions are high in bicarbonate. It is important to consider these variations in electrolyte patterns when calculating replacement requirements following gastrointestinal losses.

34. The answer is d. (*Brunicardi, pp 47-48.*) Calcium gluconate does not affect the serum potassium level but rather counteracts the myocardial effects of hyperkalemia. Reduction of an elevated serum potassium level, however, is important to avoid the cardiovascular complications that ultimately culminate in cardiac arrest. Kayexalate is a cation exchange resin that is instilled into the gastrointestinal tract and exchanges sodium for potassium ions. Its use is limited to semiacute and chronic potassium elevations. Sodium bicarbonate causes a rise in serum pH and shifts potassium intracellularly. Administration of glucose initiates glycogen synthesis and uptake of potassium. Insulin can be used in conjunction with this to aid in the shift of potassium intracellularly.

35. The answer is b. (*Brunicardi, pp 118-120.*) The determinants of a postoperative wound infection include factors predetermined by the status of the patient (eg, age, obesity, steroid dependence, multiple diagnoses [more than three], immunosuppression) and by the type of procedure (eg, contaminated versus clean, emergent versus elective). However, there are several factors that can be optimized by the surgeon. Decreasing the bacterial inoculum and virulence by limiting the patient's prehospital stay, clipping the operative site in the operating room, administering perioperative antibiotics (within a 24-hour period surrounding operation) with an appropriate antimicrobial spectrum, treating remote infections, avoiding breaks in technique, using closed drainage systems (if needed at all) that exit the skin away from the surgical incision, and minimizing the duration of the operation have all been shown to decrease postoperative infection. Making a wound less favorable to infection requires attention to basic Halstedian principles of hemostasis, anatomic dissection, and gentle handling of tissues as well as limiting the amount of foreign body and necrotic tissue in the wound. Although they are the most difficult factors to influence, host defense mechanisms can be improved by optimizing nutritional status, tissue perfusion, and oxygen delivery.

36. The answer is a. (*Townsend, pp 163-165.*) The patient has a zinc deficiency. Alopecia, poor wound healing, night blindness or photophobia, anosmia, neuritis, and skin rashes are all characteristic of patients with zinc deficiency, which often results in the setting of excessive diarrhea. Selenium deficiency is characterized by the development of a cardiomyopathy. Molybdenum deficiency is manifested by encephalopathy due to toxic accumulation of sulfur-containing amino acids. Chromium deficiency can occur in patients on long-term TPN and is characterized by difficult-to-control hyperglycemia and peripheral neuropathy and encephalopathy. Thiamine deficiency results in beriberi, which includes symptoms of encephalopathy and peripheral neuropathy; patients with beriberi can also develop cardiovascular symptoms and cardiac failure.

37. The answer is c. (*Brunicardi, pp 356-357.*) The patient is manifesting symptoms of malignant hyperthermia (fevers, rigors, and myoglobinuria), which is treated by administration of dantrolene, immediate discontinuation of offending medication (which can include succinylcholine or halothane-based inhalational anesthetics), and supportive cooling measures. While urine alkalinization, loop diuretics, and mannitol are appropriate treatment measures for rhabdomyolysis, the underlying problem in this patient is malignant hyperthermia, which, because of its associated mortality of 30% in severe cases should be treated first and foremost. Malignant hyperthermia is not a manifestation of anaphylactic shock, and, therefore, steroids and antihistamines have no role in its treatment.

38. The answer is e. *(Brunicardi, p 53; Townsend, p 98.)* Following administration of large volumes of normal saline, a non-anion-gap metabolic acidosis can result from increased chloride concentrations. Normal saline and lactated Ringer solution are examples of isotonic saline solutions, both of which can be used to replace the volume of blood lost in a ratio of 3:1. Hypotonic saline solutions such as 0.45% normal saline should not be used for acute resuscitation in hemorrhagic shock but are appropriate for postoperative fluid maintenance in the hemodynamically stable patient. The use of colloids in resuscitation of patients in hemorrhagic shock is controversial; in general, however, colloids can be used to replace blood volume lost in a ratio of 1:1. The definitive treatment of hypovolemic shock is fluid resuscitation, not initiation of vasopressors.

39. The answer is d. *(Brunicardi, p 53; Townsend, p 98.)* Isotonic saline solutions contain 154 mEq/L of both sodium and chloride ions. Each ion is in a substantially higher concentration than is found in the normal serum (Na = 142 mEq/L; Cl = 103 mEq/L). When isotonic solutions are given in large quantities, they overload the kidney's ability to excrete chloride ion, which results in a dilutional acidosis. They also may intensify preexisting acidosis by reducing the base bicarbonate–carbonic acid ratio in the body. Isotonic saline solutions are particularly useful in hyponatremic or hypochloremic states and whenever a tendency to metabolic alkalosis is present, as occurs with significant nasogastric suction losses or vomiting. Administration of lactated Ringer solution is appropriate for replacing gastrointestinal losses and correcting extracellular fluid deficits. Containing 130 mEq/L sodium, lactated Ringer is hyposmolar with respect to sodium and provides approximately 150 mL of free water with each liter given. Although this is ordinarily not a significant load, in some clinical situations it can be. Lactated Ringer is sufficiently physiological to enable administration of large amounts without significantly affecting the body's acid–base balance. It is worth noting that both isotonic saline and lactated Ringer are acidic with respect to the plasma: 0.9% NaCl/5% dextrose has a pH of 4.5, while lactated Ringer has a pH of 6.5.

40. The answer is b. *(Brunicardi, pp 56-57.)* The patient presented has the SIADH. Although this syndrome is associated primarily with diseases of the central nervous system or of the chest (eg, oat cell carcinoma of the lung), excessive amounts of antidiuretic hormone are also present in most postoperative patients. The pathophysiology of SIADH involves an inability to dilute the urine; administered water is therefore retained, which produces dilutional hyponatremia. Body sodium stores and fluid balance are normal, as evidenced by the absence of the clinical findings suggestive of abnormalities of extracellular fluid volume. While hypertonic saline infusions can transiently improve hyponatremia, the appropriate therapy is to restrict water ingestion to a level below the patient's ability to excrete water. Hypertonic saline may be dangerous, since it can shift accumulated water into the extracellular fluid and precipitate pulmonary edema in the patient who suffers from low cardiac reserves. Hyperglycemia cannot account for the hyponatremia seen in this patient because the serum osmolality, as well as the serum sodium, is depressed. Hyponatremia resulting from hyperglycemia would be associated with an elevated serum osmolality.

41. The answer is a. *(Brunicardi, pp 47-48, 54.)* The electrocardiogram demonstrates changes that are essentially diagnostic of severe hyperkalemia. Correct treatment for the affected patient includes discontinuation of exogenous sources of potassium, administration of a source of calcium ions (which will immediately oppose the myocardial effects of potassium), and administration of sodium bicarbonate (which, by producing a mild alkalosis, will shift potassium into cells); each will temporarily reduce serum potassium concentration. Infusion of glucose and insulin would also effect a temporary transcellular shift of potassium. However, these maneuvers are only temporarily effective; definitive treatment calls for removal of potassium from the body. The sodium-potassium exchange resin sodium polystyrene sulfonate (Kayexalate) would accomplish this removal, but over a period of hours and at the price of adding a sodium ion for each potassium ion that is removed. Hemodialysis or peritoneal dialysis is probably required for this patient, since these procedures also rectify the other consequences of acute renal failure, but they would not be the first line of therapy, given the acute need to reduce the potassium level. Both lidocaine and digoxin would be not only ineffective but contraindicated, since they would further depress the myocardial conduction system.

42. The answer is e. (*Brunicardi, pp 98-99.*) It is important to identify and treat occult or early sepsis before it progresses to septic shock and the associated complications of multiple organ failure. An immunocompromised host may not manifest some of the more typical signs and symptoms of infection, such as elevated temperature and white cell count; this forces the clinician to focus on more subtle signs and symptoms. Early sepsis is a physiologically hyperdynamic, hypermetabolic state representing a surge of catecholamines, cortisol, and other stress-related hormones. Changing mental status, tachypnea that leads to respiratory alkalosis, and flushed skin are often the earliest manifestations of sepsis. Intermittent hypotension requiring increased fluid resuscitation to maintain adequate urine output is characteristic of occult sepsis. Hyperglycemia and insulin resistance during sepsis are typical in diabetic as well as nondiabetic patients. This relates to the gluconeogenic state of the stress response. The cardiovascular response to early sepsis is characterized by an increased cardiac output, decreased systemic vascular resistance, and decreased peripheral utilization of oxygen, which yields a decreased arteriovenous oxygen difference.

43. The answer is d. (*Brunicardi, pp 50-51.*) The patient has a non-gap metabolic acidosis, ($[Na^+] - [Cl^- + HCO_3^-] = [128] - [102 + 20] = 6$), secondary to high output from her ileostomy with gastrointestinal losses of bicarbonate. This should be managed with fluid replacement and stool-bulking agents. The ionic composition of small-bowel fluid is Na^+ 140, K^+ 5, Cl^- 104, and HCO_3^- 30. Patients with large ileostomy outputs are at risk for dehydration with accompanying hyponatremia, hypokalemia, and non-anion-gap metabolic acidosis. While renal tubular acidosis (RTA) can be associated with a non-anion-gap metabolic acidosis, type IV RTAs are typically associated with hyperkalemia. Renal failure can result in an anion-gap, uremic acidosis and hyperkalemia, both of which may be indications for dialysis. Finally, while *C difficile* colitis should be considered in postoperative patients with diarrhea, *C difficile* enteritis is less common in a non-immunocompromised host, and Vancomycin is reserved for failures to metronidazole treatment.

44. The answer is e. (*Townsend, p 131.*) Hemolytic transfusion reactions lead to hypotension and oliguria. The increased hemoglobin in the plasma will be cleared via the kidneys, which leads to hemoglobinuria. Placement of an indwelling Foley catheter with subsequent demonstration of oliguria and hemoglobinuria not only confirms the diagnosis of a hemolytic transfusion reaction but is useful in monitoring corrective therapy. Treatment begins with discontinuation of the transfusion, followed by aggressive fluid resuscitation to support the hypotensive episode and increase urine output. Inducing diuresis through aggressive fluid resuscitation and osmotic diuretics is important to clear the hemolyzed red cell membranes, which can otherwise collect in glomeruli and cause renal damage. Alkalinization of the urine (pH > 7) helps prevent hemoglobin clumping and renal damage. Steroids do not have a role in the treatment of hemolytic transfusion reactions.

45. The answer is e. *(Brunicardi, p 1100.)* Indications for surgical treatment of *C difficile* colitis are intractable disease, failure of medical therapy, toxic megacolon, and colonic perforation; surgical therapy consists of subtotal colectomy with end ileostomy. The diagnosis can be made by either detection of the characteristic appearance of pseudomembranes on endoscopy or detection of either toxin A or toxin B in the stool. Treatment is metronidazole for first-line therapy and oral vancomycin as a second-tier agent. Recurrence appears in up to 20% of patients.

46 to 49. The answers are 46-a, 47-d, 48-e, 49-c. *(Greenfield, p 203.)* Basal metabolic rate is the energy required to maintain cell integrity in the resting state at a normal physiologic temperature. The basal energy expenditure decreases with advancing age and varies with sex and body size. The patient's clinical condition also impacts the basal energy expenditure. During starvation, the metabolic rate is decreased by 10%. Trauma, stress, sepsis, burns, and surgery all increase the metabolic rate. The basal energy expenditure can be multiplied by a stress factor to better approximate caloric requirements. The stress factor after a routine operation is 1.1, multiple organ failure or severe injury is 1.5, and less than 50% body surface area burns is 2.0.

Critical Care: Anesthesiology, Blood Gases, and Respiratory Care

Questions

50. A 75-year-old thin cachectic woman undergoes a tracheostomy for failure to wean from the ventilator. One week later, she develops significant bleeding from the tracheostomy. Which of the following would be an appropriate initial step in the management of this problem?

a. Remove the tracheostomy and place pressure over the wound.
b. Deflate the balloon cuff on the tracheostomy.
c. Attempt to reintubate the patient with an endotracheal tube.
d. Upsize the tracheostomy.
e. Perform fiberoptic evaluation immediately.

51. A 53-year-old woman has been intubated for several days after sustaining a right pulmonary contusion after a motor vehicle collision as well as multiple rib fractures. Which of the following is a reasonable indication to attempt extubation?

a. Negative inspiratory force (NIF) of −15 cm H_2O
b. PO_2 of 60 mm Hg while breathing 30% inspired FiO_2 with a positive end–expiratory pressure (PEEP) of 10 cm H_2O
c. Spontaneous respiratory rate of 35 breaths per minute
d. A rapid shallow breathing index of 80
e. Minute ventilation of 18 L/min

52. A 19-year-old male receives un-cross-matched blood during resuscitation after a gunshot wound to the abdomen. He develops fever, tachycardia, and oliguria during the transfusion and is diagnosed as having a hemolytic reaction. Which of the following is the most appropriate next step in the management of this patient?

a. Administration of a loop diuretic such as furosemide
b. Treating anuria with fluid and potassium replacement
c. Acidifying the urine to prevent hemoglobin precipitation in the renal tubules
d. Removing foreign bodies, such as Foley catheters, which may cause hemorrhagic complications
e. Stopping the transfusion immediately

53. A 74-year-old woman with a history of a previous total abdominal hysterectomy presents with abdominal pain and distention for 3 days. She is noted on plain films to have dilated small-bowel and air-fluid levels. She is taken to the operating room for a small-bowel obstruction. Which of the following inhalational anesthetics should be avoided because of accumulation in air-filled cavities during general anesthesia?

a. Diethyl ether
b. Nitrous oxide
c. Halothane
d. Methoxyflurane
e. Trichloroethylene

54. A 61-year-old alcoholic man presents with severe epigastric pain radiating to his back. His amylase and lipase are elevated, and he is diagnosed with acute pancreatitis. Over the first 48 hours, he is determined to have six Ranson's criteria, including a PO_2 less than 60 mm Hg. His chest x-ray reveals bilateral pulmonary infiltrates, and his wedge pressure is low. Which of the following major alterations in pulmonary function is associated with adult respiratory distress syndrome (ARDS)?

a. Hypoxemia
b. Increased pulmonary compliance
c. Increased resting lung volume
d. Increased functional residual capacity
e. Decreased dead-space ventilation

55. The curve depicted here plots the normal relationship of arterial P_{O_2} and percentage of hemoglobin saturation with other variables controlled at pH 7.4, Pa_{CO_2} 40 mm Hg, temperature 37°C (98.6°F), and hemoglobin 15 g/dL. Which of the following statements regarding this oxygen (O_2) dissociation relationship is true?

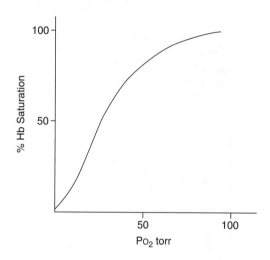

a. Modest decrements of arterial P_{O_2} have a major effect on alveolar O_2 uptake.
b. Modest decrements of hemoglobin saturation have a major effect on tissue O_2 uptake.
c. The curve shifts to the left with acidosis.
d. The curve shifts to the left following banked blood transfusion.
e. The curve is unaffected by chronic lung disease.

56. A 64-year-old man with history of severe emphysema is admitted for hematemesis. The bleeding ceases soon after admission, but the patient becomes confused and agitated. Arterial blood gases are as follows: pH 7.23; P_{O_2} 42 mm Hg; P_{CO_2} 75 mm Hg. Which of the following is the best initial therapy for this patient?

a. Correct hypoxemia with high-flow nasal O_2.
b. Correct acidosis with sodium bicarbonate.
c. Administer 10 mg intravenous dexamethasone.
d. Administer 2 mg intravenous Ativan.
e. Intubate the patient.

57. A 62-year-old woman with a history of coronary artery disease presents with a pancreatic head tumor and undergoes a pancreaticoduodenectomy. Postoperatively, she develops a leak from the pancreaticojejunostomy anastomosis and becomes septic. A Swan-Ganz catheter is placed, which demonstrates an increased cardiac output and decreased systemic vascular resistance. She also develops acute renal failure and oliguria. Dopamine is started. Which of the following effects does dopamine have?

a. At high doses it increases splanchnic flow.
b. At high doses it increases coronary flow.
c. At low doses it decreases heart rate.
d. At low doses it lowers peripheral resistance.
e. It inhibits catecholamine release.

58. A 29-year-old woman on oral contraceptives presents with abdominal pain. A computed tomography (CT) scan of the abdomen demonstrates a large hematoma of the right liver with the suggestion of an underlying liver lesion. Her hemoglobin is 6, and she is symptomatic in terms of tachycardia and light-headedness. Because of her age, the patient wishes to know more about the risk of infection with blood transfusion. Which of the following statements regarding transmission of viral illness through homologous blood transfusion is true?

a. The most common viral agent transmitted via blood transfusion in the United States is human immunodeficiency virus (HIV).
b. Blood is routinely tested for cytomegalovirus (CMV) because CMV infection is often fatal.
c. The most frequent infectious complication of blood transfusion continues to be viral meningitis.
d. Up to 10% of those who develop posttransfusion hepatitis will develop cirrhosis or hepatoma or both.
e. The etiologic agent in posttransfusion hepatitis remains undiscovered.

59. A 68-year-old hypertensive man undergoes successful repair of a ruptured abdominal aortic aneurysm. He receives 9 L Ringer lactate solution and four units of whole blood during the operation. Two hours after transfer to the surgical intensive care unit, the following hemodynamic parameters are obtained: systemic blood pressure (BP) 90/60 mm Hg, pulse 110 beats per minute, central venous pressure (CVP) 7 mm Hg, pulmonary artery pressure 28/10 mm Hg, pulmonary capillary wedge pressure (PCWP) 8 mm Hg, cardiac output 1.9 L/min, systemic vascular resistance 1400 (dyne · s)/cm^5 (normal is 900 to 1300), PaO$_2$ 140 mm Hg (FiO$_2$: 0.45), urine output 15 mL/h (specific gravity: 1.029), and hematocrit 35%. Given this data, which of the following is the most appropriate next step in management?

a. Administration of a diuretic to increase urine output
b. Administration of a vasopressor agent to increase systemic blood pressure
c. Administration of a fluid challenge to increase urine output
d. Administration of a vasodilating agent to decrease elevated systemic vascular resistance
e. A period of observation to obtain more data

60. A 59-year-old man with a history of myocardial infarction 2 years ago undergoes an uneventful aortobifemoral bypass graft for aortoiliac occlusive disease. Six hours later he develops ST segment depression, and a 12-lead electrocardiogram (ECG) shows anterolateral ischemia. His hemodynamic parameters are as follows: systemic BP 70/40 mm Hg, pulse 100 beats per minute, CVP 18 mm Hg, PCWP 25 mm Hg, cardiac output 1.5 L/min, and systemic vascular resistance 1000 (dyne · s)/cm^5. Which of the following is the single best pharmacologic intervention for this patient?

a. Sublingual nitroglycerin
b. Intravenous nitroglycerin
c. A short-acting beta blocker
d. Sodium nitroprusside
e. Dobutamine

61. A 56-year-old man undergoes a left upper lobectomy. An epidural catheter is inserted for postoperative pain relief. Ninety minutes after the first dose of epidural morphine, the patient complains of itching and becomes increasingly somnolent. Blood-gas measurement reveals the following: pH 7.24, $Paco_2$ 58, Pao_2 100, and HCO_3^- 28. Which of the following is the most appropriate initial therapy for this patient?

a. Endotracheal intubation
b. Intramuscular diphenhydramine (Benadryl)
c. Epidural naloxone
d. Intravenous naloxone
e. Alternative analgesia

62. A 71-year-old man returns from the operating room (OR) after undergoing a triple coronary bypass. His initial cardiac index is 2.8 L/(min·m²). Heart rate is then noted to be 55 beats per minute, BP is 110/80, wedge pressure is 15, and his cardiac index has dropped to 1.6 L/(min·m²). He has a normal left ventricle. Which of the following maneuvers will increase his cardiac output?

a. Increase his peripheral vascular resistance.
b. Increase his CVP.
c. Increase his heart rate to 90 by electrical pacing.
d. Increase his blood viscosity.
e. Increase his inspired O_2 concentration.

63. A 73-year-old woman with a long history of heavy smoking undergoes femoral artery–popliteal artery bypass for rest pain in her left leg. Because of serious underlying respiratory insufficiency, she continues to require ventilatory support for 4 days after her operation. As soon as her endotracheal tube is removed, she begins complaining of vague upper abdominal pain. She has daily fever spikes of 39°C (102.2°F) and a leukocyte count of 18,000/mL. An upper abdominal ultrasonogram reveals a dilated gallbladder, but no stones are seen. A presumptive diagnosis of acalculous cholecystitis is made. Which of the following is the next best step in her treatment?

a. Nasogastric suction and broad-spectrum antibiotics
b. Immediate cholecystectomy with operative cholangiogram
c. Percutaneous drainage of the gallbladder
d. Endoscopic retrograde cholangiopancreatography (ERCP) to visualize and drain the common bile duct
e. Provocation of cholecystokinin release by cautious feeding of the patient

64. A 32-year-old man undergoes a distal pancreatectomy, splenectomy, and partial colectomy for a gunshot wound to the left upper quadrant of the abdomen. One week later he develops a shaking chill in conjunction with a temperature spike of 39.4°C (103°F). His blood pressure is 70/40 mm Hg, pulse is 140 beats per minute, and respiratory rate is 45 breaths per minute. He is transferred to the intensive care unit (ICU), where he is intubated and a Swan-Ganz catheter is placed. Which of the following is consistent with the expected initial Swan-Ganz catheter readings?

a. An increase in cardiac output
b. An increase in peripheral vascular resistance
c. An increase in pulmonary artery pressure
d. An increase in PCWP
e. An increase in central venous pressure

65. A 43-year-old trauma patient develops acute respiratory distress syndrome (ARDS) and has difficulty oxygenating despite increased concentrations of inspired O_2. After the positive end-expiratory pressure (PEEP) is increased, the patient's oxygenation improves. What is the mechanism by which this occurs?

a. Decreasing dead-space ventilation
b. Decreasing the minute ventilation requirement
c. Increasing tidal volume
d. Increasing functional residual capacity
e. Redistribution of lung water from the interstitial to the alveolar space

66. A 27-year-old man was assaulted and stabbed on the left side of the chest between the areola and the sternum. He is hemodynamically unstable with jugular venous distention, distant heart sounds, and hypotension. Which of the following findings would be consistent with a diagnosis of hemodynamically significant cardiac tamponade?

a. More than a 10 mm Hg decrease in systolic blood pressure at the end of the expiratory phase of respiration
b. Decreased right atrial pressures on Swan-Ganz monitoring
c. Equalization of pressures across the four chambers on Swan-Ganz monitoring
d. Compression of the left ventricle on echocardiography
e. Overfilling of the right atrium

67. A 55-year-old woman requires a laparotomy for ovarian cancer. She has a history of stable angina. Which of the following characteristics is most likely to predict perioperative ischemic events during her noncardiac surgery?

a. Angina
b. More than three premature ventricular contractions (PVCs) per minute
c. Dyspnea on exertion
d. Tricuspid regurgitation
e. Her age

68. A woman is to undergo local excision of a suspicious nevus on her back. The surgeon intends to perform this excision with a local anesthetic. Which of the following statements regarding the use of local anesthetic agents is true?

a. When used for infiltration anesthesia, the maximal safe total dose of lidocaine is 3 mg/kg of body weight.
b. Addition of epinephrine (1:200,000) to the solution of lidocaine, procaine, or bupivacaine does not increase the maximal safe total dose but increases the duration of the block.
c. Numerous individuals are hypersensitive to local anesthetics.
d. A local anesthetic in contact with a nerve trunk will cause sensory loss but not motor paralysis in the area innervated.
e. Rapid systemic administration of local anesthetics may produce death without signs of central nervous system (CNS) stimulation.

69. A 22-year-old man sustains severe blunt trauma to the back. He notes that he cannot move his lower extremities. He is hypotensive and bradycardic. Which of the following is the best initial management of the patient?

a. Administration of phenylephrine
b. Administration of dopamine
c. Administration of epinephrine
d. Intravenous fluid bolus
e. Placement of a transcutaneous pacer

70. A 58-year-old woman with multiple comorbidities and previous cardiac surgery is in a high-speed motor vehicle collision. Because of hemodynamic instability, a Swan-Ganz catheter is placed. However, the PCWP and left ventricular end-diastolic pressure (LVEDP) do not appear to be correlating. Which of the following conditions would best explain this lack of correlation?

a. Aortic stenosis
b. Aortic regurgitation
c. Coronary artery disease
d. Positive-pressure ventilation with positive end-expiratory pressure/continuous positive airway pressure (PEEP/CPAP)
e. Bronchospasm

71. A 70-year-old man with a history of two prior strokes requires a femoral-popliteal bypass for threatened leg ischemia. His family is concerned about the risk of another perioperative stroke. Which of the following statements concerning perioperative stroke is true?

a. The mortality after postoperative stroke is high.
b. Most postoperative strokes occur directly after surgery and appear related to operative events.
c. The risk of stroke correlates with the length of time since previous stroke.
d. General state of health and severity of illness as measured by American Society of Anesthesiologists (ASA) classification are significant predictors of recurrent stroke.
e. The risk of stroke correlates with a history of multiple strokes or poststroke transient ischemic attacks (TIAs).

72. An 18-year-old woman develops urticaria and wheezing after an injection of intravenous contrast for an abdominal CT scan. Her blood pressure is 120/60 mm Hg, heart rate is 155 beats per minute, and respiratory rate is 30 breaths per minute. Which of the following is the most appropriate immediate therapy?

a. Intubation
b. Epinephrine
c. Beta blockers
d. Iodine
e. Fluid challenge

73. A patient develops a fever and tachycardia during a blood transfusion after a redo coronary artery bypass procedure. The nurse subsequently discovers that there was a mix-up in the cross-match because of a labeling error. Which of the following is diagnostic in a patient with an immediate hemolytic reaction secondary to a blood transfusion?

a. Serum haptoglobin above 50 mg/dL
b. Indirect bilirubin greater than 5 mg/dL
c. Direct bilirubin greater than 5 mg/dL
d. Positive Coombs test
e. Myoglobinuria

74. Your patient is receiving mechanical ventilation after surgery. A blood gas sample is sent to determine if weaning is possible. The P_{CO_2} is 40. Which of the following conclusions is most accurate?

a. There is probably a paradoxical aciduria.
b. Alveolar ventilation is adequate.
c. Arterial P_{O_2} will indicate the adequacy of alveolar ventilation.
d. Arterial P_{O_2} will indicate the degree of ventilation-perfusion mismatch.
e. Arterial P_{O_2} can be safely predicted to exceed 90 mm Hg on room air.

75. An obese 50-year-old woman undergoes a laparoscopic cholecystectomy. In the recovery room, she is found to be hypotensive and tachycardic. Her arterial blood gases reveal a pH of 7.29, Pa_{O_2} of 60 mm Hg, and Pa_{CO_2} of 54 mm Hg. Which of the following is the most likely cause of this patient's problem?

a. Acute pulmonary embolism
b. Carbon dioxide (CO_2) absorption from induced pneumoperitoneum
c. Alveolar hypoventilation
d. Pulmonary edema
e. Atelectasis from high diaphragm

76. A 65-year-old man who had a 25-lb weight loss over the previous 6 months is diagnosed with adenocarcinoma of the distal esophagus. He undergoes a transhiatal esophagectomy complicated by a cervical leak. He is receiving enteral feeds through a jejunostomy tube. After a week, his physicians wish to assess his nutritional resuscitation. Which of the following is the most accurate measure of adequacy of his nutritional support?

a. Urinary nitrogen excretion level
b. Total serum protein level
c. Serum albumin level
d. Serum transferrin level
e. Respiratory quotient

77. An elderly nursing home resident arrives at the emergency room moribund, with little helpful history. She is profoundly alkalotic by blood-gas measurement, and her urine shows an acid pH. Which of the following is the best possible explanation for these findings?

a. Release of inappropriate antidiuretic hormone
b. Severe crush injury
c. Acute tubular necrosis
d. Gastric outlet obstruction
e. An eosinophilic pituitary adenoma

78. A 22-year-old woman is involved in a major motor vehicle accident and receives a tracheostomy during her hospitalization. Five days after placement of the tracheostomy she has some minor bleeding around the tracheostomy site. Which of the following is the most appropriate immediate therapy?

a. Removal of tracheostomy at bedside.
b. Exchange the tracheostomy at bedside.
c. Exchange the tracheostomy in the operating room.
d. Bronchoscopic evaluation of the trachea at bedside.
e. Bronchoscopic evaluation of the trachea in the operating room.

79. A 72-year-old man undergoes resection of an abdominal aneurysm. He arrives in the ICU with a core temperature of 33°C (91.4°F) and shivering. Which of the following is a physiologic consequence of the shivering?

a. Rising mixed venous O_2 saturation
b. Increased production of CO_2
c. Decreased consumption of O_2
d. Rising base excess
e. Decreased minute ventilation

80. A 39-year-old woman with a known history of von Willebrand disease has a ventral hernia after a previous Caesarean section and desires to undergo elective repair. Which of the following should be administered preoperatively?

a. High-purity factor VIII: C concentrates
b. Low-molecular-weight dextran
c. Fresh-frozen plasma (FFP)
d. Cryoprecipitate
e. Whole blood

81. You are the physician on call for the extracorporeal membrane oxygenation (ECMO) service. There are five calls today, but only one machine and one technologist available. Which of the following patients is the most appropriate recipient of this service?

a. A 1-day-old, full-term, anencephalic 4-kg boy suffering from meconium aspiration syndrome and hypoxia
b. A 75-year-old man with Alzheimer disease, severe pneumonia, and elevated pulmonary arterial pressure
c. A neonate with a diagnosis of severe pulmonary hypoplasia who is in respiratory failure
d. A 5-year-old girl with rhabdomyosarcoma metastatic to the lungs
e. A 3-day-old boy preoperative for a congenital diaphragmatic hernia

82. A 72-year-old man has an altered sensorium after a high-speed motor vehicle collision and is placed in the intensive care unit for monitoring overnight. Which of the following strategies should be used in order to avoid the development of an aspiration pneumonia?

a. Nasogastric decompression
b. Steroids
c. Prophylactic antibiotics
d. Antacid administration
e. High positive end-expiratory pressure

83. A patient with severe neurological devastation after head trauma requires a secure long-term airway. Because of his body habitus, an open tracheostomy (as opposed to the percutaneous approach) is chosen. Which of the following is true regarding performance of the tracheostomy?

a. The strap muscles should be divided.
b. The thyroid isthmus should be preserved.
c. The trachea should be entered at the second or third cartilaginous ring.
d. Only horizontal incisions should be used.
e. Formal tracheostomy is preferable to cricothyroidotomy as an emergency procedure.

84. Shortly after the administration of an inhalational anesthetic and succinylcholine for intubation prior to an elective inguinal hernia repair in a 10-year-old boy, he becomes markedly febrile, displays a tachycardia of 160, and his urine changes color to a dark red. Which of the following is the most appropriate treatment at this time?

a. Complete the procedure but pretreat with dantrolene prior to future elective surgery.
b. Administer inhalational anesthetic agents.
c. Administer succinylcholine.
d. Hyperventilate with 100% O_2.
e. Acidify the urine to prevent myoglobin precipitation in the renal tubules.

85. A 42-year-old man has had a rocky course for the 3 days following a bowel resection for intestinal perforation due to inflammatory bowel disease. His CVP had been 12 to 14 but is now 6, in the face of diminished blood pressure and oliguria. Which of the following is the most likely etiology of his hypotension?

a. Pulmonary embolism
b. Hypervolemia
c. Positive-pressure ventilation
d. Pneumothorax
e. Gram-negative sepsis

86. Acute renal failure occurs following aortic angiography in a 72-year-old man. His weight has been rising, his lungs show rales at both bases, and he is dyspneic. His fractional excretion of sodium is greater than 1. He has eosinophilia on his peripheral smear, an elevated erythrocyte sedimentation rate, and proteinuria with microscopic hematuria. Which of the following is the most likely cause of his renal failure?

a. Hypovolemia
b. Renal artery cholesterol embolism
c. Acute tubular necrosis
d. Cardiogenic shock
e. Aortic dissection

87. A 55-year-old woman has been hospitalized because of recurrent pancreatitis, ARDS, prolonged ileus, and need for parenteral nutrition. She demonstrates weakness, lassitude, orthostatic hypotension, nausea, and fever. Which of the following abnormalities is most likely to explain these symptoms?

a. Hypothermia
b. Hypokalemia
c. Hyperglycemia
d. Hyponatremia
e. Hypervolemia

88. A 19-year-old male sustains severe lower-extremity trauma including a femur fracture and a crush injury to his foot. He requires vascular reconstruction of the popliteal artery. On the day after surgery, he becomes dyspneic and hypoxemic and requires intubation and mechanical ventilation. Which of the following is the most likely etiology of his decompensation?

a. Aspiration
b. Atelectasis
c. Fat embolism syndrome
d. Fluid overload
e. Pneumonia

89. A 33-year-old woman is brought to the emergency room from the scene of a severe motor vehicle accident. She is combative, confused, uncooperative, and appears dusky and dyspneic. Which of the following is the most appropriate management of her airway?

a. Awake endotracheal intubation is indicated in patients with penetrating ocular injury.
b. Steroids have been shown to be of value in the treatment of aspiration of acidic gastric secretions.
c. The stomach may be assumed to be empty only if a history is obtained indicating no ingestion of food or liquid during the prior 8 hours.
d. Intubation should be performed as soon as possible (in the emergency room) if the patient is unstable.
e. Cricothyroidotomy is contraindicated in the presence of maxillofacial injuries.

90. Following a boating injury in an industrial-use river, a patient begins to display fever, tachycardia, and a rapidly expanding area of erythema, blistering, and drainage from a flank wound. An x-ray shows gas in the soft tissues. Which of the following measures is most appropriate?

a. Administration of an antifungal agent
b. Administration of antitoxin
c. Wide debridement
d. Administration of hyperbaric O_2
e. Early closure of tissue defects

91. Following pelvic gynecologic surgery, a 34-year-old woman becomes dyspneic, her peripheral arterial O_2 saturation falls from 94% to 81%, and her measured PaO_2 is 52 on a 100% non-rebreathing mask. This is associated with which of the following?

a. Pulmonary thromboembolism
b. Lower abdominal surgery
c. Starvation
d. The upright position
e. Increased cardiac output

92. A 72-year-old woman who is planning to undergo ventral hernia repair is on warfarin for atrial fibrillation. She is advised to cease her warfarin several days before her surgery and is hospitalized preoperatively for heparinization. During her hospital stay, she complains of severe abdominal and flank pain. Her prothrombin time (PT) is normal, but her activated partial thromboplastin time (aPTT) is elevated. An abdominal CT scan demonstrates a large retroperitoneal hematoma. Which of the following should be administered to reverse the effects of the heparin?

a. Thrombin
b. Vitamin K
c. Protamine sulfate
d. Aprotinin
e. Platelet transfusion

93. A 42-year-old refinery worker is transferred to your burn unit. He was dyspneic and in respiratory distress at the scene and was intubated by alert paramedics. Soot is suctioned from the tube. Which of the following is characteristic of this condition?

a. Smoke inhalation is a thermal rather than a chemical injury.
b. Carbon monoxide levels are not likely to be elevated unless there is evidence of skin or oropharyngeal burns.
c. Chest x-rays during the early postinhalation period show a characteristic ground-glass appearance.
d. Damage to the upper respiratory tract is common and is usually found on laryngoscopy.
e. The mortality associated with smoke inhalation is low in the absence of cutaneous burns.

94. A young man was seen swallowing small packets containing an unknown substance during a drug bust. Which of the following would be an indication for laparotomy?

a. Refusal to take high doses of laxatives
b. Refusal to allow endoscopic retrieval
c. Refusal to allow digital rectal disimpaction
d. Intraintestinal drug packets evident on abdominal x-ray in an asymptomatic smuggler
e. Signs of toxicity from leaking drug packets

Questions 95 to 97

Match the side effects with the appropriate agent. Each lettered option may be used once, more than once, or not at all.

a. Nitrous oxide (N_2O)
b. Succinylcholine
c. Midazolam
d. Pancuronium
e. Morphine

95. A 65-year-old man with a 35% body surface area (BSA) burn develops hyperkalemia after induction.

96. An acutely injured patient becomes hypotensive shortly after induction.

97. A patient with a bowel obstruction develops increasingly distended loops of bowel after induction.

Questions 98 to 100

For each clinical problem, select the best method of physiologic monitoring necessary for the patient. Each lettered option may be used once, more than once, or not at all.

a. Central venous catheterization
b. Pulmonary artery catheterization
c. Blood-gas monitoring
d. Intracranial pressure monitoring
e. Arterial catheterization
f. Continuous ECG monitoring

98. A 74-year-old man has a 5-hour elective operation for repair of an abdominal aortic aneurysm. He had a small myocardial infarction 3 years earlier. In the ICU on the first postoperative day, he is hypotensive and is receiving dobutamine by continuous infusion.

99. A 62-year-old woman underwent a right carotid endarterectomy for symptomatic high-grade carotid artery stenosis. Postoperatively, her blood pressure is 202/105, and she is started on a nitroprusside infusion.

100. A comatose 28-year-old woman sustained a depressed skull fracture in an automobile collision. She has been unconscious for 6 weeks. Her vital signs are stable and she breathes room air. Following her initial decompressive craniotomy, she has returned to the operating room twice due to intracranial bleeding.

Questions 101 to 103

For each test, select the coagulation factor(s) whose functions are measured. Each lettered option may be used once, more than once, or not at all.

a. Factor II
b. Factor V
c. Factor VIII
d. Platelets
e. Fibrinogen

101. A patient is receiving oral warfarin to effect anticoagulation because of an artificial heart valve. Prothrombin time is 21 (INR = 2.3).

102. A patient with heparin-induced thrombocytopenia is placed on hirudin and undergoes assessment of his clotting function. Thrombin time is 30 seconds.

103. A patient is to undergo a coronary bypass. Bleeding time is 6 minutes.

Critical Care: Anesthesiology, Blood Gases, and Respiratory Care

Answers

50. The answer is c. (*Brunicardi, pp 338-339.*) The patient had a sentinel bleed from a tracheoinnominate artery fistula, which carries a greater than 50% mortality rate. If the bleeding has ceased, then immediate fiberoptic exploration in the operating room is indicated. If the bleeding is ongoing, several stopgap measures can be attempted while preparing for median sternotomy in the operating room, including inflation of the tracheostomy balloon to attempt compression of the innominate artery, reintubation of the patient with an endotracheal tube, and removal of the tracheostomy and placement of the finger through the site with anterior compression of the innominate artery.

51. The answer is d. (*Brunicardi, pp 373-374; Townsend, pp 617-618.*) There are multiple predictors that have been used to assess readiness for extubation. No single parameter is 100% predictive; attempted extubation should be based on correction of the underlying pathology, clinical status and hemodynamic stability, and a combination of the following parameters. The rapid shallow breathing index is the ratio of the respiratory rate to tidal volume. There is evidence to suggest that an index between 60 and 105 predicts successful extubation. The negative inspiratory force should be at least greater than -20 cm H_2O. The patient should be weaned to 5 cm H_2O PEEP before attempting extubation. The minute ventilation, which is the product of the tidal volume and respiratory rate, should be less than 10 L/min. The spontaneous respiratory rate should also be below 20 breaths per minute.

52. The answer is e. *(Brunicardi, pp 79-80.)* Whenever a hemolytic reaction caused by an incompatible blood transfusion is suspected, transfusion should be stopped immediately. A Foley catheter should be inserted and hourly urine output should be monitored. Renal damage caused by precipitation of hemoglobin in the renal tubules is the major serious consequence of hemolysis. This precipitation is inhibited in an alkaline environment and is promoted in an acid environment. Stimulating diuresis with mannitol and alkalinizing the urine with sodium bicarbonate intravenously are indicated procedures. Fluid and potassium intake should be restricted in the presence of severe oliguria or anuria.

53. The answer is b. *(Townsend, p 432.)* Nitrous oxide has a low solubility compared with other inhalation anesthetics; nitrous oxide is more soluble in blood than nitrogen and is the only anesthetic gas less dense than air. As a result of these properties, nitrous oxide may cause progressive distension of air-filled spaces during prolonged anesthesia. Since nitrous oxide diffuses into gas-filled compartments faster than nitrogen can diffuse out, its use can lead to worsened distention, which may be undesirable (eg, in an operation for intestinal obstruction).

54. The answer is a. *(Brunicardi, pp 344-345.)* Adult respiratory distress syndrome has been called "shock lung" or "traumatic wet lung" and occurs under a variety of circumstances. The diagnosis can be made based on bilateral pulmonary infiltrates on chest x-ray, a PaO_2/FiO_2 ratio of less than 200, and pulmonary wedge pressures of less than 18 mm Hg (low filling pressures exclude the diagnosis of pulmonary edema). Three major physiologic alterations include (1) hypoxemia usually unresponsive to elevations of inspired O_2 concentration; (2) decreased pulmonary compliance, as the lungs become progressively stiffer and harder to ventilate; and (3) decreased functional residual capacity. Progressive alveolar collapse occurs owing to leakage of protein-rich fluid into the interstitium and the alveolar spaces with the subsequent radiologic picture of diffuse fluffy infiltrates bilaterally. Ventilatory abnormalities develop that result in shunt formation, decreased resting lung volume, and increased dead-space ventilation.

55. The answer is d. *(Greenfield, pp 218-219.)* The shape of the O_2 dissociation curve translates into several physiologic advantages. The relatively flat slope above a PO_2 of 50 mm Hg means that, in this region of the curve, hemoglobin saturation decreases slightly with decrements in PO_2; loading of O_2 at the alveolar level is therefore affected minimally, with mild to moderate degrees of hypoxemia. The steeper slope at the lower end of the curve means that as the hemoglobin becomes desaturated, arterial PO_2 drops only minimally and a gradient that favors O_2 diffusion into tissue cells is maintained. Acidosis, a rise in $PaCO_2$, and elevation of temperature all shift the curve to the right, which enhances tissue O_2 uptake. Red blood cell organic phosphates, particularly 2,3-diphosphoglycerate (2,3-DPG), also affect the dissociation curve. Banked blood, being low in 2,3-DPG, shifts the curve to the left and therefore decreases tissue O_2 uptake. 2,3-DPG levels increase with chronic hypoxia. Chronic lung disease, therefore, results in a shift of the curve to the right, which enhances O_2 delivery to peripheral tissues.

56. The answer is e. *(Brunicardi, p 52.)* The patient is suffering from respiratory acidosis, caused by the accumulation of CO_2, and hypoxemia. Both disturbances can be resolved with endotracheal intubation and ventilatory support. Agitation can be an early sign of hypoxemia in an elderly patient and should never be ignored. Benzodiazepines such as Ativan in this patient will cause stupor and worsen his hypoxemia and respiratory acidosis. Bicarbonate should not be administered because buffer reserves are already adequate (serum bicarbonate is still 34 mEq/L based on the Henderson-Hasselbalch equation).

57. The answer is b. *(Townsend, pp 95-96.)* Dopamine has a variety of pharmacologic characteristics that make it useful in critically ill patients. In low doses [1-5 mg/(kg · min)], dopamine affects primarily the dopaminergic receptors. Activation of these receptors causes vasodilation of the renal and mesenteric vasculature and mild vasoconstriction of the peripheral bed, which thereby redirects blood flow to kidneys and bowel. At these low doses, the net effect on the overall vascular resistance may be slight. As the dose rises (2-10 mg/[kg · min]), β_1-receptor activity predominates and the inotropic effect on the myocardium leads to increased cardiac output and blood pressure. Above 10 mg/(kg · min), α-receptor stimulation causes peripheral vasoconstriction, shifting of blood from extremities to organs, decreased kidney function, and hypertension. At all doses, the diastolic blood pressure can be expected to rise; since coronary perfusion is largely a result of the head of pressure at the coronary ostia, coronary blood flow should be increased.

58. The answer is d. *(Goodnough, pp 602-609.)* Cytomegalovirus (CMV) is harbored in blood leukocytes. CMV infection is endemic in the United

States, and its prevalence increases steadily with age. While acute CMV infection may cause transient fever, jaundice, and hepatosplenomegaly in cases of large blood donor exposures, posttransfusion CMV infection (seroconversion) is not a significant clinical problem in immunocompetent recipients, and therefore blood is not routinely tested for the presence of CMV. Posttransfusion non-A, non-B hepatitis, however, not only represents the most frequent infectious complication of transfusion but also is associated with an incidence of chronic active hepatitis up to 16% and an 8% to 10% incidence of cirrhosis or hepatoma or both. The etiologic agent in over 90% of cases of posttransfusion hepatitis has been identified as hepatitis C.

59. The answer is c. (*Brunicardi, p 741.*) A ruptured abdominal aneurysm is a surgical emergency often accompanied by serious hypotension and vascular collapse before surgery and massive fluid shifts with renal failure after surgery. In this case, all the hemodynamic parameters indicate inadequate intravascular volume, and the patient is therefore suffering from hypovolemic shock. The low urine output indicates poor renal perfusion, while the high urine specific gravity indicates adequate renal function with compensatory free-water conservation. The administration of a vasopressor agent would certainly raise the blood pressure, but it would do so by increasing peripheral vascular resistance and thereby further decrease tissue perfusion. The deleterious effects of shock would be increased. A vasodilating agent to lower the systemic vascular resistance would lead to profound hypotension and possibly complete vascular collapse because of pooling of an already depleted vascular volume. This patient's blood pressure is critically dependent on an elevated systemic vascular resistance. To properly treat this patient, rapid fluid infusion and expansion of the intravascular volume must be undertaken. This can be easily done with lactated Ringer solution or blood (or both) until improvements in such parameters as the PCWP, urine output, and blood pressure are noted.

60. The answer is e. (*Townsend, pp 94-96.*) This patient has developed pump failure because of a combination of preexisting coronary artery occlusive disease and high preload following a fluid challenge; afterload remains moderately high as well because of systemic vasoconstriction in the presence of cardiogenic shock. Poor myocardial performance is reflected in the low cardiac output and high PCWP. Therapy must be directed at increasing cardiac output without creating too high a myocardial O_2 demand on the already failing heart. Administration of nitroglycerin could be expected to reduce both preload and afterload, but if given without an inotrope it would create unacceptable hypotension. Nitroprusside similarly would achieve afterload reduction but would result in hypotension if not accompanied by an inotropic agent. A beta blocker would act deleteriously by reducing cardiac contractility and slowing the heart rate in a setting in which cardiac output is likely to be rate-dependent. Dobutamine is a synthetic catecholamine that is becoming the inotropic agent of choice in cardiogenic shock. As a β_1-adrenergic agonist, it improves cardiac performance in pump failure both by positive inotropy and peripheral vasodilation. With minimal chronotropic effect, dobutamine only marginally increases myocardial O_2 demand.

61. The answer is d. *(Thoren, pp 687-694.)* Thoracic epidural narcotics have become an increasingly popular means of postoperative pain relief in thoracic and upper abdominal surgery. Local action on γ opiate receptors ensures pain relief and consequent improvement in respiration without vasodilation or paralysis. The less lipid-soluble opiates are effective for long periods. Their slow absorption into the circulation also ensures a low incidence of centrally mediated side effects, such as respiratory depression or generalized itching. When these do occur, the intravenous injection of an opiate antagonist is an effective antidote. The locally mediated analgesia is not affected. One poorly understood side effect, which is apparently unrelated to systemic levels, is a profound reduction in gastric activity. This may be an important consideration after thoracic surgery when an early resumption of oral intake is anticipated.

62. The answer is c. *(Brunicardi, pp 364-366.)* The cardiac index is computed by dividing the cardiac output by the body surface area; the cardiac output is the product of the stroke volume and the heart rate (CI = CO/BSA; CO = SV×HR; therefore, CI = [SV × HR]/BSA). An increased heart rate will directly increase the cardiac output and cardiac index. The remaining choices will either decrease or not affect the stroke volume and consequently will not increase the cardiac index.

63. The answer is c. *(Brunicardi, p 1208.)* The development of acute postoperative cholecystitis is an increasingly recognized complication of the severe illnesses that precipitate admissions to the ICU. The causes are obscure but probably lead to a common final pathway of gallbladder ischemia. The diagnosis is often extremely difficult because the signs and symptoms may be those of occult sepsis. Moreover, the patients are often intubated, sedated, or confused as a consequence of the other therapeutic or medical factors.

Biochemical tests, though frequently revealing abnormal liver function, are nonspecific and nondiagnostic. Bedside ultrasonography is usually strongly suggestive of the diagnosis when a thickened gallbladder wall or pericholecystic fluid is present; nonvisualization of the gallbladder on a nuclear medicine (HIDA) scan can also be diagnostic. If diagnosis is delayed, mortality and morbidity are very high. Percutaneous drainage of the gallbladder is usually curative of acalculous cholecystitis and affords stabilizing palliation if calculous cholecystitis is present. Antibiotics without drainage are too cautious a choice for a patient with a potentially fatal complication. Operative intervention is indicated only if less invasive methods of treatment (percutaneous cholecystostomy tube) have failed, and ERCP is not indicated in the absence of ductal obstruction.

64. The answer is a. *(Townsend, pp 102-107.)* The case presented is most consistent with septic shock from a postoperative intra-abdominal abscess. In the early phase of septic shock, the respiratory profile is characterized by mild hypoxia with a compensatory hyperventilation and respiratory alkalosis. Hemodynamically, a hyperdynamic state is seen with an increase in cardiac output and a decrease in peripheral vascular resistance in the face of relatively normal central pressures. Initial therapy is aimed at resuscitation and stabilization. This includes fluid replacement and vasopressors as well as antibiotic therapy aimed particularly at gram-negative rods and anaerobes for patients with presumed intra-abdominal collections, especially after bowel surgery. Laparotomy and drainage of a collection is the definitive therapy but should await stabilization of the patient and confirmation of the presence and location of such a collection.

65. The answer is d. *(Moore, pp 1267-1268.)* PEEP improves oxygenation by increasing functional residual capacity by keeping the alveoli open at the end of expiration. Extravascular lung water is shifted from the alveolar to the interstitial space. The overall result is to increase surface area for diffusive exchange of gases. Potential negative effects of increased PEEP include alveolar overdistention resulting in barotraumas (pneumothoraces), decreased venous return and decreased cardiac output, and increased minute ventilation requirements due to increased dead-space ventilation.

66. The answer is c. *(Moore, pp 172-173.)* On physical exam, cardiac tamponade may manifest with Beck triad (systemic hypotension, jugular venous distention, and distant heart sounds). Also, the patient may have pulsus paradoxus, which is manifested by a decrease in systolic blood pressure by more than 10 mm Hg at the end of the inspiratory phase of respiration. On echocardiogram, there will be pericardial fluid and right atrial collapse. On Swan-Ganz monitoring, there will be equalization of pressures across the four chambers. The right atrial pressures and central venous pressure are increased and cardiac output is decreased.

67. The answer is c. (*Charlson, pp 637-648.*) The landmark study by Goldman in 1978 identified cardiac risk factors in noncardiac surgical patients that included previous infarction (particularly infarction within 6 months, but with increased risk continuing for life), functional impairment such as dyspnea on exertion, age over 70 years, mitral regurgitation, more than five PVCs per minute, and a tortuous or calcified aorta. Angina alone was not a risk factor. Subsequent studies by others have differed regarding the importance of several of these factors, which probably reflects different comorbid characteristics in the study populations (eg, diabetes and hypertension). Additional predictors of perioperative cardiac risk that achieved significance in some studies but not in others include cardiomegaly, upper abdominal or intrathoracic surgery, and intraoperative hypotension.

68. The answer is e. (*Townsend, pp 449-451.*) The maximal safe total dose of lidocaine administered to a 70-kg man is 4.5 mg/kg, or approximately 30 to 35 mL of a 1% solution. The addition of epinephrine to lidocaine, procaine, or bupivacaine not only doubles the duration of infiltration anesthesia, but increases the maximal safe total dose by one-third by decreasing the rate of absorption of drug into the bloodstream. However, epinephrine-containing solutions should not be injected into tissues supplied by end arteries (eg, fingers, toes, ears, nose, penis). Hypersensitivity to local anesthetics is uncommon and occurs most prominently with anesthetics of the ester type (procaine, tetracaine). While small nerve fibers seem to be most susceptible to the action of local anesthetics, these agents act on any part of the nervous system and on every type of nerve fiber. CNS toxicity usually appears as stimulation followed by depression, probably because of an early selective depression of inhibitory neurons; with a massive overdose, all neurons may be depressed simultaneously.

69. The answer is d. (*Brunicardi, p 100.*) The patient is in neurogenic shock as a result of a spinal cord injury. Neurogenic shock is characterized by loss of sympathetic tone peripherally as well as bradycardia owing to loss of the reflexive increase in heart rate in response to hypotension. Initial treatment is with fluid resuscitation followed by initiation of vasoconstrictors such as dopamine or phenylephrine. Hypovolemia caused by hemorrhage should also be ruled out in trauma patients.

70. The answer is d. (*Brunicardi, pp 364-368.*) When a Swan-Ganz pulmonary artery catheter is in the wedge position, that is, isolating the pulmonary arterial system from the pulmonary capillaries, the measured PCWP is usually equivalent to both the left atrial pressure (LAP) and the left ventricular end-diastolic pressure. However, pathologic processes in the pulmonary vasculature and heart valves may alter this relationship. Pulmonary vaso-occlusive disease may elevate the PCWP independent of the LAP or LVEDP. Bronchospasm affecting the airway but not the pulmonary vasculature should not affect the validity of Swan-Ganz catheter readings. Mitral stenosis and regurgitation cause increased LAP and PCWP, which result in an overestimated LVEDP. However, aortic stenosis and regurgitation elevate the PCWP, LAP, and LVEDP equally. Accurate measurement of PCWP by a Swan-Ganz catheter may not be possible in the presence of positive airway pressure with PEEP/CPAP; transmission of the positive airway pressure to the pulmonary microvasculature via the alveoli, especially in the upper lung zones, results in measurement of alveolar pressure rather than LAP or LVEDP. Coronary artery disease does not affect the relationship between PCWP, LAP, and LVEDP.

71. The answer is a. (*Landercasper, pp 986-989.*) In an 8-year retrospective study of 173 consecutive patients with a documented medical history of stroke who underwent subsequent general anesthesia and surgery (excluding cardiac, cerebrovascular, and neurological surgery), five patients (2.9%) had documented postoperative strokes from 3 to 21 days (mean 12.2 days) after surgery. The risk of stroke did not correlate with age, sex, history of multiple strokes or poststroke TIAs, ASA classification, aspirin use, coronary artery disease, peripheral vascular disease, intraoperative blood pressure, time since previous stroke, or cause of previous stroke. The risk of recurrent stroke appears to be comparable with that for surgical patients who do not have a history of prior stroke and are undergoing cardiac and peripheral vascular surgery. Most recurrent strokes occur many hours to days following surgery and do not appear to be directly related to operative events. The mortality after postoperative stroke is high.

72. The answer is b. (*Greenfield, p 1661.*) This patient is having an anaphylactoid reaction with destabilization of the cardiovascular and respiratory systems. Anaphylactoid reactions are most commonly caused by iodinated contrast media, β-lactam antibiotics (eg, penicillin), and *Hymenoptera* stings. Manifestations of anaphylactoid reactions include both lethal (bronchospasm, laryngospasm, hypotension, dysrhythmia) and nonlethal (pruritus, urticaria, syncope, weakness, seizure) phenomena. Epinephrine is the initial treatment for laryngeal obstruction and bronchospasm, followed by histamine antagonists (H_1 and H_2 blockers), aminophylline, and hydrocortisone. Vasopressors and fluid challenges may be given for shock. Conscious patients are usually stabilized with injected or inhaled epinephrine, while unconscious patients and those with refractory hypotension or hypoxia should be intubated.

73. The answer is d. (*Brunicardi, pp 78-79.*) Most transfusion reactions are hemolytic and are due to clerical errors that result in administration of blood with major (ABO) and minor antigen incompatibility. Intravascular hemolysis results in hemoglobinemia. Because haptoglobin binds hemoglobin via a receptor located on macrophages, serum haptoglobin levels are decreased; haptoglobin level < 50 mg/dL is one criterion for a transfusion reaction. Additionally, hemoglobinuria with a free hemoglobin level greater than 5 mg/dL is another criterion. A positive Coombs test is diagnostic. Indirect hyperbilirubinemia and anemia may be seen in delayed transfusion reactions, which occur between 2 and 10 days after a transfusion. Delayed transfusion reactions can occur due to antibodies to Rh antigens and are characterized by extravascular hemolysis.

74. The answer is b. (*Brunicardi, pp 50-52.*) Because of the highly efficient diffusion characteristics of CO_2, Pa_{CO_2} levels are reliable indicators of adequacy of alveolar ventilation. A Pa_{CO_2} of 40 mm Hg is the normal value. Paradoxical aciduria occurs when hypokalemic metabolic alkalosis is present, as the kidney excretes hydrogen ion in an effort to conserve potassium ion. Though a Pa_{CO_2} of 40 mm Hg is not incompatible with metabolic alkalosis, it would ordinarily be higher, as the patient tries to conserve carbolic acid by hypoventilating to compensate. Pa_{O_2} levels are influenced by so many other variables (eg, age, concentration of inspired O_2, altitude) that no inferences can be made about adequacy of alveolar ventilation from Pa_{O_2} alone, nor can Pa_{O_2} be safely predicted by the presence of normocarbia. The ventilation-perfusion mismatch is a reflection of the gradient between alveolar and arterial O_2 tension in relationship to percentage of inspired O_2.

75. The answer is c. *(Brunicardi, p 52.)* Because of the ease with which CO_2 diffuses across the alveolar membranes, $PaCO_2$ is a highly reliable indicator of alveolar ventilation. In this postoperative patient with respiratory acidosis and hypoxemia, the hypercarbia is diagnostic of alveolar hypoventilation. Acute hypoxemia can occur with pulmonary embolism, pulmonary edema, and significant atelectasis, but in all those situations the $PaCO_2$ should be normal or reduced, as the patient hyperventilates to improve oxygenation. The absorption of gas from the peritoneal cavity may transiently affect the $PaCO_2$, but should have no effect on oxygenation.

76. The answer is c. *(Townsend, pp 1484-1485.)* The serum albumin level provides a rough estimate of protein nutritional adequacy. The accuracy of this estimate is affected by the long half-life of albumin (3 weeks) and the vagaries of hemodilution. The acute-phase serum proteins have a very short half-life (hours) and may also provide good short-term indications of nutritional status. Transferrin is one of these acute-phase proteins, but unfortunately its levels, too, are influenced by changes in intravascular volume and, along with the other acute-phase reactants, rise nonspecifically during acute illness. All the listed responses provide some useful information about nutrition and adequacy of replacement.

77. The answer is d. *(Brunicardi, pp 50-52.)* The body has elaborate mechanisms to compensate for metabolic acidosis. Not only do most body functions work better in an acidotic state, but the patient is able to move toward correction of the pH by excreting acid urine and by hyperventilating to "blow off" carbonic acid. On the other hand, we are poorly equipped to deal with metabolic alkalosis. We cannot hold our breath to save acid because the respiratory center overrides our efforts as the $PaCO_2$ rises and the PaO_2 falls. The kidney cannot make urine under any circumstance that is very far above normal pH. In the subtraction alkalosis that accompanies gastric outlet obstruction with loss of gastric acid by vomiting or suction, the potassium depletion and volume deficits provoke exchange of sodium for hydrogen ion in the distal tubule, with resultant exacerbation of the metabolic alkalosis. All the other conditions listed would be expected to produce acidosis; consequently, acid urine would not be paradoxical.

78. The answer is e. *(Brunicardi, pp 338-339.)* A rare but deadly complication of a tracheostomy is a tracheoinnominate artery fistula (TIAF); when suspected, the diagnosis should be confirmed or ruled out in the operating room. TIAFs can occur as early as 2 days after tracheostomy or as late as 2 months after the procedure. It is often associated with low placement of a tracheostomy (distal to the second and third tracheal rings). The patient may have a sentinel bleed in 50% of TIAF cases, followed by a very impressive bleed. If a sentinel bleed is suspected the patient should be transported immediately to the operating room for bronchoscopic evaluation. Initial maneuvers for management of a TIAF include overinflation of the cuff on the tracheostomy or reintubation from above followed by removal of the tracheostomy and finger compression of the innominate artery against the sternum through the tracheostomy wound.

79. The answer is b. *(Brunicardi, p 356.)* Shivering is the physiologic effort of the body to generate heat to maintain the core temperature. In healthy persons, shivering increases the metabolic rate by three to five times and results in increased O_2 consumption and CO_2 production. In critically ill patients, these metabolic consequences are almost always counterproductive and should be prevented with other means employed to correct systemic hypothermia. In the presence of vigorous shivering, O_2 debt in the muscles and lactic acidemia develop.

80. The answer is d. *(Townsend, pp 118-119.)* Von Willebrand disease is similar to true hemophilia in frequency of occurrence. It is being diagnosed more commonly today because of more reliable assays for factor VIII. This autosomal dominant disorder (recessive transmission can occur) is characterized by a diminution in factor VIII: C (procoagulant) activity. The reduction in activity is not as great as in classic hemophilia, and the clinical manifestations are more subtle. These manifestations are often overlooked until an episode of trauma or surgery makes them apparent. Treatment requires correcting the bleeding time and providing factor VIII R: WF (the von Willebrand factor). Only cryoprecipitate is reliably effective. High purity factor VIII: C concentrates, effective in hemophilia, lack the von Willebrand factor and are consequently undependable.

81. The answer is e. *(Townsend, pp 2050-2051.)* ECMO is a form of cardiopulmonary support that is useful in the setting of potentially reversible pulmonary or cardiac disease. Treatment of meconium aspiration syndrome, sepsis, pneumonia, and congenital diaphragmatic hernia (pre- or postoperatively) are thus appropriate uses. The technique is also applicable in some circumstances as a bridge to cardiac or lung transplantation since the outlook for survival is quite good if the child can be maintained in a good physiological state until donor organs are available. Hypoplastic lungs do not have enough surface area to perform adequate gas exchange and are unlikely to mature to a point where they can sustain life. Babies with hypoplastic lungs will be bypass-dependent for life and consequently are not candidates for institution of ECMO therapy.

82. The answer is a. (*Moore, pp 383-384.*) Immediate emptying of the stomach after traumatic injury and nasogastric decompression are important for the prevention of aspiration of gastric contents. Elevation of the head of the bed is also recommended for ICU patients. Prophylactic antibiotics are not indicated in high-risk patients, even after gross aspiration. Although gross aspiration results in a chemical pneumonitis, antibiotics are indicated only if pneumonia develops. Antacids result in loss of the protective effect of acidification of gastric contents and subsequent colonization with gram-negative organisms, and therefore should be avoided. Sucralfate may be a better choice for stress ulcer prophylaxis. Steroids are not indicated. High positive end expiratory pressure is not required in patients unless respiratory failure develops.

83. The answer is c. (*Brunicardi, p 338-339.*) Although tracheostomy is occasionally an emergency procedure, it can be more effectively performed in an operating room, where hemostasis and antisepsis are readily achieved. Most authorities recommend a horizontal incision; however, limited direct midline incisions have the advantage of not opening any unnecessary tissue planes and perhaps reducing the incidence of bleeding complications. Both approaches have advocates. In either case, the skin incision is made just below the cricoid cartilage, the strap muscles are spared and retracted, the thyroid isthmus is divided if necessary, and the trachea is entered at the second tracheal ring. The second and third tracheal rings are incised vertically, allowing placement of the tracheostomy tube. The first tracheal ring and the cricoid cartilage must be left intact.

84. The answer is d. (*Brunicardi, pp 356-357.*) The cause of malignant hyperthermia is unknown, but it is associated with inhalational anesthetic agents and succinylcholine. It may develop in an otherwise healthy person who has tolerated previous surgery without incident. It should be suspected in the presence of a history of unexplained fever, muscle or connective tissue disorder, or a positive family history (evidence suggests an autosomal dominant inheritance pattern). In addition to fever during anesthesia, the syndrome includes tachycardia, increased O_2 consumption, increased CO_2 production, increased serum K^+, myoglobinuria, and acidosis. Rigidity rather than relaxation following succinylcholine injection may be the first clue to its presence. Treatment of malignant hyperthermia should include prompt conclusion of the operative procedure and cessation of anesthesia, hyperventilation with 100% O_2, and administration of intravenous dantrolene. The urine should be alkalinized to protect the kidneys from myoglobin precipitation. If reoperation is necessary, the physician should premedicate heavily, alkalinize the urine, and avoid depolarizing agents such as succinylcholine. Pretreatment for 24 hours with dantrolene is helpful; it is thought to act directly on muscle fiber to attenuate calcium release.

85. The answer is e. (*Moore, pp 1196-1197.*) Determination of CVP has been helpful in the overall hemodynamic assessment of the patient. This pressure can be affected by a variety of factors including those of cardiac, noncardiac, and artifactual origin. Venous tone, right ventricular compliance, intrathoracic pressure, and blood volume all influence CVP. Vasoconstrictor drugs, positive pressure ventilation (with and without PEEP), mediastinal compression, and hypervolemia all increase CVP. Acute pulmonary embolism, when clinically significant, elevates CVP by causing right ventricular overload and increased right atrial pressure. Sepsis, on the other hand, decreases CVP through both the release of vasodilatory mediators and the loss of intravascular plasma volume due to increased capillary permeability. Trends in CVP measurement are more reliable than isolated readings.

86. The answer is b. (*Greenfield, p 1581.*) Cholesterol atheroembolism is a known complication of angiography or aortic manipulation during surgery and can result in lower extremity ischemia, acute myocardial infarction, ischemic bowel, and acute or chronic renal failure. Eosinophilia is strongly suggestive of cholesterol atheroembolization, and other laboratory findings include microscopic hematuria or proteinuria and elevated inflammatory mediators such as erythrocyte sedimentation rate. A fractional excretion of sodium (FENa) of greater than 1 suggests a renal cause of acute renal failure as opposed to prerenal causes such as hypovolemia or cardiogenic shock. Thoracic aortic dissections can result in acute renal failure if they involve the renal arteries and may present with hematuria and elevations in BUN and creatinine. However, aortic dissections are typically associated with significant chest pain.

87. The answer is d. (*Brunicardi, pp 1463-1465.*) Clinical manifestations of adrenocortical insufficiency include hyperkalemia, hyponatremia, hypoglycemia, fever, weight loss, and dehydration. There is excessive sodium loss in the urine, contraction of the plasma volume, and perhaps hypotension or shock. Classic hyperpigmentation is present in chronic Addison disease only. Addison disease may present in newborns as a congenital atrophy, as an insidious chronic state often caused by tuberculosis, as an acute dysfunction secondary to trauma or adrenal hemorrhage, or as a semiacute adrenal insufficiency seen during stress or surgery. In this last instance, signs and symptoms include nausea, lassitude, vomiting, fever, progressive salt wasting, hyperkalemia, and hypoglycemia. It may be confirmed by measurements of urinary Na^+ loss and absence of response to adrenocorticotropic hormone (ACTH).

88. The answer is c. (*Moore, p 412.*) Fat embolism syndrome is a relatively uncommon complication of long-bone fractures and is characterized by acute respiratory failure, altered mental status, and petechiae. Unfortunately, there are no reliable diagnostic tests, and management is supportive only. Pulmonary edema is unlikely in an otherwise healthy 19-year-old male without chest trauma or evidence of a cardiac contusion. Aspiration is unlikely in an awake patient with normal mental status. Pneumonias typically present with fever and/or leukocytosis, productive cough, and a new infiltrate on chest x-ray. Atelectasis in and of itself is not a cause for respiratory failure.

89. The answer is d. (*Moore, pp 189-194.*) Securing a stable airway is one of the most fundamental and important aspects of the management of the severely injured patient. The level of control required will vary from a simple oropharyngeal airway to tracheostomy, depending on the clinical situation. Full control of the airway should be secured in the emergency room if the patient is unstable. Endotracheal intubation will usually be the method chosen, but the physician should be prepared to do a tracheotomy if attempts at perioral or perinasal intubation are failing or are impractical because of maxillofacial injuries. The most dangerous period is just prior to and during the initial attempts to get control of the airway. Manipulation of the oronasopharynx may provoke combative behavior or vomiting in a patient already confused by drugs, alcohol, hypoxia, or cerebral trauma. The risk of aspiration is high during these initial attempts, and the physician should make no assumptions about the state of the contents of the patient's stomach. Antacids are recommended just prior to the intubation attempt, if feasible. Although steroids have been recommended in the past, they are no longer considered of value in the management of aspiration of acidic gastric juice. The best management requires prevention of the complication of aspiration. In a reasonably cooperative patient, awake intubation with topical anesthesia may help to prevent some of the risks of hypotension, arrhythmia, and aspiration associated with the induction of anesthesia. If awake intubation is inappropriate, then an alternative is rapid-sequence induction with a thio-barbiturate followed by muscle paralysis with succinylcholine. If elevated intracranial pressure is suspected, or if a penetrating eye injury exists, awake intubation is contraindicated.

90. The answer is c. *(Brunicardi, p 434.)* Necrotizing skin and soft tissue infections may produce insoluble gases (hydrogen, nitrogen, methane) through anaerobic bacterial metabolism. While the term "gas gangrene" has come to imply clostridial infection, gas in tissues is more likely not to be caused by *Clostridium* species but rather to other facultative and obligate anaerobes, particularly streptococci. Though fungi have also been implicated, they are less often associated with rapidly progressive infections. Treatment for necrotizing soft tissue infections includes repeated wide debridement, with wound recon-struction delayed until a stable, viable wound surface has been established. The use of hyperbaric O_2 in the treatment of gas gangrene remains controversial, due to lack of proven benefit, difficulty in transporting critically ill patients to hyperbaric facilities, and the risk of complications. Antitoxin has neither a pro-phylactic nor a therapeutic role in the treatment of necrotizing infections.

91. The answer is a. *(Townsend, pp 1743-1745.)* Abnormalities of ventila-tion-perfusion ratio result from the shunting of blood to a hypoventilated lung or from the ventilation of hypoperfused regions of lung tissue. When this imbalance is extreme, as following massive pulmonary thromboem-bolism, the effect is life-threatening hypoxemia. Other common predisposing factors in the postoperative patient that contribute to this maldistribution include the assumption of a supine position, thoracic and upper abdominal incisions, obesity, atelectasis, and reduced cardiac output.

92. The answer is c. *(Greenfield, pp 98-102.)* Heparin is reversed by the administration of protamine sulfate. Spontaneous retroperitoneal hemor-rhage is a rare but potentially fatal complication of anticoagulation. Heparin is much more frequently associated with spontaneous retroperitoneal hem-orrhage than are oral agents. Advanced patient age and poor regulation of coagulation times also increase the likelihood of bleeding complications. Most cases of retroperitoneal hemorrhage present with flank pain and signs of peritoneal irritation suggestive of an acute intraabdominal process. CT scans are most useful in confirming the diagnosis and following the course of the bleeding. Successful management is usually nonoperative and consists of the discontinuation of anticoagulants, reversal of anticoagulation, possible transfusion of clotting factors, and repletion of intravascular volume with intravenous fluids. Warfarin inhibits synthesis of vitamin K–dependent clotting factors, whereas heparin potentiates antithrombin III activity. Aprotinin is a protease inhibitor that decreases the inflammatory and fibrinolytic response and is used in patients undergoing cardiopulmonary bypass surgery to reduce bleeding complications. Lepirudin is an anticoagulant that is used in patients who develop heparin-induced thrombocytopenia. Thrombin can be used topically as a hemostatic agent.

93. The answer is e. (*Brunicardi, pp 201-204.*) The mortality from isolated smoke inhalation injuries is low in the absence of cutaneous burns. Smoke inhalation injuries, as opposed to respiratory burns (which result from thermal injury), result from epithelial injury from chemical irritation of the tracheobronchial tree and alveoli. Most patients admitted for this injury have elevated carboxyhemoglobin levels from carbon monoxide poisoning, but a minority have physical evidence of skin burns or oropharyngeal burns. Chest films initially are often negative even in those patients who subsequently develop respiratory failure from pulmonary edema or pneumonitis. Patients with elevated carboxyhemoglobin levels or evidence of smoke inhalation should be observed regardless of normal arterial blood gases and chest x-ray; hyperbaric O_2 should be considered in patients with neurologic symptoms and carbon monoxide poisoning, as it reduces the half-life of carboxyhemoglobin. Visible damage to the respiratory tract is not a frequent finding.

94. The answer is e. (*Robinson, 709-711.*) Some drug smugglers, often called body packers or mules, ingest cocaine- or heroin-filled packets and retrieve them at a later date from their stools. The drugs are usually contained in latex or plastic packets. Rupture or leakage of even one bag carries the risk of severe toxicity and death. Although conservative medical management with moderate doses of laxatives is usually safe in stable body packers, close physiologic monitoring is necessary until all packets are passed. High doses of laxatives, digital rectal disimpaction, or endoscopic removal create a high risk of rupture of the bags and therefore are generally discouraged. Emergency surgery is indicated when complications develop.

95 to 97. The answers are 95-b, 96-e, 97-a. (*Greenfield, pp 269-273.*) Nitrous oxide is a commonly used inhalation agent. Nitrous oxide is 30 times more soluble than nitrogen in the blood and enters a collection of trapped air at a rate faster than at which nitrogen leaves the collection. This leads to an increase in volume of trapped air such as loops of bowel leading to bowel distention. Succinylcholine, a depolarizing neuromuscular blocking agent, causes a rise in serum potassium of up to 1.0 mEq/L within a few minutes after administration. This is caused by efflux of potassium from the skeletal muscle at the neuromuscular junction. Patients with burns, trauma, severe infections or neuromuscular disorders have a greater than normal potassium efflux that occasionally causes severe hyperkalemia. Morphine is a narcotic agent that interacts predominantly with the opioid receptor. Rapid intravenous injections of morphine may cause hypotension. Midazolam (Versed) is a benzodiazepine and is associated with acute respiratory depression, especially in the elderly. Pancuronium is a neuromuscular blocking drug that is associated with tachycardia.

98 to 100. The answers are 98-b, 99-e, 100-d. *(Brunicardi, pp 364-374.)* This patient requires pulmonary artery catheter readings to allow his physicians to assess his volume status and need for ongoing inotropic support. Furthermore, the patient continues to be hypotensive and requires further investigation as to the etiology that would subsequently dictate treatment (volume, afterload reduction, etc). Central venous monitoring alone does not allow the physician to assess cardiac function.

A patient who is hypertensive after a carotid endarterectomy is at risk for hemorrhagic stroke and therefore requires aggressive blood pressure management, occasionally with a continuous infusion of nitroglycerin or nitroprusside. Beat-to-beat monitoring of the blood pressure is essential. A patient who has suffered blunt head trauma requiring repeated surgeries for intracranial bleeding will likely be monitored with an intracranial pressure device. Other indications for intracranial pressure monitoring include subarachnoid hemorrhage, hydrocephalus, postcraniotomy status, and Reye syndrome. Measurement of intracranial pressure (ICP) allows the physician to determine and optimize the cerebral perfusion pressure (which is the difference between the mean arterial pressure and the ICP).

101 to 103. The answers are 101-a, 102-e, 103-d. *(Brunicardi, pp 63-65; Greenfield, pp 106-107.)* Prothrombin time measures the speed of coagulation in the extrinsic pathway. A tissue source of procoagulant (thromboplastin) with calcium is added to plasma. The test will detect deficiencies in factors II, V, VII, X, and fibrinogen and is used to monitor patients receiving Coumadin derivatives. However, even small amounts of heparin will artificially prolong the clotting time, so that accurate prothrombin times can be obtained only when the patient has not received heparin for at least 5 hours.

The intrinsic pathway is measured by the partial thromboplastin time. This test is sensitive for defects in the contact and intrinsic phases of coagulation (II, V, VIII, IX, X, XI, XII, fibrinogen) and is used to monitor the status of patients on heparin.

The bleeding time assesses the interaction of platelets and the formation of the platelet plug. Therefore it will pick up deficiencies in both qualitative and quantitative platelet function. Ingestion of aspirin within 1 week of the test will alter the result.

The thrombin time assesses qualitative abnormalities in fibrinogen and the presence of inhibitors to fibrin polymerization. A standard amount of fibrin is added to a fixed volume of plasma and clotting time is measured.

Skin: Wounds, Infections, and Burns; Hands; Plastic Surgery

Questions

104. A 45-year-old woman is seen with wasting of the intrinsic muscles of the hand, weakness, and pain in the wrist. Which of the following nerves has most likely been injured?

a. Ulnar nerve
b. Radial nerve
c. Brachial nerve
d. Axillary nerve
e. Thenar and hypothenar nerves

105. A 68-year-old woman is to have a suspected melanoma excised from her trunk. It appears to be less than 1 mm deep. Which of the following is the smallest margin recommended for excision?

a. 3 mm
b. 5 mm
c. 1 cm
d. 2 cm
e. 5 cm

106. A patient has a clean incision and then closure of the incision to excise an unwanted benign nevus. With regard to the healing process, which of the following statements is correct?

a. Collagen content reaches a maximum at approximately 1 week after injury.
b. Monocytes are essential for normal wound healing.
c. Fibroblasts appear in the wound within 24 to 36 hours after the injury.
d. The function of monocytes in wound healing is limited to phagocytosis of bacteria and debris.
e. Early in wound healing, type I collagen is predominant.

107. A 3-year-old boy sustains a chemical burn after spilling bleach onto his lower extremities. Which of the following statements concerning this patient's injury is correct?

a. Alkali injuries penetrate less deeply into the tissue than acid injuries.
b. Attempts should be made to neutralize the burn wound with weak acids.
c. Initial treatment involves lavage of the burn wound with large volumes of water.
d. Wound debridement is not necessary in alkali injuries.
e. The burned area should be treated immediately with calcium gluconate gel.

108. A 35-year-old man with new diagnosis of Crohn disease presents with rapidly enlarging painful ulcerations on the lower extremities. Cultures of the lesion are negative, and skin biopsy reveals no evidence of malignancy. Which of the following is the most appropriate treatment option?

a. Surgical debridement of the wound with skin grafting
b. Local wound care with silver sulfadiazine
c. Topical corticosteroids
d. Systemic steroids and immunosuppressants
e. Saphenous vein stripping and compressive stockings

109. Following a weekend of snowmobiling, a 42-year-old man comes to the emergency department with pain, numbness, and discoloration of his right forefoot. You diagnose frostbite. Which of the following is the proper initial treatment?

a. Debridement of the affected part followed by silver sulfadiazine dressings
b. Administration of corticosteroids
c. Administration of vasodilators
d. Immersion of the affected part in water at 40°C to 44°C (104°F-111.2°F)
e. Rewarming of the affected part at room temperature

110. A 54-year-old woman cuts her hand with a kitchen knife. There is evidence of tendon injury. Which of the following is true regarding the muscles of the hand?

a. The flexor digitorum superficialis inserts on the distal phalanx.
b. The flexor digitorum profundus inserts on the middle phalanx.
c. The tendons of the flexor digitorum superficialis arise from a common muscle belly.
d. The best results for repair of a flexor tendon are obtained with injuries in the fibroosseous tunnel (zone 2).
e. The process of healing a tendon injury involves formation of a tenoma.

III. A 35-year-old woman undergoes an elective laparoscopic cholecystectomy for symptomatic cholelithiasis. Which of the following wound classes best describes her procedure?

a. Class I, Clean
b. Class II, Clean/contaminated
c. Class III, Contaminated
d. Class IV, Dirty
e. None of the above

112. A 65-year-old woman presents with a 1-cm lesion with a pearly border on her nose, and punch biopsy is consistent with a basal cell carcinoma. She is scheduled to undergo Mohs surgery. Which of the following statements is true regarding this technique?

a. Mohs surgery results in a larger cosmetic defect because of the emphasis on obtaining negative margins circumferentially.
b. The major benefit of Mohs surgery is a shorter operating time.
c. Mohs surgery is indicated for all basal and squamous cell carcinomas.
d. Frozen sections are not necessary if Mohs surgery is performed.
e. There is no difference in cure rates between wide local excision and Mohs surgery.

113. A 60-year-old woman presents with the skin lesion shown here, which has been present for 10 years. She reports a history of radiation treatments to that hand for eczema. Which of the following statements is true concerning this lesion?

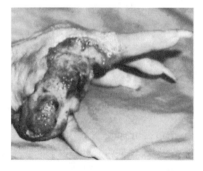

a. It is more malignant than basal cell carcinoma.
b. It occurs more frequently in brunettes.
c. It rarely metastasizes to regional lymph nodes.
d. It should be treated by radiation therapy.
e. It is rarely associated with chronic sun exposure.

114. A 25-year-old man is brought to the emergency room after sustaining burns during a fire in his apartment. He has blistering and erythema of his face, left upper extremity, and chest, with frank charring of his right upper extremity. He is agitated, hypotensive, and tachycardic. Which of the following statements concerning this patient's initial wound management is correct?

a. Topical antibiotics should not be used, as they will encourage growth of resistant organisms.
b. Early excision of facial and hand burns is especially important.
c. Escharotomy should be performed only if neurologic impairment is imminent.
d. Excision of areas of third-degree or deep second-degree burns usually takes place three to seven days after injury.
e. Split-thickness skin grafts over the eschar of third-degree burns should be performed immediately in order to prevent fluid loss.

115. A 24-year-old firefighter sustains 30% total body surface area (TBSA) burns to his torso, face, and extremities. His wounds are treated topically with silver nitrate. Which of the following complications is associated with use of this agent?

a. Hypernatremia
b. Metabolic acidosis
c. Hyperchloremia
d. Neutropenia
e. Hyponatremia

116. A 54-year-old man sees you because of a growth on his lip. He works in construction and is usually outdoors. The biopsy report confirms squamous cell carcinoma. Which of the following is true?

a. The lesion often arises in areas of persistent hyperkeratosis.
b. More than 90% of cases occur on the upper lip.
c. The lesion constitutes 30% of all cancers of the oral cavity.
d. Radiotherapy is considered inappropriate treatment for these lesions.
e. Initial metastases are to the ipsilateral posterior cervical lymph nodes.

117. A 40-year-old woman complains of pain in her right wrist. There are also paresthesias in her hand. With regard to her diagnosis, which of the following statements is correct?

a. It is rarely secondary to trauma.
b. It may be associated with pregnancy.
c. It most often causes dysesthesia during waking hours.
d. It is often associated with vascular compromise.
e. Surgical treatment involves release of the extensor retinaculum.

118. A 60-year-old diabetic man undergoes incision and drainage of an infected boil on his back. The wound is left open for packing and cleansing. Week by week, the wound grows smaller. Which of the following is true concerning wound contracture?

a. It is the primary process affecting closure of an open surgical wound.
b. Bacterial colonization significantly slows the process of contraction.
c. It may account for a maximum of 50% decrease in the size of a wound.
d. It is based on specialized leukocytes which prevent infection.
e. The percentage reduction of wound size is increased with increased adherence of skin to underlying tissue.

119. A 70-year-old man is concerned when his dentist finds a white patch on his oral mucosa during a routine exam. Proper management should include which of the following?

a. Excisional biopsy of all lesions
b. Application of topical antibiotics
c. Low-dose radiation therapy
d. Strict oral hygiene and avoidance of alcohol and tobacco
e. Application of topical chemotherapeutic agents

120. An 8-lb infant, born following uncomplicated labor and delivery, is noted to have a unilateral cleft lip and palate. Which of the following is true?

a. The child almost certainly has other congenital anomalies.
b. Rehabilitation requires adjunctive speech therapy.
c. Lip repair is indicated at 1 year of age.
d. Palate repair is indicated prior to 6 months of age.
e. Cosmetic revisions to the nose should be performed at the same time as cleft lip repair.

121. A 40-year-old woman undergoes wide excision of a pigmented lesion of her thigh. Pathologic examination reveals malignant melanoma, Clark level IV. Findings on examination of the groin are normal. Which of the following is true regarding treatment of her melanoma?

a. Radiotherapy will be an important part of subsequent therapy.
b. The likelihood of groin node metastases is remote.
c. Immunotherapy is an effective form of adjunctive treatment for metastatic malignant melanoma.
d. Lymph node dissection in melanoma is reserved for patients with a positive sentinel lymph node or clinically positive lymph nodes.
e. Intralesional bacille Calmette-Guérin (BCG) administration has been found to aid in local control in the majority of patients.

122. A 42-year-old woman has a childhood history of a third-degree scald burn to her right lower extremity that did not require skin grafting. She states that she experienced trauma to the wound 1 year ago and since then she has had persistent nonhealing of the area. A biopsy of the wound is performed. Which of the following is the most likely diagnosis?

a. Angiosarcoma
b. Malignant melanoma
c. Squamous cell carcinoma
d. Kaposi sarcoma
e. Keloid

123. A 13-year-old male is in a motor vehicle collision in which the car caught fire. He sustained a circumferential burn but no fractures or other soft tissue trauma to his left lower extremity during extrication from the burning vehicle. Several hours after admission, he complains of numbness and severe pain in his left calf. On examination, he has a palpable, although weak, dorsalis pedis pulse. Which of the following is the most appropriate management?

a. Four-compartment fasciotomies
b. Medial and lateral escharotomies
c. Computed tomography (CT) scan of the left lower extremity
d. Magnetic resonance imaging (MRI) of the left lower extremity
e. Left lower extremity angiogram

124. During a bar brawl, a 19-year-old male sustains a 4-in laceration on his left arm from glass and presents to the emergency room the following morning, 10 hours later. He is neurovascularly intact and the wound is deep, extending down to fascia. Which of the following is the most appropriate management of the wound?

a. Closure of the skin only and administration of oral antibiotics for 1 week
b. Closure of the skin and subcutaneous tissue and administration of oral antibiotics for 1 week
c. A single dose of intravenous antibiotics and closure of the skin only
d. A single dose of intravenous antibiotics and closure of the skin and subcutaneous tissue
e. Local wound care without wound closure or antibiotics

125. A 59-year-old woman undergoes an exploratory laparotomy for peritonitis and is found to have perforated diverticulitis. She undergoes a sigmoid resection with an end colostomy. She is administered a third-generation cephalosporin within 1 hour prior to the incision and the antibiotic is continued postoperatively. One week later, she develops an intra-abdominal abscess, which is percutaneously drained. *Bacteroides fragilis* is isolated from the cultures. Which of the following statements regarding her perioperative antibiotic regimen is most accurate?

a. The preoperative dose of antibiotics should have been given closer to the time of incision.
b. The patient should have received several doses of antibiotics prior to laparotomy.
c. The patient should have received a first-generation cephalosporin.
d. The patient did not have adequate gram-negative coverage.
e. The patient did not have adequate anaerobic coverage.

126. A 30-year-old man with a history of Crohn disease develops an enterocutaneous fistula and is placed on total parenteral nutrition through a right subclavian central venous catheter. After 5 days, the patient develops a fever and leukocytosis; CT scan of the abdomen reveals no intra-abdominal abscess. The subclavian catheter insertion site is inspected and noted to be erythematous and painful. Blood cultures are positive. Which of the following organisms is the most likely cause of his fever?

a. Coagulase-positive staphylococci
b. Coagulase-negative staphylococci
c. Group A streptococcus
d. Enterococcus
e. *Escherichia coli*

127. A 65-year-old man sustains a 50% TBSA burn while burning trash in the backyard. The patient is resuscitated with lactated Ringer (LR) solution using the Parkland formula and a weight of 80 kg. What is the rate of LR given in the first 8 hours?

a. 100 mL/h
b. 500 mL/h
c. 1000 mL/h
d. 5000 mL/h
e. 10,000 mL/h

128. A 47-year-old woman presents to her primary care physician with a skin lesion on her left cheek. On examination, it has a waxy appearance with rolled, pearly borders. Which of the following statements is true concerning this lesion?

a. It is the second most common type of skin cancer.
b. It is associated with a precursor skin lesion.
c. It has a fast growth rate and metastasizes frequently.
d. 70% are nodulocystic or noduloulcerative type.
e. 80% are shades of blue and black.

Questions 129 to 131

Match each lower extremity lesion with its correct etiology. Each lettered option may be used once, more than once, or not at all.

a. Ischemic ulcer
b. Venous stasis ulcer
c. Diabetic ulcer
d. Pyoderma gangrenosum
e. Marjolin ulcer

129. A 43-year-old man with a painless ulceration over the left medial malleolus with surrounding brawny induration

130. A 69-year-old man with a history of diabetes mellitus with pain in the balls of his feet at night with an ulcer over the lateral aspect of his right fifth toe

131. A 52-year-old woman with a history of diabetes mellitus with an ulcer on the plantar surface of her right heel

Skin: Wounds, Infections, and Burns; Hands; Plastic Surgery

Answers

104. The answer is a. *(Townsend, pp 2154-2158.)* The ulnar nerve innervates 15 of the 20 intrinsic muscles of the hand. The musculocutaneous, radial, ulnar, and median nerves are all important to hand function. The musculocutaneous and radial nerves allow forearm supination; the radial nerve alone innervates the extensor muscles. The median nerve is the "eye of the hand" because of its extensive contribution to sensory perception; it also maintains most of the long flexors, the pronators of the forearm, and the thenar muscles.

105. The answer is c. *(Brunicardi, pp 442-445.)* The appropriate margin for wide excision of melanomas is dependent on the depth of the lesion. For thin lesions, less than or equal to 1 mm in depth, a 1-cm margin is adequate. For intermediate (1-4 mm) and thick (>4 mm) lesions, a 2-cm margin is recommended.

106. The answer is b. *(Brunicardi, pp 224-230.)* Wound healing is an overlapping sequence of inflammation, proliferation, and remodeling. The inflammatory phase is characterized by a rapid influx of neutrophils, followed in about 2 days by an influx of mononuclear cells. These monocytes act not only by phagocytosing debris and bacteria, but also by secreting numerous growth factors including tumor necrosis factor (TNF), transforming growth factor, platelet-derived growth factor (PDGF), and fibroblast growth factor, which are essential to normal wound healing. Angiogenesis and collagen formation take place during the proliferative phase of wound healing. Fibroblasts, which enter the wound at about day 3, continue to proliferate with increasing collagen deposition. Throughout the proliferative phase, type III collagen predominates. Collagen content is maximal at 2 to 3 weeks, at which time the remodeling phase begins. Type III collagen, which is elastic fibrils, is gradually replaced by rigid fibrils, or type I collagen, at this time. During remodeling, collagen deposition and degradation reach a steady state, which may continue for up to 1 year.

107. The answer is c. (*Brunicardi, pp 214-215*) Treatment of alkali chemical burns involves immediate removal of the alkali agent with large volumes of water lavage. Alkalis dissolve and unite with the proteins of the tissues to form alkaline proteinates which contain hydroxide ions. These ions cause further chemical reactions, penetrating deeper into the tissue. Attempts to neutralize the alkali with weak acids are not recommended because the heat released by neutralization reactions induces further injury. Particularly strong bases should undergo wound debridement in the operating room. Tangential removal of affected areas is performed until the tissues removed are of normal pH. Calcium gluconate is used to treat wounds exposed to hydrofluoric acid.

108. The answer is d. (*Brunicardi, p 436.*) The patient has pyoderma gangrenosum, which is a rare cause of cutaneous ulcerations that can be associated with inflammatory bowel disease as well as other immune disorders. The mainstay of treatment is systemic steroids and immunosuppressants such as cyclosporine. Surgical debridement without medical therapy is not recommended, and local wound care alone or topical steroids are not therapeutic. Saphenous vein ligation and compressive stockings would be more appropriate treatment options in patients with venous stasis ulcers.

109. The answer is d. (*Moore, pp 1071-1072.*) Many methods of treating frostbite have been tried throughout the years. These include massage, warm-water immersion, and covering the affected area. Rapid warming by immersion in water slightly above normal body temperature (40°C-44°C, or 104°F-111.2°F), is the most effective method; however, because the frostbitten region is numb and especially vulnerable, it should be protected from trauma or excessive heat during treatment. Further treatment may include elevation to minimize edema, administration of antibiotics and tetanus toxoid, and debridement of necrotic skin as needed.

110. The answer is e. (*Brunicardi, pp 2025-2056.*) Each digit has two long flexors, called "superficial" and "deep," according to the relative position of the muscle bellies. In the fingers, each superficial flexor tendon divides around the corresponding deep tendon to reach its insertion on the base of the middle phalanx. The deep flexor tendon continues to its insertion on the base of the distal phalanx. Only the deep flexors can flex the distal interphalangeal joint. Since the tendons of the deep flexors share a common muscle belly, only the superficial flexors can move a finger when the adjacent fingers are immobilized. These tendons are prevented from bowstringing across the joints by the flexor retinaculum of the wrists and the fibro-osseous tunnels, which extend from the distal palmar crease to the middle phalanx. They run within synovial sheaths and are nourished by vincula tendinum (short mesenteries). The process of healing a tendon injury involves the formation of a tenoma, which tends to become adherent to the surrounding sheath. A difficult balance has to be struck between the desire to prevent adhesions by early mobilization and the risk of rupturing an unhealed tendon. Verdan has divided the hand into six regions according to the anatomy surrounding the tendons. Zone 2, sometimes referred to as no-man's land, refers to the fibro-osseous tunnels. Repair in this region is fraught with difficulty.

111. The answer is b. *(Brunicardi, pp 118-120.)* Clean wounds are those in which no part of the respiratory, gastrointestinal, or genitourinary tract is entered. Examples include herniorrhaphy and breast surgery. Clean-contaminated wounds encompass those cases in which these systems are entered, but without evidence of active infection or gross spillage. Examples include elective cholecystectomy or elective colon resection with adequate bowel preparation. Contaminated wounds include open accidental wounds encountered early after injury, those with extensive introduction of bacteria into a normally sterile area of the body, or gross spillage of viscus contents such as from the intestine. Examples include penetrating abdominal trauma, large tissue injury, and enterotomy during bowel obstruction. Dirty wounds include traumatic wounds in which a significant delay in treatment has occurred and in which necrotic tissue is present, those created in the presence of purulent material, and those involving a perforated viscus accompanied by a high degree of contamination. Examples include perforated diverticulitis and necrotizing soft tissue infections.

112. The answer is e. *(Brunicardi, p 440.)* There is no difference in cure rate between Mohs surgery and wide local excision of a basal cell carcinoma. Mohs surgery describes a technique for resecting either basal or squamous cell carcinomas on the face or near the nose or eye in order to achieve the optimal cosmetic result. Resection of the tumor is performed in small increments with immediate frozen section analysis in order to ensure negative margins. The disadvantage of the Mohs technique is the longer time required.

113. The answer is a. (*Brunicardi, p 440.*) Squamous cell carcinoma occurs in people who have had chronic sun exposure, chronic ulcers or sinus tracts (draining osteomyelitis), or a history of radiation or thermal injury (Marjolin ulcer). It is more invasive, grows more rapidly, and metastasizes more frequently than basal cell carcinoma. It occurs more frequently in blondes and fair-skinned people. A radiation-induced carcinoma, or one arising in a burn scar, should not be treated with radiation therapy for fear of further damage.

114. The answer is d. (*Brunicardi, pp 204-209.*) Early wound management is characterized by early excision of areas of devitalized tissue, with the exception of deep wounds of the palms, soles, genitals, and face. Staged excision of deep partial-thickness or full-thickness burns occurs between 3 and 7 days after the injury. There are several proven advantages to early excision, including decreased hospital stay and lower cost. This is especially true of burns encompassing more than 30% to 40% of the total body surface area. In conjunction with early excision, topical antimicrobials such as silver sulfadiazine are extremely important in delaying colonization of the newly excised or fresh burn wounds. Permanent coverage through split-thickness skin grafting usually occurs more than 1 week after injury. Skin autograft requires a vascular bed and therefore cannot be placed over eschar. Meticulous attention to deep circumferential burns is crucial in the management of burn patients. Progressive tissue edema may lead to progressive vascular and neurologic compromise. Because the blood supply is the initial system affected, frequent assessment of flow is vital, with longitudinal escharotomy performed at the first sign of vascular compromise. A low threshold should be maintained in performing an escharotomy in the setting of severely burned limbs.

115. The answer is e. (*Brunicardi, pp 212-213.*) The three main topical agents used to treat burns include silver nitrate, silver sulfadiazine, and mafenide acetate. Complications of silver nitrate are electrolyte abnormalities (hyponatremia, hypokalemia, hypocalcemia, hypochloremia) and methemoglobinemia. The main complication with silver sulfadiazine is neutropenia; mafenide acetate causes metabolic acidosis secondary to inhibition of carbonic anhydrase.

116. The answer is a. (*Brunicardi, pp 518-519.*) Squamous cell carcinoma of the lip is the most common malignant tumor of the lip and constitutes 15% of all malignancies of the oral cavity. Basal cell carcinomas do occur on the lip, but much less frequently. There is a strong association between squamous cell tumors of the lip and sun exposure. Therefore, these lesions are more common in the southern United States and in occupational groups who work outdoors. Because of its greater sun exposure, the lower lip is the site of more than 90% of such lesions. Persistent hyperkeratosis precedes 35% to 40% of these lesions. The incidence of metastases increases with the size of the lesion, and spread is usually via lymphatics to the ipsilateral submental node. Contralateral nodal metastases are rare unless the lesion crosses the midline. Approximately 10% to 15% of all patients have metastases at the time of diagnosis. These lip tumors are very responsive to radiotherapy, which works well for small- to medium-sized lesions. Large lesions treated with radiotherapy usually require surgical reconstruction. Radiotherapy should not be used in patients who will have ongoing sun exposure to the area because radiation therapy sensitizes the tissues to solar trauma.

117. The answer is b. (*Townsend, p 2186.*) Signs and symptoms of carpal tunnel syndrome are related to the distribution of the median nerve. This nerve, which passes through the carpal tunnel in the wrist with the finger flexor tendons, may suffer compression from fibrous scarring or malalignment following a fracture of the wrist. Nerve compression may also occur in patients with rheumatoid arthritis who develop flexor tenosynovitis. In women, the syndrome frequently first appears during pregnancy and recurs during the premenstrual phase of subsequent menstrual cycles. In these cases, symptoms are presumably the result of the effects of fluid retention and pressure on the median nerve owing to tissue swelling. In many instances, symptoms are limited to nocturnal pain and paresthesias. If conservative treatment of carpal tunnel syndrome is unsuccessful, surgical treatment may be required. Open and endoscopic techniques have been employed, both of which release adhesions of the median nerve and divide the transverse carpal ligament. The extensor retinaculum is located on the dorsal aspect of the wrist and contains the six compartments of extensor tendons.

118. The answer is a. (*Brunicardi, pp 224-230.*) While epithelialization is responsible for the healing of a closed incision, wound contraction is the primary method of closure in open wounds. During this process, the skin surrounding the wound is pulled over the wound surface and may account for up to a 90% reduction in the size of an open wound. In areas of greater adherence of skin to underlying tissue, the ability of contraction to close the wound is hindered due to the decreased mobility of the skin. Therefore, in areas of tight skin adherence such as the leg, contraction may only account for 30% to 40% reduction in wound size. Fibroblasts in the open wound, which predominate during the proliferative phase, contain increasing numbers of actin microfilaments, thereby becoming myofibroblasts. These specialized fibroblasts are thought to be responsible for wound contraction either through intrinsic cellular contraction or attachment to collagen strands. Bacterial colonization does not harm the process of wound contraction and surgical wound healing. While wound infection is often difficult to diagnose in open wounds, it is generally accepted that bacterial counts of 1 million bacteria per gram of tissue are deleterious to wound closure.

119. The answer is d. (*Townsend, pp 813-814.*) White patches in the oral cavity (leukoplakia) sometimes are incorrectly interpreted as a premalignant condition. Microscopic examination of leukoplakia may reveal hyperplasia, keratosis, or dyskeratosis, of which the last finding is the most serious because of its association with malignancy. Approximately 50% of all oral cancers occur in patients who have associated areas of hyperkeratosis and dyskeratosis. Only about 5% of patients with leukoplakia develop cancer. A suggested treatment protocol for patients with leukoplakia advocates a program of strict oral hygiene and avoidance of the source of irritants such as alcohol and tobacco. Biopsy is reserved only for those with thick lesions or those in whom the lesion does not resolve after avoidance therapy (to rule out malignancy). Radiation therapy is contraindicated.

120. The answer is b. (*Townsend, pp 2138-2139.*) Clefts of the lip and palate occur relatively frequently (1 in 750 live births); they may be unilateral or bilateral and can vary from a small notch to a complete cleft of the lip and palate. Most clefts occur as isolated anomalies, but occasionally they are associated with neurologic, orthopedic, or cardiac anomalies. A frequently recommended protocol for management is lip repair in the first 3 months of life and palate repair at 12 to 18 months. Other cosmetic procedures can be performed late in childhood and adolescence. Palate repair after 2 years of age is associated with a high incidence of speech impairment, often requiring speech therapy; repair in the early months of life can lead to a hazardous loss of blood that is poorly tolerated by the infant. Repair of the lip usually should be accomplished as soon as the infant is sufficiently stabilized to tolerate anesthesia with reasonable safety. Ten to twelve weeks is often recommended as the time for lip repair. At this age, the affected baby usually can be converted to dropper or cup feedings in the postoperative period, which thereby facilitates healing of the lip by reducing the need for suckling with the freshly wounded tissues.

121. The answer is d. (*Townsend, pp 767-779.*) The survival of patients with malignant melanoma correlates with the depth of invasion (Clark) and the thickness of the lesion (Breslow). It is widely held that patients with thin lesions (<0.76 mm) and Clark level I and II lesions are adequately managed by wide local excision. The incidence of nodal metastases rises with increasing Clark level of invasion such that a level IV lesion has a 30% to 50% incidence of nodal metastases. Lymph node dissection for melanoma is generally reserved for patients with a positive sentinel lymph node or clinically positive lymph nodes. The sentinel lymph node is the first node that drains a particular nodal basin and can be identified with preoperative injection of ^{99m}Tc sulfur colloid around the lesion and detection with a gamma counter intraoperatively and/or intraoperative injection of blue dye. Sentinel lymph node biopsy is performed for lesions greater than 1 mm in depth, and the topic is controversial for thinner lesions, given the low likelihood of metastasis. The sentinel lymph node is analyzed using histologic staining, immunostaining, and reverse transcription polymerase chain-reaction testing. Immunotherapy has not been successful in controlling widespread metastatic melanoma even when added to chemotherapy. Intralesional administration of BCG has been demonstrated to control local skin lesions in only 20% of patients. Dinitrochlorobenzene (DNCB) can also be used.

122. The answer is c. (*Brunicardi, pp 216, 446.*) A Marjolin ulcer refers to a squamous cell carcinoma that develops in a chronic wound such as a previous burn scar or a sinus tract secondary to osteomyelitis. Although basal cell carcinoma, melanoma, and other malignancies can develop in a chronic wound, squamous cell carcinoma is the most common. The mainstay of treatment is surgical excision or amputation. Kaposi sarcoma usually presents as multifocal lesions on the extremities that may be associated with immunocompromised individuals, and the mainstay of therapy is radiation. Keloids can occur in areas of previous burn and represent an overexuberance of wound healing. Surgical excision alone of a keloid is associated with a high recurrence rate, and other adjunctive modalities that have been utilized include injection of steroids, radiation, external compression, and topical retinoids.

123. The answer is b. (*Townsend, p 569.*) The patient should undergo medial and lateral escharotomies of his left lower extremity. Based on his clinical history of a circumferential, full-thickness burn and on his symptoms of numbness and pain, the patient has compartment syndrome. The presence of pedal pulses does not preclude the diagnosis of compartment syndrome. If the diagnosis is in question, compartment pressures can be measured, and a pressure of greater than 30 to 40 mm Hg is diagnostic. Compartment syndromes secondary to burns are a result of increased pressure secondary to tissue edema and lack of elasticity of the burnt skin (eschar), causing compression of the blood vessels. Fasciotomies are rarely required.

124. The answer is e. *(Townsend, p 590.)* The wound should not be closed because the elapsed time to presentation was greater than 6 hours. Wounds that are dirty or contaminated (eg, animal bites), that are traumatically induced by a puncture, gunshot, or crush injury, or that are older than 6 hours should be left open. Prophylactic antibiotics have not been demonstrated to prevent wound infections.

125. The answer is e. *(Townsend, pp 265-267.)* Third-generation cephaosporins provide good coverage against most gram-negative bacteria, but have poor activity against anaerobic bacteria (eg, *B fragilis*). Clindamycin or metronidazole can be used in addition to a third-generation cephalosporin to provide anaerobic coverage. Other alternatives include a combination of a penicillin/β-lactamase inhibitor or a cefoxitin or cefotetan, both of which are second-generation cephalosporins. Prophylactic antibiotics against anaerobic organisms are indicated only in cases where they are likely to be encountered (eg, bowel cases). Prophylactic antibiotics should optimally be administered intravenously within 1 hour prior to incision. Continuation of postoperative antibiotics for more than 24 hours is indicated in patients with preexisting infection, for example, secondary to perforated viscera, but not after routine elective operations.

126. The answer is b. *(Townsend, p 312-313.)* The most common organism in patients with nosocomial bacteremia is coagulase-negative staphylococcus.

127. The answer is c. *(Brunicardi, p 198.)* The Parkland formula recommends 4 mL LR/kg for each percent TBSA burned over the first 24 hours, with 1 half of the amount administered in the first 8 hours, and the remaining half over the next 16 hours.

$$4 \text{ mL/kg} \times 80 \text{ (kg)} \times 50\% \text{ TBSA} = 16,000$$
$$16,000/2 = 8000$$
$$8000 \text{ (mL)}/8 \text{ (hours)} = 1000 \text{ mL/h}$$

128. The answer is d. *(Brunicardi, pp 439-440.)* Basal cell carcinomas (BCCs) are the most common type of skin cancer. There is no precursor skin lesion. Most BCCs are pink or skin colored and have a slow growth rate. BCCs commonly infiltrate locally but rarely metastasize. The nodulocystic or noduloulcerative type accounts for 70% of BCCs.

129 to 131. The answers are 129-b, 130-a, 131-c. *(Townsend, pp 1376, 2009, 2148.)* Venous stasis ulcers are typically located over the medial malleolus, are painless, and may be associated with brawny induration. Treatment consists of leg elevation, compression stockings, local wound care, and occasionally surgical debridement. Ischemic ulcers are often associated with other symptoms of severe peripheral vascular disease such as rest pain, and are commonly located on the dorsum of the foot or the lateral first or fifth toes. Patients with ischemic ulcers should undergo urgent evaluation for lower extremity revascularization. Diabetic ulcers are often associated with trauma or pressure secondary to sensory neuropathy and typically occur on the plantar surface of the foot. Treatment should include optimization of the patient's blood sugars, protective shoe wear, and debridement of necrotic tissue. Pyoderma gangrenosum can be associated with underlying disorders such as inflammatory bowel disease, rheumatic heart disease, or malignancy. The lesions are painful ulcerations surrounded by erythema. Treatment consists primarily of corticosteroids and immunosuppressants. A Marjolin ulcer is a squamous cell carcinoma that arises in a chronic wound and is treated with surgical excision.

Trauma and Shock

Questions

132. A teenage boy falls from his bicycle and is run over by a truck. On arrival in the emergency room (ER), he is awake and alert and appears frightened but in no distress. The chest radiograph suggests an air-fluid level in the left lower lung field and the nasogastric tube seems to coil upward into the left chest. Which of the following is the next best step in his management?

a. Placement of a left chest tube
b. Thoracotomy
c. Laparotomy
d. Esophagogastroscopy
e. Diagnostic peritoneal lavage

133. A 10-year-old boy was the backseat belted passenger in a high-speed motor vehicle collision. On presentation to the ER, he is awake, alert, and hemodynamically stable. He is complaining of abdominal pain and has an ecchymosis on his anterior abdominal wall where the seatbelt was located. Which of the following statements is true regarding need for additional workup?

a. The boy can be safely discharged home without any other workup, since his abdominal pain is probably secondary to his abdominal wall ecchymosis.
b. The boy can be safely discharged home if his amylase level is normal.
c. The boy can be safely discharged home if abdominal plain films are negative for the presence of free air.
d. The boy can be safely discharged home if an abdominal computed tomography (CT) scan is negative.
e. The boy should be observed regardless of negative test results.

134. A 65-year-old man who smokes cigarettes and has chronic obstructive pulmonary disease falls and fractures the third, fourth, and fifth ribs in the left anterolateral chest. Chest x-ray is otherwise normal. Which of the following would be the most appropriate next step in his management?

a. Strapping the chest with adhesive tape
b. Admission to the hospital and treatment with oral analgesia
c. Tube thoracostomy
d. Placement of an epidural for pain management
e. Surgical fixation of the fractured ribs

135. A 36-year-old man who was hit by a car presents to the ER with hypotension. On examination, he has tenderness and bruising over his left lateral chest below the nipple. An ultrasound examination is performed and reveals free fluid in the abdomen. What is the most likely organ to have been injured in this patient?

a. Liver
b. Kidney
c. Spleen
d. Intestine
e. Pancreas

136. A 52-year-old man is pinned against a loading dock. The patient has a fractured femur, a pelvic fracture, a tender abdomen, and no pulses in the right foot with minimal tissue damage to the right leg. Angiography discloses a popliteal artery injury with obstruction. At surgery, the popliteal vein is also transected. His blood pressure is 85/60 mm Hg. Which of the following is the best management strategy for his vascular injuries?

a. Repair of the popliteal vein with simple closure
b. Repair of the popliteal vein with saphenous vein patch
c. Repair of the popliteal vein with a synthetic interposition graft
d. Ligation of the popliteal vein
e. Amputation of the right lower extremity above the knee

137. A 27-year-old man sustains a single gunshot wound to the left thigh. In the ER, he is noted to have a large hematoma of his medial thigh. He complains of paresthesias in his left foot. On examination, there are weak pulses palpable distal to the injury and the patient is unable to move his foot. Which of the following is the most appropriate initial management of this patient?

a. Angiography
b. Immediate exploration and repair in the operating room
c. Fasciotomy of the anterior compartment of the calf
d. Observation for resolution of spasm
e. Local wound exploration at the bedside

138. A 25-year-old woman arrives in the ER following an automobile accident. She is acutely dyspneic with a respiratory rate of 60 breaths per minute. Breath sounds are markedly diminished on the right side. Which of the following is the best first step in the management of this patient?

a. Take a chest x-ray
b. Draw arterial blood for blood-gas determination
c. Decompress the right pleural space
d. Perform pericardiocentesis
e. Administer intravenous fluids

139. A 17-year-old male is stabbed in the left seventh intercostal space, midaxillary line. He presents to the ER with a heart rate of 86 beats per minute, blood pressure of 125/74 mm Hg, and oxygen saturation of 98%. Breath sounds are equal bilaterally. Which of the following is the most appropriate next step in his workup?

a. Local exploration of the wound
b. Left tube thoracostomy
c. Diagnostic laparoscopy
d. CT scan of the abdomen
e. Echocardiography

140. Your hospital is conducting an ongoing research study involving the hormonal response to trauma. Blood is drawn regularly (with Institutional Review Board [IRB] approval) for various studies. Which of the following values are likely to be seen after a healthy 36-year-old man is hit by a bus and sustains a ruptured spleen and a lacerated small bowel?

a. Increased secretion of insulin
b. Increased secretion of thyroxine
c. Decreased secretion of vasopressin (antidiuretic hormone [ADH])
d. Decreased secretion of glucagon
e. Decreased secretion of aldosterone

141. A 29-year-old man sustained a gunshot wound to the right upper quadrant. He is taken to the operating room and, after management of a liver injury, is found to have a complete transection of the common bile duct with significant tissue loss. Which of the following is the optimal surgical management of this patient's injury?

a. Choledochoduodenostomy
b. Loop choledochojejunostomy
c. Primary end-to-end anastomosis of the transected bile duct
d. Roux-en-Y choledochojejunostomy
e. Bridging of the injury with a T tube

142. You evaluate an 18-year-old male who sustained a right-sided cervical laceration during a gang fight. Your intern suggests nonoperative management and observation. Which of the following is a relative, rather than an absolute, indication for neck exploration?

a. Expanding hematoma
b. Dysphagia
c. Dysphonia
d. Pneumothorax
e. Hemoptysis

143. Following blunt abdominal trauma, a 12-year-old girl develops upper abdominal pain, nausea, and vomiting. An upper gastrointestinal series reveals a total obstruction of the duodenum with a coiled spring appearance in the second and third portions. In the absence of other suspected injuries, which of the following is the most appropriate management of this patient?

a. Gastrojejunostomy
b. Nasogastric suction and observation
c. Duodenal resection
d. TPN (total parental nutrition) to increase the size of the retroperitoneal fat pad
e. Duodenojejunostomy

144. A 29-year-old man sustains a closed humeral shaft fracture and on examination in the ER is noted to have a radial nerve injury. Which of the following statements is true regarding his treatment and prognosis?

a. Immediate exploration with primary repair of the radial nerve should be undertaken.
b. Fracture reduction and observation is the initial management strategy of choice.
c. Delayed exploration after 6 to 8 weeks with sural nerve graft results in the best long-term function.
d. The incidence of recovery from a closed radial nerve palsy is only 50% with nonoperative management.
e. Nerve regeneration occurs at the rate of approximately 0.1 mm/day.

145. An 18-year-old male was assaulted and sustained significant head and facial trauma. Which of the following is the most common initial manifestation of increased intracranial pressure?

a. Change in level of consciousness
b. Ipsilateral (side of hemorrhage) pupillary dilation
c. Contralateral pupillary dilation
d. Hemiparesis
e. Hypertension

146. A 28-year-old man is brought to the ER for a severe head injury after a fall. He was intubated in the field for his decreased level of consciousness. He is tachycardic and hypotensive. On examination, he is noted to have an obvious skull fracture and his right pupil is dilated. Which of the following is the most appropriate method for initially reducing his intracranial pressure?

a. Elevation of the head of the bed
b. Saline-furosemide (Lasix) infusion
c. Mannitol infusion
d. Intravenous dexamethasone (Decadron)
e. Hyperventilation

147. A 45-year-old man was an unhelmeted motorcyclist involved in a high-speed collision. He was ejected from the motorcycle and was noted to be apneic at the scene. After being intubated, he was brought to the ER, where he is noted to have a left dilated pupil that responds only sluggishly. What is the pathophysiology of his dilated pupil?

a. Infection within the cavernous sinus
b. Herniation of the uncal process of the temporal lobe
c. Laceration of the corpus callosum by the falx cerebri
d. Occult damage to the superior cervical ganglion
e. Cerebellar hypoxia

148. A 31-year-old man is brought to the ER following an automobile accident in which his chest struck the steering wheel. Examination reveals stable vital signs and no evidence of respiratory distress, but the patient exhibits multiple palpable rib fractures and paradoxical movement of the right side of the chest. Chest x-ray shows no evidence of pneumothorax or hemothorax. Which of the following is the most appropriate initial management of this patient?

a. Intubation, mechanical ventilation, and positive end-expiratory pressure
b. Stabilization of the chest wall with sandbags
c. Stabilization with towel clips
d. Immediate operative stabilization
e. Pain control, chest physiotherapy, and close observation

149. A 30-year-old man is stabbed in the arm. There is no evidence of vascular injury, but he cannot flex his three radial digits. Which of the following structures has he most likely injured?

a. Flexor pollicis longus and flexor digitus medius tendons
b. Radial nerve
c. Median nerve
d. Thenar and digital nerves at the wrist
e. Ulnar nerve

150. Following a 2-hour firefighting episode, a 36-year-old fireman begins complaining of a throbbing headache, nausea, dizziness, and visual disturbances. He is taken to the ER, where his carboxyhemoglobin (COHb) level is found to be 31%. Which of the following is the most appropriate next step in his treatment?

a. Begin an immediate exchange transfusion.
b. Transfer the patient to a hyperbaric oxygen chamber.
c. Begin bicarbonate infusion and give 250 mg acetazolamide (Diamox) intravenously.
d. Administer 100% oxygen by mask.
e. Perform flexible bronchoscopy with further therapy determined by findings.

151. A 75-year-old man with a history of coronary artery disease, hypertension, and diabetes mellitus undergoes a right hemicolectomy for colon cancer. On the second postoperative day, he complains of shortness of breath and chest pain. He becomes hypotensive with depressed mental status and is immediately transferred to the intensive care unit. After intubation and placement on mechanical ventilation, an echocardiogram confirms cardiogenic shock. A central venous catheter is placed that demonstrates a central venous pressure of 18 mm Hg. Which of the following is the most appropriate initial management strategy?

a. Additional liter fluid bolus
b. Inotropic support
c. Mechanical circulatory support with intra-aortic balloon pump (IABP)
d. Cardiac catheterization
e. Heart transplant

152. An 18-year-old male climbs up a utility pole to retrieve his younger brother's kite. An electrical spark jumps from the wire to his metal belt buckle and burns his abdominal wall, knocking him to the ground. Which of the following should guide your treatment of this patient?

a. Injuries are generally more superficial than those from thermal burns.
b. Intravenous fluid replacement is based on the percentage of body surface area burned.
c. Electric burns often result in a transient traumatic optic neuropathy.
d. Evaluation for fracture of the other extremities and visceral injury is indicated.
e. Cardiac conduction abnormalities are unlikely.

153. A 22-year-old man is examined following a motor vehicle accident. His right leg is injured, as are his elbow and clavicle. Which of the following fractures or dislocations is most likely to result in an associated vascular injury?

a. Knee dislocation
b. Closed posterior elbow dislocation
c. Midclavicular fracture
d. Supracondylar femur fracture
e. Tibial plateau fracture

154. A 23-year-old, previously healthy man presents to the ER after sustaining a single gunshot wound to the left chest. The entrance wound is 3 cm inferior to the nipple and the exit wound is just below the scapula. A chest tube is placed that drains 400 mL of blood and continues to drain 50 to 75 mL/h during the initial resuscitation. Initial blood pressure of 70/0 mm Hg has responded to 2 L crystalloid and is now 100/70 mm Hg. Abdominal examination is unremarkable. Chest x-ray reveals a reexpanded lung and no free air under the diaphragm. Which of the following is the best next step in his management?

a. Admission and observation
b. Peritoneal lavage
c. Exploratory thoracotomy
d. Exploratory celiotomy
e. Local wound exploration

155. A patient is brought to the ER after a motor vehicle accident. He is unconscious and has a deep scalp laceration and one dilated pupil. His heart rate is 120 beats per minute, blood pressure is 80/40 mm Hg, and respiratory rate is 35 breaths per minute. Despite rapid administration of 2 L normal saline, the patient's vital signs do not change significantly. Which of the following is the most appropriate next step in the workup of his hypotension?

a. Neurosurgical consultation for emergent ventriculostomy to manage his intracranial pressure
b. Neurosurgical consultation for emergent craniotomy for suspected subdural hematoma
c. Emergent burr hole drainage at the bedside for suspected epidural hematoma
d. Administration of mannitol and hyperventilation to treat his elevated intracranial pressure
e. Abdominal ultrasound (focused assessment with sonography in trauma, or FAST)

156. A 25-year-old man is involved in a gang shoot-out and sustains an abdominal gunshot wound from a .22 pistol. At laparotomy, it is discovered that the left transverse colon has incurred a through-and-through injury with minimal fecal soilage of the peritoneum. Which of the following is the most appropriate management of this patient?

a. A colostomy should be performed regardless of the patient's hemodynamic status to decrease the risk of an intraabdominal infection.
b. Primary repair should be performed, but only in the absence of hemodynamic instability.
c. Primary repair should be performed with placement of an intraabdominal drain next to the repair.
d. Primary repair should be performed and intravenous antibiotics administered for 14 days.
e. The patient should undergo a two-stage procedure with resection of the injured portion and reanastomosis 48 hours later when clinically stabilized.

157. A 34-year-old prostitute with a history of long-term intravenous drug use is admitted with a 48-hour history of pain in her left arm. She is tachycardic to 130 and her systolic blood pressure is 80 mm Hg. Physical examination is remarkable for crepitus surrounding needle track marks in the antecubital space with a serous exudate. The plain x-ray of the arm is shown here. Which of the following is the most appropriate next step in her management?

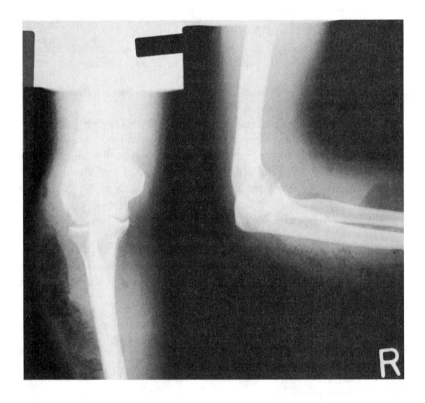

a. Treatment with penicillin G and close observation
b. MRI of the arm
c. CT scan of the arm
d. Surgical exploration and debridement
e. Hyperbaric oxygen therapy

158. A 47-year-old man is extracted from an automobile after a motor vehicle accident. The patient has a steering wheel bruise on the anterior chest. His electrocardiogram (ECG) shows some premature ventricular complexes, and his cardiac isoenzymes are elevated. There is suspicion of a cardiac contusion. Which of the following is true regarding a cardiac contusion?

a. Elevated cardiac isoenzyme levels sensitively identify patients at risk for life-threatening arrhythmias.
b. The majority of patients have abnormalities on the initial ECG after injury.
c. Cardiac imaging such as echocardiography is sensitive in detecting wall motion abnormalities or valvular dysfunction.
d. Echocardiography is a good predictor of subsequent cardiac complications such as arrhythmias and pump failure.
e. All patients diagnosed with myocardial contusion should be monitored in an intensive care unit setting for 72 hours.

159. A 70-year-old man presents to the ER with several fractures and a ruptured spleen after falling 20 ft. Which of the following best represents his body's response to the injury?

a. Decreased liver gluconeogenesis
b. Inhibition of skeletal muscle breakdown by interleukin 1 and tumor necrosis factor (TNF, cachectin)
c. Decreased urinary nitrogen loss
d. Hepatic synthesis of acute-phase reactants
e. Decreased glutamine consumption by fibroblasts, lymphocytes, and intestinal epithelial cells

160. A 36-year-old man sustains a gunshot wound to the left buttock. He is hemodynamically stable. There is no exit wound, and an x-ray of the abdomen shows the bullet to be located in the right lower quadrant. Which of the following is most appropriate in the management of his suspected rectal injury?

a. Barium studies of the colon and rectum
b. Barium studies of the bullet track
c. CT scan of the abdomen and pelvis
d. Angiography
e. Sigmoidoscopy in the ER

161. A 27-year-old man presents to the ER after a high-speed motor vehicle collision with chest pain and marked respiratory distress. On physical examination, he is hypotensive with distended neck veins and absence of breath sounds in the left chest. Which of the following is the proper initial treatment?

a. Intubation
b. Chest x-ray
c. Pericardiocentesis
d. Chest decompression with a needle
e. Emergent thoracotomy

162. A 48-year-old man sustains a gunshot wound to the right upper thigh just distal to the inguinal crease. He is immediately brought to the ER. Peripheral pulses are palpable in the foot, but the foot is pale, cool, and hypesthetic. The motor examination is normal. Which of the following statements is the most appropriate next step in the patient's management?

a. The patient should be taken to the operating room immediately to evaluate for a significant arterial injury.
b. A neurosurgical consult should be obtained and somatosensory evoked potential monitoring performed.
c. A fasciotomy should be performed prophylactically in the emergency room.
d. A duplex examination should be obtained to rule out a venous injury.
e. The patient should be observed for at least 6 hours and then reexamined for changes in the physical examination.

163. A 62-year-old woman is seen after a 3-day history of fever, abdominal pain, nausea, and anorexia. She has not urinated for 24 hours. She has a history of previous abdominal surgery for inflammatory bowel disease. Her blood pressure is 85/64 mm Hg, and her pulse is 136. Her response to this physiologic state includes which of the following?

a. Increase in sodium and water excretion
b. Increase in renal perfusion
c. Decrease in cortisol levels
d. Hyperkalemia
e. Hypoglycemia

164. A 20-year-old man presents after being punched in the right eye and assaulted to the head. On a facial CT scan, he is noted to have a blowout fracture of the right orbital floor. Which of the following findings mandates immediate surgical intervention?

a. A fracture 25% of the orbital floor
b. 1 mm of enophthalmos
c. Periorbital ecchymosis
d. Inability to move the right eye upward
e. Traumatic optic neuropathy

165. A 33-year-old woman is seen in the ER with severe rectal bleeding. She has a history of ulcerative colitis. Her blood pressure is 78/56 mm Hg, her pulse is 144, and she is pale and clammy. Which of the following responses is likely to occur after administration of Ringer lactate solution?

a. Increase in serum lactate concentration
b. Impairment of liver function
c. Improvement in hemodynamics by alleviating the deficit in the interstitial fluid compartment
d. Increase in metabolic acidosis
e. Increase in the need for blood transfusion

166. An 18-year-old high school football player is kicked in the left flank. Three hours later he develops hematuria. His vital signs are stable. A CT scan demonstrates a Grade II renal injury based on the Urologic Injury Scale of the American Association for the Surgery of Trauma. Which of the following is the most appropriate treatment for this patient?

a. Resumption of normal daily activity excluding sports
b. Exploration and suture of the laceration
c. Exploration and wedge resection of the left kidney
d. Nephrostomy
e. Strict bed rest with serial hemoglobin levels

167. A 32-year-old man is in a high-speed motorcycle collision and presents with an obvious pelvic fracture. On examination, he has a scrotal hematoma and blood at his urethral meatus. Which of the following is the most appropriate next step in his management?

a. Placement of a Foley catheter
b. Cystoscopy
c. CT of the pelvis
d. Retrograde urethrogram
e. Nephrostomy tube placement

168. A 17-year-old male sustains a small-caliber gunshot wound to the mid-epigastrium with no obvious exit wound. His abdomen is very tender; he is taken to the operating room and the bullet appears to have tracked through the midpancreas. Which of the following is correct regarding this type of injury?

a. Most injuries do not involve adjacent organs.
b. Management of a ductal injury to the left of the mesenteric vessels is Roux-en-Y pancreaticojejunostomy.
c. Management of a ductal injury in the head of the pancreas is pancreaticoduodenectomy.
d. Small peripancreatic hematomas need not be explored to search for pancreatic injury.
e. The major cause of death is exsanguination from associated vascular injuries.

169. A 43-year-old man is examined in the trauma bay after being stabbed in the chest with a long kitchen knife. A chest tube is placed and 800 mL of blood is recovered, with subsequent drainage of approximately 50 mL/h. Resuscitation is best facilitated by which of the following?

a. Placement of long 18-gauge subclavian vein catheters
b. Placement of percutaneous femoral vein catheters
c. Bilateral saphenous vein cutdowns
d. Placement of short, large-bore percutaneous peripheral intravenous catheters
e. Infusion of cold whole blood

170. The victim of a motor vehicle accident who was in shock is delivered to your trauma center by a rural ambulance service with the pneumatic antishock garment (PASG) in place and inflated. Blood pressure is 110/86 mm Hg. X-rays reveal a pelvic fracture. Which of the following statements is true regarding the use of this garment?

a. Elevates blood pressure by an autotransfusion effect, with augmentation of venous return and cardiac output
b. Is not recommended for control of persistent bleeding in the setting of severe pelvic fracture
c. Increases peripheral vascular resistance
d. Expedites assessment of lower body injuries in the trauma patient
e. Should be terminated by means of prompt deflation as soon as the trauma patient reaches the emergency department

171. A radio transmission is received in your trauma unit stating that a victim of a motor vehicle collision is en route to your ER with no vital signs. The ambulance is 3 minutes away. As you formulate your plan, which of the following situations would constitute an indication for ER thoracotomy?

a. Massive hemothorax following blunt trauma to the chest
b. Blunt trauma to multiple organ systems with obtainable vital signs in the field, but none on arrival in the ER
c. Rapidly deteriorating patient with cardiac tamponade from penetrating thoracic trauma
d. Penetrating thoracic trauma and no signs of life in the field
e. Penetrating abdominal trauma and no signs of life in the field

172. A 22-year-old man sustains a gunshot wound to the abdomen. At exploration, an apparently solitary distal small-bowel injury is treated with resection and primary anastomosis. On postoperative day 7, small-bowel fluid drains through the operative incision. The fascia remains intact. The fistula output is 300 mL/day and there is no evidence of intra-abdominal sepsis. Which of the following is the most appropriate treatment strategy?

a. Early reoperation to close the fistula tract
b. Broad-spectrum antibiotics
c. Total parenteral nutrition
d. Somatostatin to lower fistula output
e. Loperamide to inhibit gut motility

173. A 26-year-old man sustains a gunshot wound to the left thigh. Exploration reveals that a 5-cm portion of superficial femoral artery is destroyed. Which of the following is the most appropriate regarding his management?

a. Debridement and end-to-end anastomosis
b. Debridement and repair with an interposition prosthetic graft
c. Debridement and repair with an interposition arterial graft
d. Debridement and repair with an interposition vein graft
e. Ligation and observation

174. The patient shown in this chest x-ray film and contrast study was hospitalized after a car collision in which he suffered blunt trauma to the abdomen. He sustained several left rib fractures, but was hemodynamically stable. Which of the following statements is true regarding the injury demonstrated in the films?

a. The injury depicted is the most frequent organ injury in the setting of blunt trauma to the abdomen.

b. Delayed operative repair is indicated after the patient's rib fractures are allowed to stabilize.

c. Surgical treatment of this injury is indicated during this hospitalization.

d. Early repair of this injury is preferably accomplished through a left posterolateral thoracotomy.

e. If this injury is incidentally discovered during a surgical exploration, it should not be repaired.

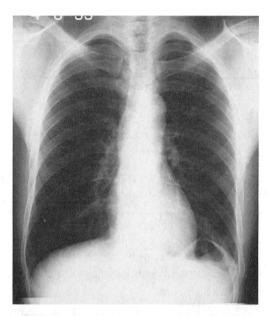

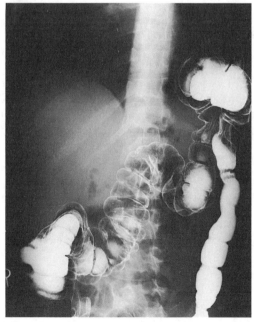

175. A 56-year-old woman sustains blunt abdominal trauma from an assault. Her blood pressure is 107/56 mm Hg and her pulse is 92. She complains of abdominal pain. She undergoes CT scanning of the abdomen and pelvis, which demonstrates a splenic injury. Which of the following would preclude an attempt at nonoperative management of the patient?

a. Presence of a subcapsular hematoma involving more than 25% of the surface area of the spleen
b. Presence of a subcapsular hematoma involving more than 50% of the surface area of the spleen
c. Evidence of a blush on CT scan
d. A red blood cell (RBC) count of 120,000/μL on diagnostic peritoneal lavage
e. Peritoneal signs on abdominal examination

176. A 49-year-old man was the restrained driver in a motor vehicle collision. He decelerated rapidly in order to avoid hitting another car and swerved into a ditch. He complains of chest pain. Which of the following findings on chest x-ray would be most suspicious for an aortic injury?

a. Multiple right-sided rib fractures
b. A left pulmonary contusion
c. A left pneumothorax
d. Widening of the mediastinum greater than 8 cm
e. Pneumomediastinum

177. A 29-year-old woman was hit by a car while crossing the street. She is hemodynamically unstable with a heart rate of 124 beats per minute and a systolic blood pressure of 82/45 mm Hg. The ultrasound machine is broken, and therefore a diagnostic peritoneal lavage (DPL) is performed. Which of the following findings on DPL is an indication for exploratory laparotomy in this patient?

a. Aspiration of 5 cc of gross blood initially
b. Greater than 50,000/μL red blood cells (RBCs)
c. Greater than 100,000/μL RBCs
d. Greater than 100/μL white blood cells (WBCs)
e. Greater than 250/μL WBCs

178. A 27-year-old construction worker falls about 30 ft from a scaffold. At the scene, he complains of inability to move his lower extremities. On arrival in the ER, he has a heart rate of 45 beats per minute and a blood pressure of 78/39 mm Hg. His extremities are warm and pink. His blood pressure improves with 1 L of crystalloid. A central venous catheter is placed for further resuscitation and his central venous pressure is 2 mm Hg. Which of the following is the best initial treatment strategy for improving his blood pressure?

a. Immediate celiotomy
b. Fluid resuscitation with crystalloids
c. Administration of O-negative blood
d. Administration of a peripheral vasoconstrictor
e. Administration of intravenous corticosteroids

179. A 22-year-old man undergoes an exploratory laparotomy after a gunshot wound to the abdomen. The patient has multiple injuries including a significant liver laceration, multiple small-bowel and colon injuries, and an injury to the infrahepatic vena cava. The patient receives 35 units of packed RBCs, 15 L of crystalloid, 12 units of fresh-frozen plasma (FFP), and a 12-pack of platelets. The patient's abdomen is packed closed and he is taken to the intensive care unit for further resuscitation. Which of the following warrants a decompressive laparotomy?

a. Increased peak airway pressure
b. Increased cardiac output
c. Decreased systemic vascular resistance
d. Decreased plasma renin and aldosterone
e. Increased cerebral perfusion pressure

180. A 10-year-old girl is the unrestrained backseat passenger in a high-speed motor vehicle collision. She is intubated in the field for unresponsiveness and on presentation to the ER, her heart rate is 160 beats per minute and her blood pressure is 60/35 mm Hg. She weighs 40 kg. Which of the following is the most appropriate recommendation for her fluid resuscitation?

a. Bolus 1 L of normal saline initially.
b. Bolus 1 L of 5% albumin initially.
c. Bolus 400 cc of packed RBCs initially.
d. Blood transfusion should be initiated if there is only a transient response to the first bolus.
e. Blood transfusion should be initiated after one repeat bolus if there is no response to the first bolus.

181. A 21-year-old woman sustains a stab wound to the middle of the chest. Upon arrival to the ER she has equal breath sounds, blood pressure of 85/46 mm Hg, distended neck veins, and pulsus paradoxus. Which of the following is the most appropriate management of this patient?

a. Emergent intubation and mechanical ventilation in the ER
b. Emergent pericardiocentesis in the ER
c. Emergent thoracotomy in the ER
d. Emergent pericardiocentesis or subxiphoid pericardial drainage after anesthetic induction in the operating room
e. Emergent pericardiocentesis or subxiphoid pericardial drainage under local anesthesia in the operating room

182. A 58-year-old man presents to the ER after falling 10 ft from a ladder. Examination reveals stable vital signs, no evidence of respiratory distress, and multiple right-sided rib fractures. Chest x-ray shows a hemothorax on the right side and a right tube thoracostomy is performed in the ER. Approximately 700 mL of blood is immediately drained with placement of the thoracostomy tube. Over the next 4 hours he continues to drain 300 mL/h after the original evacuation. Which of the following is the definitive treatment for this patient?

a. Platelets
b. Fresh frozen plasma
c. Second tube thoracostomy
d. Thoracotomy in the operating room
e. Thoracotomy in the ER

183. A 65-year-old woman is involved in a motor vehicle collision and sustains multiple left-sided rib fractures. Upon presentation to the ER her vital signs are stable and she is in no respiratory distress. Chest x-ray reveals fractures of ribs 4 to 7 on the left side without evidence of hemothorax or pneumothorax. She is admitted for observation and a few hours later she develops shortness of breath. A repeat chest x-ray demonstrates a well-defined infiltrate in her left lung. What is the most likely diagnosis?

a. Pulmonary contusion
b. Pulmonary embolus
c. Pneumonia
d. Myocardial infarction
e. Cardiac tamponade

184. Following a head-on motor vehicle collision, a 21-year-old unrestrained passenger presents to the ER with dyspnea and respiratory distress. She is intubated and physical examination reveals subcutaneous emphysema and decreased breath sounds. Chest x-ray reveals cervical emphysema, pneumomediastinum, and a right-sided pneumothorax. What is the most likely diagnosis?

a. Tension pneumothorax
b. Open pneumothorax
c. Tracheobronchial injury
d. Esophageal injury
e. Pulmonary contusion

185. An intoxicated 22-year-old man is a restrained driver in a high-speed motor vehicle collision. Examination reveals normal vital signs but the rest of the examination is unreliable secondary to the patient's intoxicated state from alcohol. Which of the following sole finding on a CT scan of the abdomen and pelvis mandates an exploratory laparotomy?

a. Free fluid in the pelvis
b. Pelvic fracture
c. Liver hematoma
d. Splenic hematoma
e. Renal hematoma

186. A 23-year-old man arrives in the ER after a motor vehicle collision. Examination reveals an unstable pelvis and blood at the urethral meatus. Which of the following studies would most accurately identify a urethral injury?

a. CT scan of the pelvis
b. Intravenous pyelogram
c. Stress cystogram
d. Antegrade urethrogram
e. Retrograde urethrogram

Questions 187 to 191

An 18-year-old female is transported to your trauma unit after sustaining a side-impact collision on her side of the car. She is hypotensive and in respiratory distress, and has distended neck veins. For each immediately life-threatening injury of the chest, select the proper intervention. Each lettered option may be used once, more than once, or not at all.

a. Endotracheal intubation
b. Cricothyroidotomy
c. Subxiphoid window
d. Tube thoracostomy
e. Occlusive dressing

187. Laryngeal obstruction

188. Open pneumothorax

189. Flail chest

190. Tension pneumothorax

191. Pericardial tamponade

Trauma and Shock

Answers

132. The answer is c. (*Townsend, pp 500-501.*) The patient has an acute diaphragmatic rupture, which occurs in about 4% of patients who sustain either blunt abdominal or chest trauma, and should be treated with immediate laparotomy, which allows both for examination of the intra-abdominal solid and hollow viscera for associated injuries and for adequate exposure of the diaphragm to allow secure repair. Because of the risk of vascular compromise of the contents of the hernia, exacerbated by the negative thoracic pressure, acute diaphragmatic rupture should be repaired immediately. Diagnosis may be difficult. The finding of an air-fluid level in the left lower chest, with a nasogastric tube entering it after blunt trauma to the abdomen, is diagnostic of diaphragmatic rupture with gastric herniation into the chest. Esophagogastroscopy is of limited value. CT scanning and MRI may be useful adjuncts, but neither can definitively rule out diaphragmatic rupture. Diagnostic peritoneal lavage is neither sensitive nor specific for diaphragmatic injuries, particularly in the absence of significant hemorrhage. Diaphragmatic repair can be accomplished via the left chest, but laparotomy is the procedure of choice for acute traumatic rupture for the stated reasons.

133. The answer is e. (*Townsend, pp 503-504.*) The presence of an abdominal wall ecchymosis from a seatbelt, or a "seatbelt sign," should raise suspicion for an enteric or mesenteric injury. Therefore, these patients should be observed closely for worsening abdominal pain, fevers, or signs of sepsis, even in the face of negative diagnostic tests. Serum amylase levels, plain films of the abdomen, abdominal CT scans, and DPL all have low sensitivity for small-bowel injuries. CT scan findings of free air, or thickening of the small-bowel wall or mesentery, or free fluid in the absence of solid organ injury should raise suspicion of a hollow viscus injury. DPL findings of a WBC count greater than 500/μL, an elevated amylase value, or detection of bile, bacteria, or food fibers should prompt exploratory laparotomy to rule out a bowel injury.

134. The answer is d. (*Townsend, pp 495-496.*) Patients with lower rib fractures may have associated abdominal injuries and should undergo appropriate evaluation (eg, ultrasound examination, CT scanning, or peritoneal lavage). Epidural catheters, continuous narcotic infusions, and patient-controlled analgesia are the most effective methods for ensuring pain control in hospitalized patients with rib fractures. Patients who are elderly, have multiple rib fractures, demonstrate ventilatory compromise, or have underlying respiratory problems (such as chronic obstructive pulmonary disease or smoking) are at increased risk for pulmonary complications (atelectasis, pneumonia, respiratory failure) and should be hospitalized. Patients with minor fracture injuries and no significant comorbidities may be managed at home with oral analgesics and appropriate instructions for coughing and deep breathing. Attempts to relieve pain by immobilization or splinting, such as strapping the chest, merely compound the problem of inadequate ventilation. Tube thoracostomy is indicated only if pneumothorax is diagnosed. Intercostal nerve blocks often provide prolonged periods of pain relief, but have been largely replaced by epidural catheters and intravenous narcotic administration. Rib fractures heal spontaneously, without need for surgical fixation.

135. The answer is c. (*Townsend, pp 502-504, 513-515.*) The spleen is the organ most likely to be damaged in blunt abdominal trauma, and splenic and liver injuries combined account for 75% of all blunt intra-abdominal injuries. The diagnosis of injuries resulting from blunt abdominal trauma is difficult; injuries are often masked by associated injuries. Thus, trauma to the head or chest, together with fractures, frequently conceals intra-abdominal injury. Apparently trivial injuries may rupture abdominal viscera in spite of the protection offered by the rib cage. Abdominal ultrasound (or FAST) is a rapid diagnostic test used to evaluate for free intraperitoneal fluid and has largely replaced DPL as the test of choice for evaluation for abdominal injury after blunt trauma. Abdominal CT scans are more specific than either ultrasound or DPL for hepatic, splenic, and renal injuries and can be performed in hemodynamically stable patients, who are candidates for nonoperative therapy.

136. The answer is d. (*Townsend, pp 542-544.*) Ligation rather than venous repair is the treatment of choice in hemodynamically unstable patients. However, the role of venous repair in hemodynamically stable patients with combined arterial and venous extremity injuries is controversial. Proximal veins should be repaired to avoid the sequelae of chronic venous insufficiency. Repairs can be performed primarily with suture closure, using saphenous vein patches, or using synthetic interposition grafts. Amputation may be necessary in the setting of extensive soft tissue and skeletal injuries in conjunction with the vascular injury.

137. The answer is b. (*Townsend, pp 542-544.*) Immediate exploration and repair is mandated for acute arterial insufficiency in the presence of neurologic symptoms. The five P's of arterial injury include pain, paresthesias, pallor, pulselessness, and paralysis. In the extremities, the tissues most sensitive to anoxia are the peripheral nerves and striated muscle. The early developments of paresthesias and paralysis are signals that there is significant ischemia present, and immediate exploration and repair are warranted. The presence of palpable pulses does not exclude an arterial injury because this presence may represent a transmitted pulsation through a blood clot. When severe ischemia is present, the repair must be completed within 6 to 8 hours to prevent irreversible muscle ischemia and loss of limb function. Delay to obtain an angiogram or to observe for change needlessly prolongs the ischemic time. Fasciotomy may be required, but should be done in conjunction with and after reestablishment of arterial flow. Local wound exploration at the bedside is not recommended because brisk hemorrhage may be encountered without the securing of prior proximal and distal vascular control.

138. The answer is c. (*Townsend, pp 1671-1672.*) Tension pneumothorax is a life-threatening problem requiring immediate treatment. A lung wound that behaves as a ball or flap valve allows escaped air to build up pressure in the intrapleural space. This causes collapse of the ipsilateral lung and shifting of the mediastinum and trachea to the contralateral side, in addition to compression of the vena cava and contralateral lung. Sudden death may ensue because of a decrease in cardiac output, hypoxemia, and ventricular arrhythmias. To accomplish rapid decompression of the pleural space, a large-gauge needle should be passed into the intrapleural cavity through the second intercostal space at the midclavicular line just above the third rib. This may be attached temporarily to an underwater seal with subsequent insertion of a chest tube after the life-threatening urgency has been relieved. Tension pneumothorax produces characteristic x-ray findings of ipsilateral lung collapse, mediastinal and tracheal shift, and compression of the contralateral lung. Occasionally, adhesions prevent complete lung collapse, but the tension pneumothorax is evident because of the mediastinal displacement.

139. The answer is c. (*Townsend, pp 500-501, 502-504.*) Diaphragmatic or abdominal injuries should be suspected in patients with a penetrating injury below the nipples. Diagnostic laparoscopy is appropriate to evaluate for an abdominal injury in penetrating trauma to the thoracoabdominal transition area. CT scan has a low sensitivity for diagnosing abdominal injuries in the setting of penetrating trauma. Local wound exploration is contraindicated in penetrating trauma to the chest, given the risk of creating a pneumothorax. An immediate tube thoracostomy is indicated in patients with a suspected tension pneumothorax or in the hemodynamically unstable patient with a suspected pneumo- or hemothorax (eg, decreased breath sounds). In hemodynamically stable patients without clinical evidence of a pneumothorax, a chest x-ray should be obtained prior to tube thoracostomy. Echocardiography is appropriate for the evaluation for a pericardial effusion in the setting of a penetrating cardiac injury and should be performed for penetrating wounds between the clavicle and costal margin and medial to the midclavicular line.

140. The answer is a. (*Brunicardi, pp 5-9.*) Though the immediate release of catecholamines causes a transient drop in insulin levels, shortly thereafter there is a significant rise in plasma insulin levels in injured humans. Because of increased peripheral insulin resistance in conjunction with increased insulin production, the overall net effect after severe injury is that of hyperglycemia. Since injured patients are highly hypermetabolic, it might be expected that the activity of the thyroid hormones would be increased following injury. This is not the case, however, and increased levels of the thyroid hormones are not seen. Vasopressin (ADH) is regulated by serum osmolality. In the post-injury period, many factors are at play that provoke the excretion of vasopressin. Glucagon secretion is normal or increased after injury; not only are aldosterone levels elevated, but the diurnal fluctuations ordinarily seen are lost.

141. The answer is d. (*Moore, pp 654-656.*) Traumatic injury to the common bile duct must be considered in two separate categories. Complete transection of the common bile duct can be handled in many ways. If the patient is unstable and time is limited, simply placing a T tube in either end of the open common bile duct and staging the repair is the treatment of choice. In a stable patient with a transected bile duct and a loss of tissue, a biliary enteric bypass is preferred. This can be accomplished by Roux-en-Y choledochojejunostomy or cholecystojejunostomy. The jejunum is favored over the duodenum because a lateral duodenal fistula is avoided if the anastomosis leaks. For similar reasons, the defunctionalizing of the jejunal limb is also preferable. This can be accomplished by creating a Roux-en-Y limb of jejunum. Primary end-to-end repair of a completely transected common bile duct can be performed if there is no significant tissue loss and an anastomosis can be performed without significant tension. Primary repair under tension is associated with an increased likelihood of a subsequent stricture. Primary repair is the procedure of choice if the common bile duct is lacerated or only partially transected.

142. The answer is a. (*Townsend, pp 489-493.*) Acute signs of airway distress (stridor, hoarseness, dysphonia), visceral injury (subcutaneous air, hemoptysis, dysphagia), hemorrhage (expanding hematoma, unchecked external bleeding), and neurologic symptoms referable to carotid injury (stroke or altered mental status) or lower cranial nerve or brachial plexus injury requires formal neck exploration. Pneumothorax would mandate a chest tube; the necessity for exploration would depend on clinical judgment and institutional policy. Additionally, all hemodynamically unstable patients with a penetrating neck wound should be explored, while management of asymptomatic, stable patients with neck injuries that penetrate the platysma is more controversial. In the past, treatment of asymptomatic, stable patients with zone II (between the lower border of the cricoid cartilage to the angle of the mandible) injuries was mandatory operative exploration. However, proponents for selective management of these patients argue that there is a high rate of negative explorations of the neck (40%-60%) and that serious injuries can be overlooked despite operative exploration. Furthermore, studies have demonstrated similar incidences of overall mortality with either selective or mandatory exploration. Stable patients with zone III (between the angle of the mandible and the skull), zone I (between the sternal notch and the lower border of the cricoid cartilage), or multiple neck wounds, should undergo initial angiography irrespective of the ultimate treatment plan. For zone II injuries, algorithms exist for nonoperative management of asymptomatic patients that employ observation alone or combinations of vascular and aerodigestive contrast studies and endoscopy.

143. The answer is b. (*Townsend, pp 505-506.*) Duodenal hematomas result from blunt abdominal trauma, and they should be managed initially with observation in patients not undergoing laparotomy to rule out other associated injuries. They present as a proximal bowel obstruction with abdominal pain and occasionally a palpable right upper quadrant mass. An upper gastrointestinal series is almost always diagnostic, with the classic coiled spring appearance of the second and third portions of the duodenum secondary to the crowding of the valvulae conniventes (circular folds) by the hematoma. Observation is the initial management strategy in patients with no other injuries, since the vast majority of duodenal hematomas resolve spontaneously. However, in patients undergoing immediate laparotomy for other associated injuries, duodenal exploration with drainage of the hematoma is indicated. Also, patients whose obstructive symptoms do not resolve after 2 weeks should undergo exploration and evacuation of the hematoma in order to rule out a perforation or injury to the head of the pancreas. Surgical bypass and duodenal resection are not indicated in the initial management of a duodenal hematoma.

144. The answer is b. (*Townsend, pp 2172-2175.*) The initial management of choice for closed radial nerve palsies is fracture reduction and observation, since the prognosis is excellent—the incidence of recovery is close to 90%. Operative intervention may be indicated after several months if function does not appear to be returning; either primary repair or reconstruction with sural nerve graft can be employed at that time.

Transection of a peripheral nerve results in hemorrhage and in retraction of the severed nerve ends. Almost immediately, degeneration of the axon distal to the injury begins. Degeneration also occurs in the proximal fragment back to the first node of Ranvier. Phagocytosis of the degenerated axonal fragments leaves a neurilemmal sheath with empty cylindrical spaces where the axons were. Several days following the injury, axons from the proximal fragment begin to regrow. If they make contact with the distal neurilemmal sheath, regrowth occurs at about the rate of 1 mm/day. However, if associated trauma, fracture, infection, or separation of neurilemmal sheath ends precludes contact between axons, growth is haphazard and a traumatic neuroma is formed.

145. The answer is a. (*Townsend, pp 485-487.*) Closed head injuries may result in cerebral concussion owing to depression of the reticular formation of the brainstem. This type of injury is usually reversible. A characteristic symptom pattern occurs and it is initiated by progressive depression of mental status. Local bleeding and swelling (intracranial or extracranial) produce an increase in intracranial pressure. Patients may develop Cushing triad (hypertension, bradycardia, and irregular respirations) as a sign of increased intracranial pressure. Lateralizing signs (motor or pupillary) are relatively uncommon and are highly suggestive of focal intracranial lesions.

146. The answer is e. (*Townsend, pp 486-487.*) Emergency measures to reduce intracranial pressure include hyperventilation, mannitol infusion, and elevation of the head of the bed (reverse Trendelenburg position). However, in the face of inadequate volume resuscitation, osmotic diuresis with mannitol and placement of the patient in reverse Trendelenburg may exacerbate the patient's hypotension. CT scanning should be performed as soon as possible along with neurosurgical evaluation in order to determine the need for operative drainage or decompression.

147. The answer is b. (*Townsend, pp 485-487.*) Increasing intracranial pressure tends to displace brain tissue away from the source of the pressure; if the pressure is sufficient, herniation of the uncal process through the tentorium cerebri occurs. Pupillary dilation is caused by compression of the ipsilateral oculomotor nerve and its parasympathetic fibers. If the pressure is not relieved, the brainstem will herniate through the foramen magnum and cause death. Hypertension and bradycardia are preterminal events.

148. The answer is e. (*Townsend, pp 496-497.*) Management of flail chest consists of adequate analgesia, chest physiotherapy, and mechanical ventilation if respiratory compromise develops. Flail chest is diagnosed in the presence of paradoxical respiratory movement in a portion of the chest wall. At least two fractures in each of three adjacent rib or costal cartilages are required to produce this condition. The complications of flail chest are no longer believed to arise from this paradoxical motion, but rather the underlying pulmonary parenchymal injury with resultant hypoventilation can lead to atelectasis, pneumonia, and respiratory failure. Indications for mechanical ventilation include significant impedance to ventilation by the flail segment, large pulmonary contusion, an uncooperative patient (eg, owing to head injury), general anesthesia for another indication, and the development of respiratory failure. Chest stabilization with sandbags or towel clips is no longer used. Surgical stabilization is performed only if thoracotomy is to be performed for another indication.

149. The answer is c. (*Brunicardi, pp 1764-1770.*) The motor components of the median nerve maintain the muscular function of most of the long flexors of the hand as well as the pronators of the forearm and the thenar muscles. The median nerve is also an extremely important sensory inner-vator of the hand and is commonly described as the "eye of the hand" because the palm, the thumb, and the index and middle fingers all receive their sensation via the median nerve.

150. The answer is d. *(Brunicardi, pp 200-201.)* Carbon monoxide (CO) is the leading cause of toxin-related death in the United States. Tobacco smoke—particularly smoke released from the tip of the cigarette, which has 2.5 times more CO than inhaled smoke—produces a significant amount of the gas; nonsmokers working in closed quarters with smokers may have carboxyhemoglobin levels as high as 15%, easily enough to cause headache and some impairment of judgment. Firefighters are at particularly high risk for CO intoxication. The pathophysiology of CO poisoning is unclear. It is known to cause an adverse shift in the oxygen-hemoglobin dissociation curve, to cause direct cardiovascular depression, and to inhibit cytochrome a_3. Tissue hypoxia is the result. Treatment is directed toward increasing the partial pressures of O_2 to which the transalveolar hemoglobin is exposed. In most cases, administering 100% oxygen through a tightly fitted face mask will result in a serum elimination half-life of COHb of 80 minutes (compared with 520 minutes when breathing room air). In severe cases, where coma, seizures, or respiratory failure are present, the partial pressure of O_2 is increased by administering it in a hyperbaric chamber with an atmospheric pressure of 2.8. In this situation, the serum elimination half-life is reduced to 23 minutes. In any case, the oxygen therapy should continue until the COHb levels reach 10%.

151. The answer is b. *(Brunicardi, pp 96-98.)* Cardiogenic shock is a cir-culatory pump failure leading to substantial reduction in cardiac output and resulting tissue hypoxia in the setting of adequate intravascular volume. Acute myocardial infarction is the most common cause of cardiogenic shock. Treatment of cardiac dysfunction includes maintenance of adequate oxy-genation and judicious fluid administration to avoid fluid overload and development of cardiogenic pulmonary edema. The patient in this scenario has evidence of volume overload based on the elevated central venous pres-sure; therefore, further fluid administration is contraindicated. Inotropic support is indicated when profound cardiac dysfunction exists to improve cardiac contractility and cardiac output. Dobutamine and dopamine are commonly used inotropes in cardiogenic shock. Patients who are refractory to inotropes may require mechanical circulatory support with an intra-aortic

balloon pump. This balloon pump increases coronary blood flow by reduction of systolic afterload and augmentation of diastolic perfusion pressure.
Cardiac catheterization and heart transplantation have no role in the management of cardiogenic shock.

152. The answer is d. (*Moore, p 1056.*) The treatment of electrical injury
should be modified from that of thermal burns because tissue damage is
much deeper than is apparent at first inspection. The heat generated is proportional to the resistance to the flow of current. Bone, fat, and tendons offer
the greatest resistance. Therefore, the tissue deep within the center of an
extremity may be injured while more superficial tissues are spared. For this
reason, the quantification of fluid requirements cannot be based on the percentage of body surface area involved, as in the Parkland, Brooke, or Baxter
formulas used to calculate fluid replacement after thermal burns. Massive
fluid replacement is usually essential. A brisk urine output is desirable because
of the likelihood of myonecrosis with consequent myoglobinuria and renal
damage. As with deep thermal burns, debridement, skin grafting, and
amputation of extremities may be required following electrical injury. However, fasciotomy is more frequently required than escharotomy with electrical
injury because deep myonecrosis results in increased intracompartmental
pressures and compromised limb perfusion. In addition, distant fractures
may result, owing to vigorous muscle contraction during the accident or if
subsequent falls occur. Cardiac or respiratory arrest may occur if the pathway of the current includes the heart or brain. An electrical current can also
damage the pulmonary alveoli and capillaries and lead to respiratory infections, a major cause of death in these victims. Electrical burns can also result
in cataract development even months after the injury, and therefore these
patients require ophthalmologic follow-up.

153. The answer is a. (*Bunt, pp 226-228.*) The highest rate of vascular
injury occurs with knee dislocations because of the extreme force required
to dislocate the joint. Angiograms and vascular surgical consultations
should be obtained when vascular compromise is suspected, owing to clinical
examination or Doppler confirmation of flow abnormalities. While vascular
injuries due to fractures on either side of a joint (eg, supracondylar femur
fracture or tibial plateau fracture) are uncommon, major joint dislocations
are more commonly associated with vascular injury. An exception to this
rule is the type III supracondylar humerus fracture, where displacement of
bone may injure or entrap the tethered brachial artery. Clavicular fractures

are rarely associated with significant vascular injury. In open elbow dislocations, the brachial artery is often disrupted by forcible hyperextension of the joint; closed elbow dislocations are rarely associated with vascular injury unless the dislocation is anterior.

154. The answer is d. *(Townsend, pp 495-496, 500-504.)* Gunshot wounds to the lower chest are often associated with intra-abdominal injuries; any patient with a gunshot wound below the level of T4 should be subjected to abdominal exploration. The domes of the diaphragm are at the level of the nipples, and the diaphragm can rise to the level of T4 during maximal expiration. Exploratory thoracotomy is not automatically indicated because most parenchymal lung injuries will stop bleeding and heal spontaneously with tube thoracostomy alone. Indications for thoracic exploration for bleeding are 1500 mL of blood on initial chest tube placement or persistent bleeding at a rate of 200 mL/h for 4 hours or 100 mL/h for 8 hours. Peritoneal lavage is not indicated even when the abdominal examination is unremarkable. As many as 25% of patients with negative physical findings and negative peritoneal lavage will have significant intra-abdominal injuries in this setting. These injuries include damage to the colon, kidney, pancreas, aorta, and diaphragm. Local wound exploration is not recommended because the determination of diaphragmatic injury with this technique is unreliable.

155. The answer is e. *(Moore, pp 174-179.)* Except in the rare circumstance, hypotension in a trauma patient should be presumed to be secondary to hypovolemia and not the head injury. When cardiovascular collapse occurs as a result of rising intracranial pressure, it is generally accompanied by hypertension, bradycardia, and respiratory depression. On the other hand, loss of consciousness following head trauma should be assumed to be because of intracranial hemorrhage until proved otherwise. A thorough evaluation of the head-injured patient includes assessment for other potentially life-threatening injuries including abdominal, thoracic, and pelvic hemorrhage. Appropriate workup should be initiated (chest and pelvic x-rays, abdominal evaluation with FAST examination or DPL). Rarely, a patient may have sufficient hemorrhage from a scalp laceration to cause hypotension, but caution should be used in attributing hypotension and tachycardia solely to such an injury.

156. The answer is b. *(Townsend, pp 508-509.)* Primary repair of traumatic colon injuries can be safely performed in the absence of risk factors such as gross fecal contamination, shock on presentation, multiple other injuries, or delayed intervention. Alternatives to primary repair include end colostomy with mucous fistula or Hartmann pouch and protection of a primary repair in the distal colon by formation of a proximal colostomy or ileostomy.

157. The answer is d. *(Townsend, pp 307-309.)* Crepitus in a soft tissue infection implies anaerobic metabolism. Since human tissue cannot survive in an anaerobic environment, gas associated with an infection implies dead tissue and therefore a surgical infection. Necrotizing fasciitis is associated with high rates of morbidity and mortality and prompt surgical exploration is mandatory. While CT and MRI may be useful adjuncts in the diagnosis of necrotizing fasciitis, they should not be performed in unstable patients or patients in whom the diagnosis is likely. Treatment consists of prompt surgical debridement and intravenous antibiotics. Most of these infections are polymicrobial, although monomicrobial necrotizing soft tissue infections can be caused by *Group A beta-hemolytic Streptococcus* or *Clostridium*. If the latter is suspected, high-dose penicillin G should be administered. Hyperbaric oxygen may be used as an adjunct; however, its efficacy has never been proven in clinical trials.

158. The answer is c. *(Townsend, pp 499-500.)* Echocardiography provides a sensitive assessment of ventricular wall motion and ejection fraction after blunt chest trauma, but is a poor predictor of the significant cardiac complications of pump failure and arrhythmia. On the other hand, although fewer than 10% of patients have an abnormal initial ECG, virtually all patients who develop cardiac complications display ECG abnormalities on arrival in the ER or within the first 24 hours. The spectrum of blunt cardiac injuries includes myocardial contusion, rupture, and internal (chamber and septal) disruptions such as traumatic septal defects, papillary muscle tears, and valvular tears. Myocardial contusions are by far the most common of these injuries. They usually occur in persons who sustain a direct blow to the sternum, as seen in a driver whose sternum is forcibly compressed by the steering column in a deceleration injury. They may have external signs of thoracic trauma, including sternal tenderness, abrasions, ecchymosis, palpable crepitus, rib fractures, or flail segments. Overall, fewer than 10% of patients have conduction abnormalities, dysrhythmias, or ischemic patterns on the initial ECG. Elevated cardiac isoenzyme levels are specific for myocardial injury, but they lack clinical significance in patients without

ECG abnormalities or hemodynamic instability. Patients without evidence of ECG abnormalities on presentation and who are hemodynamically stable do not require extended ICU monitoring. Stable patients with possible myocardial contusions but with a normal ECG tracing may be placed on telemetry for 24 hours rather than monitored in an ICU.

159. The answer is d. (*Weissman, pp 308-327.*) Injury and sepsis result in accelerated protein breakdown with increased urinary nitrogen loss and increased peripheral release of amino acids. The negative nitrogen balance represents the net result of breakdown and synthesis (with breakdown increased and synthesis increased or diminished). Amino acids such as alanine are released by muscle and transported to the liver for incorporation into acute-phase proteins including fibrinogen, complement, haptoglobin, and ferritin. The amino acids also undergo gluconeogenesis to glucose, which is utilized primarily by the brain and other glycolytic tissues such as peripheral nerves, erythrocytes, and bone marrow. Other tissues receive energy from fat in the form of fatty acids or ketone bodies during starvation following major trauma; this helps to conserve body protein. Glutamine is the most abundant amino acid in the blood, and its levels in muscle and blood decrease following injury and sepsis, as it is consumed rapidly by replicating fibroblasts, lymphocytes, and intestinal endothelial cells. The use of glutamine may decrease protein catabolism in the intestine and may help prevent atrophy of the gastrointestinal tract in starved and parenterally nourished patients. Along with the counter regulatory hormones (glucagon, epinephrine, cortisol), interleukin 1 appears to mediate muscle breakdown. Recent studies have indicated that TNF (also called cachectin because of the role it plays in muscle wasting in septic or oncologic patients) also may be a principal catabolic cytokine in the traumatized patient. This protein is secreted by macrophages and further affects metabolism by inducing secretion of interleukin 1 and inhibiting synthesis and activity of lipogenic enzymes.

160. The answer is c. (*Moore, pp 728-729.*) A CT scan should be routinely requested for suspected rectal perforation. The use of rectal contrast with water-soluble radiopaque medium such as Gastrografin is helpful when reconstructing a bullet trajectory. The use of barium is contraindicated because its spillage in the peritoneal cavity mixed with feces would increase the likelihood of subsequent intra-abdominal abscesses. Instrumentation of the bullet track is also contraindicated because of the risk of injury to adjacent structures (eg, bladder, ureters, iliac vessels). Angiography is not a sensitive method for demonstrating injury of the intestinal wall. Rigid sigmoidoscopy should be used if the CT scan is suggestive but ambiguous.

161. The answer is d. *(Moore, p 173.)* The patient has a tension pneumothorax caused by blunt trauma from the motor vehicle collision, which should be treated with emergent needle decompression. A tension pneumothorax develops when air continuously enters the pleural space from the lung or through the chest wall, cannot escape, and causes the lung to collapse. This air is under pressure and causes a shift of the mediastinum toward the opposite side with compression of the vena cava, leading to decreased venous return to the heart and hypotension. The diagnosis of a tension pneumothorax is a clinical one and should never wait for chest x-ray confirmation. This will delay life-saving intervention with emergent needle decompression of the chest (14-gauge catheter-over-needle inserted into the second intercostal space in the midclavicular line). Hypotension and distended neck veins are also seen in cardiac tamponade, but breath sounds are usually symmetric. An emergent thoracotomy is not indicated for a tension pneumothorax.

162. The answer is a. *(Townsend, pp 542-544.)* The presence of ischemic changes following vascular trauma is an indication for emergency exploration and repair. Nonsurgical management of arterial trauma when distal pulses are palpable may lead to delayed sequelae of embolization, occlusion, secondary hemorrhage, false aneurysm, and traumatic arteriovenous fistula. The presence of palpable pulses does not reliably exclude significant arterial injury. Injuries that may be missed if exploration is not performed include lacerations and partial transections containing hematomas, intramural or intraluminal thromboses, and intimal disruptions or tears. Injury to motor nerves would be apparent on neurologic examination. Injury to bone would be diagnosed by x-ray. Adjacent venous injury, in the absence of an expanding hematoma, would not by itself mandate exploration because there are numerous collateral venous channels in the extremities.

Prophylactic fasciotomy is not routinely performed for all arterial injuries but is indicated in the presence of an ischemic period exceeding 4 to 6 hours, combined arterial and major venous injury, prolonged periods of hypotension, massive associated soft tissue trauma, and massive edema.

163. The answer is d. (*Townsend, pp 93-94.*) The biochemical changes associated with shock result from tissue hypoperfusion, endocrine response to stress, and specific organ system failure. During shock, the sympathetic nervous system and adrenal medulla are stimulated to release catecholamines. Renin, angiotensin, antidiuretic hormone, adrenocorticotropin, and cortisol levels increase. Resultant changes include sodium and water retention and an increase in potassium excretion, protein catabolism, and gluconeogenesis. Potassium levels rise as a result of increased tissue release, anaerobic metabolism, and decreased renal perfusion. If renal function is maintained, potassium excretion is high and normal plasma potassium levels are restored.

164. The answer is d. (*Moore, p 432.*) Blowout orbital fractures require immediate operative intervention in the event of extraocular muscle entrapment. Inability to move the eye upward suggests entrapment of the inferior rectus muscle and mandates surgical release of the muscle. Patients with blowout fractures can have periorbital ecchymoses, pain, or diplopia. Surgery is indicated in patients with enophthalmos greater than 2 mm, diplopia on primary or inferior gaze, entrapment of extraocular muscles, or fracture greater than 50% of the orbital floor.

165. The answer is c. (*Townsend, p 100.*) Infusion of lactated Ringer solution is an effective immediate step, both clinically and experimentally, in managing hypovolemic shock. Use of this balanced salt solution helps correct the fluid deficit (in the extracellular, extravascular compartment), resulting from hypovolemic shock. This procedure may decrease requirements for whole blood in patients with hemorrhagic shock. If blood loss has been minimal and is controlled, whole blood transfusion may be avoided entirely. The lactate in lactated Ringer is metabolized to bicarbonate in the liver. Along with the hemodynamic improvement that follows volume restitution, liver function improves, lactate metabolism is improved, excess lactate levels drop, and metabolic acidosis improves.

166. The answer is e. (*Moore, pp 790-803.*) The organ injury scale utilizes five grades of injury, ranging from contusion or subcapsular hematoma (I) to shattered kidney or avulsion of the hilum (V). Grade II consists of a non-expanding perirenal hematoma confined to the renal retroperitoneum or laceration less than 1 cm of parenchymal depth of renal cortex without urinary extravasation. Low-grade renal injuries can be managed nonoperatively with a high success rate. The patient is placed on strict bed rest for the first 24 to 72 hours with serial hemoglobins. If nonoperative management is successful the patient is instructed to avoid significant physical exertion until follow-up imaging reveals adequate healing. Indications for renal exploration following injury include hemodynamic instability, ongoing hemorrhage requiring significant transfusion, or avulsion of the pedicle.

167. The answer is d. *(Moore, pp 805-806.)* If a urethral injury is suspected, a retrograde urethrogram should be performed before attempting to place a Foley catheter. If there is a urethral disruption, a suprapubic catheter should be placed. Urethral injuries can be associated with pelvic fractures, and suspicion of a urethral injury should be increased if any of the following signs are present: blood at the urethral meatus, a scrotal hematoma, or a free-floating prostate on rectal examination.

168. The answer is e. *(Moore, pp 713-716.)* Complications of pancreatic injury include fistula, pseudocyst, and abscess, but the cause of death in patients with pancreatic injury is most frequently exsanguination from associated injury to major vascular structures such as the splenic vessels, mesenteric vessels, aorta, or inferior vena cava. The majority of penetrating pancreatic injuries can be managed with simple drainage. Injury to the major pancreatic duct to the left of the mesenteric vessels is effectively treated with a distal pancreatectomy. The high morbidity and mortality of pancreaticoduodenectomy for trauma limit its use to extensive blunt injuries to both pancreatic head and duodenum. For ductal injury in the region of the head of the pancreas (to the right of the mesenteric vessels), a Roux-en-Y limb of jejunum can be brought up and used to drain the transected duct. Finally, however small, all peripancreatic hematomas should be explored to search for pancreatic injury.

169. The answer is d. *(Dutky, pp 856-860.)* Rapid fluid administration is often the key to successful trauma resuscitation. Some of the important factors affecting the rate of fluid resuscitation include the diameter of the intravenous tubing, the size and length of the venous cannulas, the fluid viscosity, and the site of administration. According to Poiseuille law, flow is proportional to the fourth power of the radius of a catheter and inversely proportional to its length. Therefore, the shorter a catheter and the larger its diameter, the faster a solution can be infused through it. Central venous placement alone does not ensure rapid flow. Importantly, the diameter of the intravenous tubing employed may be the rate-determining factor in fluid delivery: blood infusion tubing allows twice the flow of standard intravenous tubing and should be used when rapid fluid resuscitation is needed. Any patient suspected of having a major abdominal injury should immediately have at least two short, large-bore (16-gauge or larger) intravenous cannulas placed in peripheral veins. Longer, smaller catheters, such as standard 18-gauge central venous catheters, may take more time to place and will have lower flow rates. Once fluid resuscitation is under way, the physician may elect to place an 8- or 9-French pulmonary artery catheter-introducer via a central venous approach for further volume administration, as well as for measurement of central venous pressure or for Swan-Ganz catheter insertion. Lower extremity venous cannulas, placed by saphenous vein cutdown or percutaneously into the femoral veins, are no longer advised as primary access for patients with abdominal trauma, since possible disruption of iliac veins or the inferior vena cava will render volume infusion ineffective. Studies have demonstrated that the flow rate of cold whole blood is roughly two-thirds that of whole blood at room temperature. Diluting and warming the blood by "piggybacking" it into infusion lines that are delivering crystalloid will decrease the blood's viscosity, enhance flow, and minimize hypothermia.

170. The answer is c. *(Flint, pp 703-707; Trunkey, pp 479-486.)* The PASG is composed of inflatable overalls with three compartments, two for the legs and one for the abdomen. It has now been convincingly demonstrated that the PASG elevates blood pressure by increasing peripheral vascular resistance rather than by an autotransfusion effect on venous return and increased cardiac output. The PASG is beneficial for controlling bleeding from pelvic fractures by reduction of pelvic volume and immobilization to restrict fracture movement. The suit pressure must be released very slowly because rapid deflation can lead to sudden, irreversible hypotension. This is probably caused by a sudden decrease in peripheral vascular resistance and to the effects of vasodilation and washout of accumulated metabolites of capillary beds under the suit. On reperfusion of the lower body, a systemic metabolic acidemia with hyperkalemia may result and must be closely monitored. For these reasons, satisfactory intravenous volume must be attained prior to decompression of the PASG, a delay that may prevent adequate early evaluation of concealed injuries to the lower body.

171. The answer is c. *(Moore, pp 515-516.)* Although indications for thoracotomy in the ER are controversial, the procedure appears to be most beneficial when it is employed to (1) release cardiac tamponade in patients with penetrating thoracic trauma who are deteriorating too rapidly for a subxiphoid pericardial window to be created; (2) allow cross-clamping of the descending aorta in patients with intra-abdominal bleeding for whom other measures are not effective in maintaining blood pressure; or (3) allow effective internal cardiac massage in patients who arrive in the ER with faint or absent pulses and distant heart sounds, and for whom other resuscitative efforts are unsuccessful. By contrast, existing evidence suggests that patients who are unsalvageable and do not benefit from ER thoracotomy include (1) those with no vital signs (pulse, pupillary reaction, spontaneous respiration) in the field and (2) those with blunt trauma to multiple organ systems and absent vital signs on arrival in the ER.

172. The answer is c. *(Way, p 189.)* In the absence of sepsis, patients with enterocutaneous fistulas should be treated initially nonoperatively with bowel rest, TPN, and correction of electrolyte abnormalities. Most enterocutaneous fistulas result from trauma sustained during surgical procedures. Irradiated, obstructed, and inflamed intestine is prone to fistulization. Complications of fistulas include fluid and electrolyte depletion, skin necrosis, and malnutrition. Fistulas are classified according to their location and the volume of output, because these factors influence prognosis and treatment. When the patient is stable, a small-bowel follow-through study can be obtained to determine (1) the location of the fistula, (2) the relation of the fistula to other hollow intra-abdominal organs, and (3) whether there is distal obstruction. Proximal small-bowel fistulas (from the stomach to mid-ileum) tend to produce a high output of intestinal fluid and are less likely to close with conservative management than are distal, low-output fistulas (distal ileum or colon). Small-bowel fistulas that communicate with other organs (eg, bladder) may need aggressive surgical repair because of the risk of associated infections. When these poor prognostic factors for stabilization and spontaneous closure are observed, early surgical intervention must be undertaken. The patient in the question, however, appears to have a low-output, distal enterocutaneous fistula. Antispasmodic drugs have not been proved effective; somatostatin has been used with mixed success in the setting of high-output fistulas. There is no indication for antibiotics in the absence of sepsis. TPN is given to maintain or restore the patient's nutritional balance while minimizing the quantity of dietary fluids and endogenous secretions in the gastrointestinal tract. Initial TPN therapy is warranted to allow for spontaneous closure of a low-output distal fistula, but often these patients can be subsequently placed on a low-residue diet. Should conservative management fail, surgical closure of the fistula is performed.

173. The answer is d. (*Moore, pp 955-956.*) Traumatic arterial injuries can be handled with several techniques. The basic principles of debridement of injured tissue and reestablishment of flow should be observed. Primary end-to-end anastomosis is preferable if this can be accomplished without tension. When 5 cm of artery has been destroyed, it is impossible to perform a tension-free primary anastomosis, and a reversed saphenous vein graft is the repair of choice. Ligation of the artery is to be avoided in order to prevent gangrene and limb loss. The use of prosthetic material (Gore-Tex) in a potentially infected field is also to be avoided, as infection at the suture line often leads to delayed hemorrhage. Harvesting an arterial graft of similar diameter from elsewhere in the body is hazardous and unnecessary when vein is available.

174. The answer is c. (*Moore, pp 623-633.*) Traumatic injuries to the diaphragm are associated with both blunt and penetrating trauma. The spleen, kidneys, intestines, and liver are the most frequently injured abdominal organs in blunt trauma; the diaphragm is the least. Missed injuries lead to problems with herniation and bowel strangulation with sufficient frequency that repair should not be delayed. All such injuries require repair once the diagnosis is made and the patient has been stabilized. Most acute defects in the diaphragm can be repaired via an abdominal approach, which allows exploration for coexisting injuries.

175. The answer is e. (*Moore, pp 666-672.*) Nonoperative management of a splenic injury is contraindicated if the physical examination is suggestive of an associated injury, requiring operative intervention such as a blunt intestinal injury. The severity of the splenic injury can be graded based on the CT scan, but the grade of splenic injury does not always correlate to the need for operative intervention. Therefore, even the presence of a grade V injury (completely shattered spleen or hilar vascular injury) does not preclude a trial of nonoperative therapy. However, the opposite may also be true in that an apparently minor injury on CT scan may be much more significant on exploration. There may be a role for angiographic embolization of the splenic artery in the presence of a blush on CT scan, and there is evidence to suggest that the presence of a blush decreases the likelihood of success with nonoperative management. Patients who are hemodynamically unstable or who demonstrate clinical deterioration should undergo exploratory laparotomy. Although an RBC count greater than 100,000/μL constitutes a positive DPL in blunt abdominal trauma, a positive DPL in and of itself (ie, in a hemodynamically stable patient) does not require exploratory laparotomy.

176. The answer is d. (*Moore, pp 590-595.*) There are multiple findings on chest x-ray that are suggestive of a thoracic aortic injury, such as widening of the mediastinum more than 8 cm (because of the presence of a mediastinal hematoma), loss of the aortic knob, deviation of the nasogastric tube in the esophagus, depression of the left mainstem bronchus, an apical cap (apical pleural hematoma), sternal or scapular fracture, multiple left-sided rib fractures, and massive left hemothorax. However, a normal chest x-ray does not rule out a diagnosis of a thoracic great vessel injury. If clinical suspicion is high, then further diagnostic workup should be pursued. Aortography, CT angiography, and transesophageal echocardiography may establish the diagnosis. Traumatic aortic injuries are deceleration injuries because of differential forces to the fixed and mobile parts of the thoracic aorta; most aortic injuries are located near the ligamentum arteriosus.

177. The answer is c. (*Moore, pp 608-609.*) A positive DPL or a positive ultrasound examination in the hemodynamically unstable patient mandates exploratory laparotomy. A positive DPL for blunt abdominal trauma is characterized by aspiration of 10 cc of gross blood initially or more than 100,000/μL RBC, more than 500/μL WBC, or elevated amylase, bilirubin, or alkaline phosphatase.

178. The answer is b. (*Moore, p 224.*) The patient is in neurogenic shock secondary to a spinal cord injury. In patients with cervical or thoracic injuries, loss of sympathetic regulation results in loss of vasomotor tone and hypotension. Patients with neurogenic shock are warm and pink, as opposed to patients who are hypovolemic, and who are cold and clammy. Because of loss of the reflexive tachycardic response to hypotension, these patients are usually also bradycardic. Treatment is with fluid resuscitation initially and vasoconstrictors after the intravascular volume have been restored. Central venous pressure (CVP) is used to assess right ventricular function and systemic fluid status. Normal CVP is 2 to 6 mm Hg. The patient in this scenario has a low CVP suggesting intravascular volume depletion. Therefore, the patient requires further fluid resuscitation.

179. The answer is e. (*Moore, pp 858-860.*) There are multiple sequelae of increased abdominal pressure or abdominal compartment syndrome.

Compartment syndrome results in increased peak airway pressures, decreased venous return and decreased cardiac output, increased systemic vascular resistance, decreased renal blood flow and glomerular filtration rate, and decreased portal venous flow with decreased liver function. Because of decreased venous return, the intracranial pressure increases and cerebral perfusion pressure decreases. Treatment requires decompressive laparotomy.

180. The answer is e. (*Moore, pp 989-990.*) Initial management should consist of isotonic crystalloid resuscitation with either normal saline or lactated Ringer at a dose of 20 mL/kg body weight (800 mL). If the patient transiently responds, a second bolus should be administered. If the patient has a sustained response, fluids can be decreased to maintenance. If the patient does not respond, the bolus should be repeated and then blood transfusion initiated.

181. The answer is e. (*Moore, p 356.*) The clinical presentation is consistent with cardiac tamponade. In most cases of trauma-related cardiac tamponade, patients need surgical exploration to relieve the tamponade and repair the wound in the heart that caused it. It is advisable to perform pericardiocentesis or subxiphoid pericardial drainage under local anesthesia before anesthetic induction in these unstable patients. Cardiac tamponade is a reversible cause of shock that occurs when fluid or blood accumulates between the pericardium and the heart. If the pericardial fluid develops under significant pressure, filling of the heart cannot occur during diastole, and the amount of blood ejected during systole decreases. Cardiac tamponade is mainly seen in patients with penetrating trauma in proximity to the sternum. The diagnosis should be considered in patients with pulsus paradoxus, which is a greater than 10 mm Hg fall in arterial systolic blood pressure with inspiration. Echocardiography is the preferred diagnostic tool for identification of fluid or blood in the pericardium.

182. The answer is d. (*Moore, pp 173-174.*) The recommended guidelines for a thoracotomy in patients with a hemothorax are greater than or equal to 1500 mL of immediate drainage of blood through the thoracostomy tube after placement or greater than 200 mL/h of continuous drainage of blood for several hours after the original evacuation. The patient's physiology and blood transfusion requirements should also factor into a decision for operative intervention.

183. The answer is a. (*Moore, p 542.*) Pulmonary contusion is hemorrhage and edema of the lung parenchyma without parenchymal disruption. It occurs more frequently after blunt chest trauma and radiologic findings may not be present on admission, developing several hours after the initial injury. The management of pulmonary contusion is almost entirely supportive with maintenance of good oxygenation and adequate pulmonary toilette. Patients with persistent low PaO$_2$ levels who do not respond to supplemental oxygen, pulmonary toilette, and pain control should be intubated and mechanically ventilated. The findings of rib fractures and an underlying well-defined infiltrate is less supportive of the diagnosis of pulmonary embolus, pneumonia, myocardial infarction, or cardiac tamponade.

184. The answer is c. (*Moore, pp 553-557.*) Tracheobronchial injuries are uncommon and can occur with blunt or penetrating trauma. Blunt injuries to the tracheobronchial tree occur after direct compression of the airway with a closed glottis or after decelerating injuries causing partial or complete avulsion of the right mainstem bronchus from the carina or tracheal lacerations. Patients may present with pneumothorax, subcutaneous emphysema, pneumomediastinum, hemoptysis, and respiratory distress. Small injuries usually heal spontaneously with supportive care but are associated with late complications such as stricture formation at the site of injury and recurrent pulmonary infection. More extensive wounds are primarily repaired in the operating room. The patient does not have physical examination findings of a sucking chest wound to support an open pneumothorax. A tension pneumothorax would not involve air in the subcutaneous space or mediastinum. An esophageal injury would not present with the large amount of emphysema or respiratory distress. A pulmonary contusion is not associated with a pneumothorax.

185. The answer is a. (*Moore, pp 686-688, 693.*) Free fluid in the abdomen or pelvis in the absence of solid organ injury warrants an exploratory laparotomy to evaluate for small-bowel or mesenteric injury. DPL to evaluate the fluid for WBCs, amylase levels, or bacteria on gram stain could be performed alternatively. However, DPL is being used less frequently because of its invasiveness. Furthermore, the lavage WBC count was found to be nonspecific for hollow viscus injuries. Findings seen on CT scan suggestive of small-bowel injury include bowel wall thickening, pneumoperitoneum, mesenteric fat streaking, and extravasation of either luminal or vascular contrast. Exploratory laparotomy is not indicated in solid organ injury (liver, spleen, kidney) in patients with hemodynamic stability and no evidence of contrast extravasation. A pelvic fracture requires internal or external fixation if it is unstable.

186. The answer is e. (*Moore, pp 796-799.*) A retrograde urethrogram is essential for diagnosis of a urethral injury. A Foley catheter is inserted into the distal urethra and minimally inflated. This is followed by instillation of 30 mL of water-soluble contrast and a plain radiograph is obtained. No attempt at insertion of a bladder catheter should be made until a negative retrograde urethrogram is obtained to avoid further damaging a urethral injury. A stress cystogram is useful in diagnosing a bladder injury. An intravenous pyelogram is obtained to evaluate the kidneys, ureter, and bladder. A CT scan of the pelvis does not evaluate the urethra.

187 to 191. The answers are 187-b, 188-e, 189-a, 190-d, 191-c. (*Moore, pp 532-538, 553-560, 569-572.*) Flail chest describes the paradoxical motion of the chest wall that occurs when consecutive ribs are broken in more than one place, usually following blunt trauma to the thorax. Respiratory distress may ensue when the noncompliant flail segment interferes with generation of adequate positive and negative intrathoracic pressure needed to move air through the trachea. In addition, a blow sufficiently violent to cause a flail chest may also contuse the underlying pulmonary parenchyma, which compounds the respiratory distress. Treatment consists of pain control and treatment of the underlying pulmonary contusion.

Airway obstruction denotes partial or complete occlusion of the tracheobronchial tree by foreign bodies, secretions, or crush injuries of the upper respiratory tract. Patients may present with symptoms ranging from cough and mild dyspnea to stridor and hypoxic cardiac arrest. An initial effort should be made to digitally clear the airway and to suction visible secretions; in selected stable patients, fiberoptic endoscopy may be employed to determine the cause of obstruction and to retrieve foreign objects. Unstable patients whose airways cannot be quickly reestablished by clearing the oropharynx must be intubated. An endotracheal intubation may be attempted, but cricothyroidotomy is indicated in the presence of proximal obstruction or severe maxillofacial trauma.

Blunt or penetrating trauma to the pericardium and heart will result in pericardial tamponade when fluid pressure in the pericardial space exceeds central venous pressure and thus prevents venous return to the heart. The result is shock, despite adequate volume and myocardial function. The treatment is pericardial decompression. A subxiphoid, supradiaphragmatic incision and creation of a pericardial window, ideally performed in the operating room, provides a rapid, safe means of confirming the diagnosis of tamponade and of relieving venous obstruction. If bleeding is encountered on opening the pericardial window, a sternotomy should be performed.

Tension pneumothorax occurs when a laceration of the visceral pulmonary pleura acts as a one-way valve that allows air to enter the pleural space from an underlying parenchymal injury but not to escape. Increasing intrapleural pressure causes collapse of the ipsilateral lung, compression of the contralateral lung due to mediastinal shift toward the opposite hemithorax, and diminished venous return. Treatment consists of relieving the pneumothorax. This is best accomplished via tube thoracostomy.

Open pneumothorax occurs when a traumatic defect in the chest wall permits free communication of the pleural space with atmospheric pressure. If the defect is larger than two-thirds of the tracheal diameter, respiratory efforts will move air in and out through the defect in the chest wall rather than through the trachea. The immediate treatment is placement of an occlusive dressing over the defect; subsequent interventions include placement of a thoracostomy tube (preferably through a separate incision), formal closure of the chest wall, and ventilatory assistance if needed.

Transplants, Immunology, and Oncology

Questions

192. A 43-year-old man with a gangrenous gallbladder and gram-negative sepsis agrees to participate in a research study. An assay of tumor necrosis factor (TNF) is performed. Which of the following is the origin of this peptide?

a. Fibroblasts
b. Damaged vascular endothelial cells
c. Monocytes/macrophages
d. Activated T lymphocytes
e. Activated killer lymphocytes

193. A 49-year-old man who underwent liver transplantation 5 years ago for alcoholic cirrhosis presents with a gradually increasing bilirubin level. He undergoes a liver biopsy, which demonstrates a paucity of bile ducts. Which of the following is his best option for treatment?

a. Increase his immunosuppression
b. Administration of a monoclonal antibody against T cells
c. Exploratory laparotomy with hepatic arterial reconstruction
d. Exploratory laparotomy with thrombectomy of the portal vein
e. Retransplantation

194. A 52-year-old woman in renal failure is listed as a transplant candidate. In order to assess the propriety of the transplant, which of the following combinations represents how a cross-match is performed?

a. Donor serum with recipient lymphocytes and complement
b. Donor lymphocytes with recipient serum and complement
c. Donor lymphocytes with recipient lymphocytes
d. Recipient serum with a known panel of multiple donor lymphocytes
e. Recipient serum with donor red blood cells and complement

195. A 39-year-old woman presents with generalized malaise and lymphadenopathy. Biopsy of a supraclavicular lymph node reveals non-Hodgkin lymphoma. Forty-eight hours after initiation of chemotherapy, she develops a high-grade fever and her laboratory studies demonstrate hyperkalemia, hyperphosphatemia, and hypocalcemia. Which of the following cells mediate this syndrome?

a. Macrophages
b. Cytotoxic T lymphocytes
c. Natural killer cells
d. Polymorphonuclear leukocytes
e. Helper T lymphocytes

196. A 33-year-old diabetic man receives a renal allograft. The physicians choose cyclosporine as one of the antirejection medications. Which of the following functions does cyclosporine A primarily inhibit?

a. Macrophage function
b. Antibody production
c. Interleukin 1 production
d. Interleukin 2 production
e. Cytotoxic T-cell effectiveness

197. A 24-year-old woman presents with lethargy, anorexia, tachypnea, and weakness. Laboratory studies reveal a BUN of 150 mg/dL, serum creatinine of 16 mg/dL, and potassium of 6.2 mEq/L. Chest x-ray shows increased pulmonary vascularity and a dilated heart. Which of the following is the most appropriate management of this patient?

a. Emergency kidney transplantation
b. Creation and immediate use of a forearm arteriovenous fistula
c. Placement of a catheter in the internal jugular vein and initiation of hemodialysis
d. A 100-g protein diet
e. Renal biopsy

198. A hypertensive 47-year-old man is proposed for kidney transplantation. He is anemic but is otherwise functional. Which of the following would preclude renal transplantation?

a. Positive cross-match
b. Donor blood type O
c. Two-antigen HLA match with donor
d. Blood pressure of 180/100 mm Hg
e. Hemoglobin level of 8.2 g/dL

199. A 56-year-old woman is undergoing a cadaveric renal transplant. After revascularization of the transplanted kidney the transplanted renal parenchyma becomes swollen and blue. Which of the following statements is true regarding her transplanted kidney?

a. The donor had preformed antibodies against the recipient's HLA antigens.
b. It is characterized pathologically by fibrin and platelet thrombosis of renal arterioles and small arteries and necrosis of the glomerular tufts.
c. Biopsies should not be obtained intraoperatively.
d. This form of rejection is associated with disseminated intravascular coagulation (DIC).
e. The rejection process can be treated with a steroid bolus and OKT3.

200. A 57-year-old man has end-stage heart failure due to atherosclerosis. He is first on the transplant list, and a donor becomes available. The harvest team is dispatched. Which of the following statements regarding heart transplantation is true?

a. Heart transplants are matched by size and ABO blood type rather than tissue typing.
b. Cadaveric graft survival is significantly lower with heart transplants as compared with renal transplants.
c. Cold ischemia time for donor hearts does not affect outcome.
d. The upper age limit for heart transplant eligibility is 55 years.
e. The leading cause of death after the first year of cardiac transplantation is chronic rejection.

201. A 47-year-old man with hypertensive nephropathy develops fever, graft tenderness, and oliguria 4 weeks following cadaveric renal transplantation. Serum creatinine is 3.1 mg/dL. A renal ultrasound reveals mild edema of the renal papillae but normal flow in both the renal artery and the renal vein. Nuclear scan demonstrates sluggish uptake and excretion. Which of the following is the most appropriate next step?

a. Performing an angiogram
b. Decreasing steroid and cyclosporine dose
c. Beginning intravenous antibiotics
d. Performing renal biopsy, steroid boost, and immunoglobulin therapy
e. Beginning FK 506

202. Approximately 6 weeks following a heart transplant, a 59-year-old woman develops fever, malaise, and myalgias and is found to have a cytomegalovirus (CMV) infection. Which of the following is a potential sequela of CMV infection?

a. Pyelonephritis
b. Gastrointestinal (GI) ulceration and hemorrhage
c. Cholecystitis
d. Intra-abdominal abscess
e. Parotitis

203. A 55-year-old man presents with worsening cirrhosis. After evaluation by a hepatologist, he presents to you with questions about an MELD (model for end-stage liver disease) score. Which of the following is true regarding the MELD score?

a. A statistical model with high predictive capacity in identifying patients with end-stage liver disease at greatest risk for mortality within 1 year
b. A scoring system developed for allocation of liver transplants to give priority to the sickest patients using a system based on objective variables
c. A scoring system based on total bilirubin, International Normalized Ratio, creatinine, and ascites
d. A scoring system based on bilirubin, International Normalized Ratio, albumin, ascites, and encephalopathy
e. A scoring system based on ascites and encephalopathy

204. A young woman who has received a transplant has posttransplant fever and malaise. Graft-versus-host disease (GVHD) is diagnosed. This has occurred most commonly with the transplantation of which of the following?

a. Kidney
b. Lung
c. Heart
d. Bone marrow
e. Pancreas

205. A brain-dead potential donor has become available. You must plan for the dispersal of the thoracic organs. Which of the following will necessitate a heart-lung transplant?

a. Primary pulmonary hypertension
b. Cystic fibrosis
c. End-stage emphysema
d. Idiopathic dilated cardiomyopathy with long-standing secondary pulmonary hypertension
e. End-stage pulmonary fibrosis secondary to sarcoidosis

206. A 19-year-old male who has had type I diabetes for many years has several stigmata, such as renal failure and retinopathy. Which of the following is true regarding successful whole-organ pancreas transplantation in type I diabetes?

a. It results in maintenance of normal serum glucose levels.
b. Recurrence of diabetic nephropathy in simultaneously transplanted kidneys is not prevented.
c. Oral glucose tolerance tests remain abnormal.
d. The pathologic changes of diabetic retinopathy are reversed.
e. The rate of diabetic ulcers and amputations in the lower extremities is reduced.

207. A 55-year-old woman who has end-stage liver disease is referred to a hepatologist for evaluation. Which of the following would prevent her from being a transplantation candidate?

a. Use of alcohol 3 months ago
b. Two 2-cm hepatocellular carcinomas (HCCs) in the right lobe of the liver
c. A 4-cm hepatocellular carcinoma in the right lobe of the liver
d. Development of hepatorenal syndrome requiring hemodialysis
e. History of breast cancer 5 years ago with no evidence of disease currently

208. A kidney transplant recipient presents with severe acute rejection that does not respond to steroid treatment. She is started on OKT3, which is a monoclonal antibody directed against the CD3 antigen complex on T cells. Which of the following statements is true regarding OKT3?

a. Binding of OKT3 to the CD3 antigen complex stimulates the T cells to proliferate.
b. The most severe side effects of OKT3 are fever, chills, and headaches from cytokine release.
c. OKT3 is an effective drug for acute rejection but cannot be used to prevent rejection.
d. OKT3 should be used cautiously in patients with fluid overload because of the risk of pulmonary edema.
e. OKT3 efficacy should be measured by checking drug levels in the blood

209. A 19-year-old college student presents with a testicular mass, and after treatment he returns for regular follow-up visits. Which of the following is the most useful serum marker for detecting recurrent disease after treatment of nonseminomatous testicular cancer?

a. Carcinoembryonic antigen (CEA)
b. Human chorionic gonadotropin (hCG)
c. Prostate-specific antigen (PSA)
d. CA125
e. p53 oncogene

210. An edentulous 72-year-old man with a 50-year history of cigarette smoking presents with a nontender, hard mass in the lateral neck. Which of the following is the best diagnostic test for establishing a diagnosis of malignancy?

a. Fine-needle aspiration cytology
b. Bone marrow biopsy
c. Nasopharyngoscopy
d. Computed tomography (CT) scan of the head and neck
e. Sinus x-ray

211. A 49-year-old woman undergoes surgical resection of a malignancy. The family asks about the prognosis. The histopathology is available for review. For which of the following malignancies does histologic grade best correlate with prognosis?

a. Lung cancer
b. Melanoma
c. Colonic adenocarcinoma
d. Hepatocellular carcinoma
e. Soft tissue sarcoma

212. A mother notices an abdominal mass in her 3-year-old son while giving him a bath. There is no history of any symptoms, but the boy's blood pressure is elevated at 105/85 mm Hg. Metastatic workup is negative and the patient is explored. The mass shown here is found within the left kidney. Which of the following statements concerning this disease is correct?

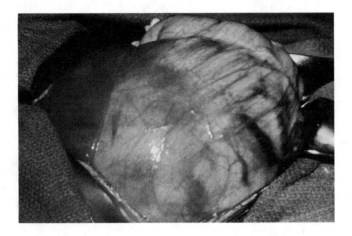

a. This tumor is associated with aniridia, hemihypertrophy, and cryptorchidism.
b. The majority of patients present with an asymptomatic abdominal mass and hematuria.
c. Treatment with surgical excision, radiation, and chemotherapy results in survival of less than 60% even in histologically low-grade tumors.
d. Surgical excision is curative and no further treatment is ordinarily advised.
e. This tumor is the most common abdominal malignancy of childhood.

213. An 11-year-old girl presents to your office because of a family history of medullary carcinoma of the thyroid. Physical examination is normal. Which of the following tests should you perform?

a. Urine vanillylmandelic acid (VMA) level
b. Serum insulin level
c. Serum gastrin level
d. Serum glucagon level
e. Serum somatostatin level

214. A 37-year-old woman has developed a 6-cm mass on her anterior thigh over the past 10 months. The mass appears to be fixed to the underlying muscle, but the overlying skin is movable. Which of the following is the most appropriate next step in her management?

a. Above-knee amputation
b. Excisional biopsy
c. Incisional biopsy
d. Bone scan
e. Abdominal CT scan

215. A 50-year-old man is incidentally discovered to have non-Hodgkin lymphoma confined to the submucosa of the stomach during esophagogastroduodenoscopy for dyspepsia. Which of the following statements is true regarding his condition?

a. Surgery alone cannot be considered adequate treatment.
b. Combined chemotherapy and radiation therapy, without prior resection, are not effective.
c. Combined chemotherapy and radiation therapy, without prior resection, result in a high risk of severe hemorrhage and perforation.
d. Outcome (freedom from progression and overall survival) is related to the histologic grade of the tumor.
e. The stomach is the most common site for non-Hodgkin lymphoma of the gastrointestinal tract.

216. A 33-year-old woman seeks assistance because of a swelling of her right parotid gland. Biopsy is performed and reveals acinar carcinoma. In your discussion regarding surgery, which of the following statements regarding malignant parotid tumors is correct?

a. Acinar carcinoma is a highly aggressive malignant tumor of the parotid gland.
b. Squamous carcinoma of the parotid gland exhibits only moderately malignant behavior.
c. Regional node dissection for occult metastases is not indicated for malignant parotid tumors because of their low incidence and the morbidity of lymphadenectomy.
d. Facial nerve preservation should be attempted when the surgical margins of resection are free of tumor.
e. Total parotidectomy (superficial and deep portions of the gland) is indicated for malignant tumors.

217. A 42-year-old man is undergoing chemotherapy after resection of a cecal adenocarcinoma with positive lymph nodes. You are asked to see him regarding a potential surgical complication. Which of the following potentially operable complications is a common occurrence among patients receiving systemic chemotherapy?

a. Acute cholecystitis
b. Perirectal abscess
c. Appendicitis
d. Incarcerated femoral hernia
e. Diverticulitis

218. A 28-year-old medical student seeks your attention because of a testicular mass. You recommend a biopsy. Subsequently, you must plan for optimal operative and perioperative therapy. Which of the following statements regarding testicular cancer is true?

a. Lymph node dissection after radical orchiectomy is useful for staging, but does not increase survival.
b. Seminomas and choriocarcinomas are best treated with orchiectomy and retroperitoneal lymph node dissection.
c. Seminomas are extremely resistant to radiotherapy.
d. Orchiectomy for a testicular mass is approached via the scrotum.
e. Cryptorchidism is associated with an increased risk of testicular cancer.

219. A 25-year-old woman with end-stage renal disease is exploring the benefits of renal transplantation. Which of the following is an advantage of dialysis over renal transplantation?

a. Better patient survival
b. More cost effective longterm
c. Improved quality of life
d. No need for lifelong immunosuppression
e. More cost effective if the renal transplant functions for less than 2 years

220. A 30-year-old previously healthy man presents with refractory hypertension on four medications. Urinalysis is positive for metanephrines. He was adopted as an infant and therefore does not know his family history. Which of the following inherited syndromes is not associated with this disease?

a. MEN IIA
b. MEN IIB
c. von Hippel-Lindau disease
d. Neurofibromatosis I
e. Neurofibromatosis II

221. A 45-year-old man presents to his family physician to discuss screening colonoscopy. Which of the following is true about colorectal cancer screening?

a. In the absence of any family or personal history of colon cancer, he should begin screening at age 40.
b. If a polyp is detected on screening colonoscopy, the patient should undergo repeat colonoscopy in 1 year.
c. If no polyps are detected on screening colonoscopy, the patient should undergo repeat colonoscopy in 3 years.
d. The sensitivity of air contrast barium enema for detecting polyps greater than 1 cm is only 70% and therefore should not be used in colorectal cancer screening.
e. In patients with hereditary nonpolyposis colorectal cancer (HNPCC), screening colonoscopy should begin at either age 20 to 25 or 10 years younger than the youngest age of diagnosis in the family.

222. A 53-year-old woman is submitted for breast lumpectomy and radiation therapy for breast cancer. You discuss this treatment with the radiation oncology attending in order to better understand the mechanism of action on your patient. Which of the following statements is true concerning radiation therapy?

a. Damage to DNA occurs primarily by the direct effect of ionizing radiation.
b. Cellular hypoxia decreases sensitivity to radiation.
c. Cells in the S phase of the cell cycle are most radiosensitive.
d. Radiation therapy following lumpectomy of a breast cancer results in decreased survival when compared to modified radical mastectomy.
e. Skin, GI mucosa, and bone marrow are relatively insensitive to radiotherapy.

223. You are asked to provide a 1-hour lecture to medical residents on the general topic of nutrition and cancer. You review a number of areas of interest. Which of the following statements concerning cancer and nutrition is correct?

a. Levels of nitrates in food and drinking water are positively correlated with the incidence of bladder cancer.

b. Regular ingestion of vitamin D from childhood probably inhibits formation of carcinogens.

c. Consumption of excessive amounts of animal dietary fats is associated with increased incidence of colon cancer.

d. Nutritional support of cancer patients improves response of the tumor to chemotherapy.

e. Alcohol ingestion is associated with pancreatic cancer.

224. A patient requires both cardiac and renal transplantation. Preparation for the procedures has begun. How do cardiac allografts differ from renal allografts?

a. Cardiac allografts are matched by HLA tissue typing and renal allografts are not.

b. Cardiac allografts can tolerate a longer period of cold ischemia than renal allografts.

c. One-year graft survival for cardiac allografts is substantially lower than that for renal allografts.

d. Cardiac allografts are matched only by size and ABO blood type.

e. Cyclosporine is a critical component of the immunosuppressive regimen for cardiac allografts but not renal allografts.

225. A patient with colon cancer has a mass in the upper lobe of his left lung 2.5 years following resection of his colon cancer and subsequent 12 months of chemotherapy. His CEA level is rising. Which of the following predicts a 5-year survival rate of greater than 20% following resection of pulmonary metastases?

a. Other organ metastases are present.

b. Lung lesions are solitary.

c. Local tumor recurrence is found.

d. The tumor doubling time is less than 20 days.

e. The patient has received prior chemotherapy.

226. Preoperative preparations with your scrub team are under way prior to performing a thoracotomy for persistent pneumothorax on a patient who is known to have AIDS. Which of the following statements about transmission of HIV in the health care setting is true?

a. A freshly prepared solution of dilute chlorine bleach will not adequately decontaminate clothing.
b. All needles should be capped immediately after use.
c. Cuts and other open skin wounds are believed to act as portals of entry for HIV.
d. Double gloving reduces the risk of intraoperative needle sticks.
e. The risk of seroconversion following a needle stick with a contaminated needle is greater for HIV than for hepatitis B.

227. A 57-year-old woman discovers a breast mass, which is biopsied and found to be carcinoma. After her treatment, she assembles her family and attempts to encourage them to obtain regular examinations and mammograms. Regarding the risk of breast cancer, which of the following statements is true?

a. Breast cancer occurs more commonly among women of the lower social classes.
b. A history of breast cancer in a first-degree family relative is associated with a fourfold increase in risk.
c. Women with a first birth after age 30 have increased risk compared to women with a first birth before age 18.
d. Cigarette smoking increases the risk of breast cancer.
e. Hair dyes have been shown to increase the risk of breast cancer.

228. A 42-year-old man is diagnosed with an osteosarcoma. His family history is significant for a 37-year-old sister with breast cancer and an uncle with adrenocortical carcinoma. His family physician suspects that he may have Li-Fraumeni syndrome and suggests genetic testing. Which of the following genes is most likely to be mutated if he has the syndrome?

a. Adenomatous polyposis coli (APC) gene
b. RET
c. p53
d. Phosphatase and tensin homologue (PTEN)
e. p16

229. A patient with a solid malignancy is discussing chemotherapy with his oncologist. He is interested in the risks of the treatment. What is the primary toxicity of doxorubicin (Adriamycin)?

a. Cardiomyopathy
b. Pulmonary fibrosis
c. Peripheral neuropathy
d. Uric acid nephropathy
e. Hepatic dysfunction

230. A 25-year-old woman is diagnosed with bilateral breast cancer. She undergoes genetic testing to assess whether she has a mutation in either *BRCA1* or *BRCA2*. Which of the following statements is true regarding *BRCA* mutations?

a. Her risk, as a woman under the age of 40, for having a mutation in *BRCA1* or 2 is 40%.
b. *BRCA1* tumors are more likely to be estrogen-receptor positive.
c. A mutation in *BRCA2* is associated with an increased risk of colon cancer.
d. A mutation in *BRCA1* is associated with an increased risk for pancreatic, bile duct, and gallbladder cancers.
e. Both *BRCA1* and *BRCA2* are associated with an increased risk of ovarian cancer by age 70.

231. A 56-year-old woman is undergoing chemotherapy. She presents today with complaints of burning on urination and bloody urine. Which of the following agents causes hemorrhagic cystitis?

a. Bleomycin
b. 5-fluorouracil
c. Cisplatin
d. Vincristine
e. Cyclophosphamide

232. A 38-year-old woman who underwent a cadaveric renal transplant 8 years previously presents with fevers, fatigue, and weight loss. Evaluation included CT scans of the head, neck, chest, abdomen, and pelvis; she is noted to have diffuse lymphadenopathy and pulmonary nodules. A biopsy and histologic examination of a lymph node is performed. Which of the following viruses is most likely to be present in the lymph node?

a. Cytomegalovirus
b. Human papillomavirus
c. Human herpesvirus 8
d. Epstein-Barr virus
e. Coxsackie virus

233. A 41-year-old man underwent a successful living related kidney transplantation 1 year previously with good results. Preoperatively, he was noted to have an elevated calcium level; posttransplantation, he continues to have elevated calcium levels and associated symptoms. Which of the following is the most appropriate next step in management?

a. ^{99m}Tc sestamibi scanning
b. Ultrasound of the neck
c. CT scan of the neck and mediastinum
d. Total parathyroidectomy with autotransplantation of a portion of a gland into the forearm
e. Measurement of urinary calcium levels

234. A 53-year-old man presents with constipation and a 20-lb weight loss over the course of 6 months. Colonoscopy reveals a fungating mass in the sigmoid colon; biopsy is consistent with adenocarcinoma. His metastatic workup is negative. A CEA level is obtained and is fourfold greater than normal. Which of the following is the appropriate use of this test?

a. As an indication for neoadjuvant chemotherapy
b. As an indication for postoperative radiation therapy
c. As an indication for preoperative PET scanning
d. As an indication for a more aggressive sigmoid resection
e. As a baseline measurement prior to monitoring postoperatively for recurrence

Questions 235 to 237

For each stage in the patient's treatment, select the appropriate next step. Each lettered option may be used once, more than once, or not at all.

a. Left hemicolectomy
b. Right hemicolectomy
c. Subtotal colectomy
d. Total colectomy
e. Hepatic resection
f. External beam irradiation
g. 5-fluorouracil and leucovorin
h. External beam irradiation and chemotherapy
i. Abdominal MRI
j. No further treatment

235. A 65-year-old man presents to his primary care physician with complaints of intermittent constipation and is found to have microcytic anemia. Colonoscopy reveals a fungating mass in the proximal sigmoid colon with no other synchronous lesions. Biopsy of the mass confirms adenocarcinoma.

236. The patient undergoes surgery and recovers uneventfully. Pathology of the resected specimen is reported as T3, N1 with negative surgical margins.

237. At 6-month follow-up, an abdominal CT scan shows a 2-cm isolated lesion in the right lobe of the liver. Repeat colonoscopy shows no evidence of recurrent or metachronous lesions. Chest x-ray and bone scan are normal.

Questions 238 to 241

A 32-year-old man with diabetic nephropathy undergoes an uneventful renal transplant from his sister (two-haplotype match). His immunosuppressive regimen includes azathioprine, steroids, and cyclosporine. For each development in the postoperative period, select the most appropriate next step. Each lettered option may be used once, more than once, or not at all.

a. Begin gancyclovir
b. Administer steroid boost
c. Withhold steroids
d. Decrease cyclosporine
e. Increase cyclosporine
f. Decrease azathioprine
g. Obtain renal ultrasound
h. Begin broad-spectrum antibiotics
i. Administer filgrastim (Neupogen)
j. Administer FK50

238. On postoperative day 3 the patient is doing well, but you notice on his routine laboratory tests that his white blood cell count is 2.0.

239. The patient's WBC count gradually returns to normal, but on postoperative day 7 he develops a fever of 39.4°C (103°F) and a nonproductive cough. A chest x-ray reveals diffuse interstitial infiltrates, and a buffy coat is positive for viral inclusions.

240. The patient recovers from this illness and is discharged home on postoperative day 18. At 3-month follow-up he is doing well, but you notice that his creatinine is 2.8 mg/dL. He has no fever, his graft is not tender, and his renal ultrasound is normal.

241. Six months following his transplant, the patient begins to develop fever, malaise, and pain of the right lower quadrant. On palpation, the graft is tender. Chest x-ray and urine and blood cultures are normal. Renal ultrasound shows an edematous graft.

Transplants, Immunology, and Oncology

Answers

192. The answer is c. (*Greenfield, pp 139-140.*) TNF is a peptide hormone produced by endotoxin-activated monocytes/macrophages and has been postulated to be the principal cytokine mediator in gram-negative shock and sepsis-related organ damage. Biologic actions of TNF include polymorphonuclear neutrophil (PMN) activation and degranulation; increased nonspecific host resistance; increased vascular permeability; lymphopenia; promotion of interleukins 1, 2, and 6; capillary leak syndrome; microvascular thrombosis; anorexia and cachexia; and numerous other protective and adverse effects in sepsis. Its role in sepsis provides a fertile field for research in critical care.

193. The answer is e. (*Brunicardi, pp 320-322.*) Chronic rejection is a late complication that manifests months to years after transplantation and is characterized by a paucity of bile ducts on biopsy due to immune-mediated injury to the biliary epithelium—the "vanishing bile duct syndrome." Treatment options are limited, and the best option for treatment is retransplantation. Portal venous thrombosis that occurs early after transplantation should be treated with exploratory laparotomy and thrombectomy, but late portal venous thrombosis does not necessitate operative intervention due to the formation of collaterals. Hepatic arterial thrombosis (HAT), when detected early, should be treated with reexploration and thrombectomy with revision of the anastomosis. A late sequela of HAT is biliary strictures secondary to ischemia.

194. The answer is b. (*Greenfield, pp 557-558.*) The purpose of a cross-match is to determine whether the recipient has circulating antibodies against donor HLA antigens. Such antibodies do not occur naturally, but rather are the result of prior sensitization during pregnancy, blood transfusions, or previous transplantation. A complement-dependent lymphocytotoxicity cross-match is performed by adding recipient serum and complement to donor cells (T cells,

B cells, or monocytes). If specific antidonor antibodies are present, antibody binding results in complement fixation and cell lysis. This is detected by addition of a vital dye, which is taken up by the damaged cell membrane, resulting in a positive cross-match. If a positive cross-match is detected to donor T cells (HLA class I), transplantation will result in hyperacute rejection.

195. The answer is b. (*Greenfield, p 545.*) The patient is manifesting symptoms of tumor lysis syndrome, which is mediated by cytotoxic T cells. Hyperkalemia and hyperphosphatemia are a result of tumor cell lysis, and hypocalcemia is a result of precipitation of phosphate and calcium. Unlike the granulocyte line, T lymphocytes express the T-cell receptor. This receptor imparts antigen specificity to T cells. The helper T cell, when stimulated by interleukin 1 and antigens, produces various lymphokines that ultimately produce effector cells. One of these effector cells is the cytotoxic T cell, which kills cells that express specific antigens, including viral, tumor, and nonbiologic antigens. Macrophages and natural killer cells have some tumoricidal activity; however, this is not specific for tumors.

196. The answer is d. (*Greenfield, pp 552-553.*) Cyclosporine is a highly effective immunosuppressive agent produced by fungi. It is more specific than the anti-inflammatory agents such as steroids or the antiproliferative agents such as azathioprine. The effectiveness of cyclosporine in preventing allograft rejection is related to its ability to inhibit interleukin 2 production. Without interleukin 2 from helper T cells, there is no clonal expansion of alloantigen-directed cytotoxic T cells and no stimulation of antibody production by B cells.

197. The answer is c. (*Townsend, pp 692-693.*) Hemodialysis, rather than management by dietary manipulation alone, should be considered for patients with Stage 5 kidney disease defined as an estimated glomerular filtration rate of less than 15 mL/min/1.73 m^2 or earlier in patients with complications due to renal failure according to National Kidney Foundation guidelines. These complications include hyperkalemia, congestive heart failure, peripheral neuropathy, severe hypertension, pericarditis, bleeding, and severe anemia. The uremic hyperkalemic patient in congestive heart failure may require emergency dialysis in addition to the standard conservative measures, which include (1) limitation of protein intake to less than 60 g/day and restriction of fluid intake and (2) reduction of elevated serum potassium levels by insulin-glucose or sodium polystyrene sulfonate (Kayexalate) enema treatment. Arteriovenous fistulas require several weeks to months to develop adequate size and flow. While awaiting maturation, temporary dialysis can be satis-factorily performed using a catheter placed in a central vein. Renal biopsy would be performed in an attempt to obtain a diagnosis of the underlying renal disease. Patients who are acceptable candidates for kidney transplan-tation usually should undergo this form of treatment, after they are stabilized, rather than chronic hemodialysis, the mortality for which is now higher than for transplantation. Despite adequate dialysis, problems of neuropathy, bone disease, anemia, and hypertension remain difficult to manage. Compared with chronic dialysis, transplantation restores more patients to happier and more productive lives.

198. The answer is a. (*Townsend, pp 693-694.*) A positive cross-match means that the recipient has circulating antibodies that are cytotoxic to donor-strain lymphocytes. This incompatibility, which almost always leads to an acute humoral rejection of the graft, precludes transplantation. Blood type matching prior to organ allograft is similar to cross-matching prior to trans-fusion; O is the universal donor and AB the universal recipient. Minor blood group factors do not appear to act as histocompatibility antigens. Matching of HLA antigens in cadaveric renal transplants may improve graft survival, but the impact is relatively minor. While attempts are made to pair recipient and donor by tissue typing, a two-antigen match is perfectly acceptable and even zero-antigen matches can be transplanted with good results. Neither hypertension nor anemia is a contraindication to transplantation; indeed, hypertension may be cured or ameliorated following successful transplantation. Patients with end-stage renal failure generally are anemic and can be transfused, if necessary, intraoperatively or postoperatively. Anemia generally also improves following transplantation because of increased erythropoietin production by the graft.

199. The answer is c. (*Townsend, p 713.*) Hyperacute rejection occurs within minutes after transplantation and is mediated primarily by preformed antibody. It usually occurs during surgery after the clamps are released from the vascular anastomosis and the recipient's antibodies are exposed to the donor's passenger lymphocytes and kidney tissue. Typically, the kidney will become swollen and bluish. Intraoperative biopsies of the transplanted kidney should be performed to evaluate for signs of hyperacute rejection such as extensive intravascular deposits of fibrin and platelets and intraglomerular accumulation of polymorphonuclear leukocytes, fibrin, platelets, and red blood cells. The intravascular coagulation rarely results in a systemic coagulopathy.

Careful cross-matching can test for cytotoxic antibodies and prevent hyper-acute rejections. Hyperacute rejection is refractory to immunosuppressive or anticoagulant therapy and inevitably leads to rapid destruction of the transplanted kidney.

200. The answer is a. (*Greenfield, pp 557-558.*) Cardiac transplantation is a treatment modality for selected patients with end-stage cardiac failure. Allograft survivals are approximately 80% at 1 year, while survival is about 96% at 1 year for renal cadaveric grafts. Although kidneys can be safely preserved by either hypothermic storage or hypothermic perfusion for periods up to 48 hours, donor hearts protected by simple hypothermia should be transplanted within 4 hours. Increased ischemic time is a significant predictor of poor outcome in heart transplant recipients. For this reason the usual tissue-typing procedures used in kidney transplantation are impractical in cardiac transplantation, and indeed there is no correlation between match and outcome. In pairing donor and recipient for heart transplants, there must be at least ABO blood group compatibility. Cyclosporine has improved results in both cardiac and renal transplantation despite its major drawback of dose-related nephrotoxicity. Eligibility for cardiac transplantation has evolved from strict age criteria to more flexible guidelines based on a patient's likelihood of surviving and resuming a normally functional life after transplantation. Many centers, however, observe age 65 as the upper limit for transplantation. The leading causes of death in patients surviving more than 1 year after transplantation are infection and rejection.

201. The answer is d. (*Greenfield, pp 547-548.*) The patient is experiencing an acute rejection episode. Acute rejection typically occurs between 1 week and 3 months posttransplantation and is characterized by an increasing creatinine, decreased urine output, and possible fevers or tenderness over the graft. Diagnosis is confirmed with a biopsy of the graft, and treatment includes high-dose steroids and an anti-T-cell antibody (eg, OKT3, which is a murine monoclonal antibody to the human CD3 complex).

202. The answer is b. (*Greenfield, pp 556-557.*) The most common posttransplantation viral infections are DNA viruses of the herpesvirus family and include cytomegalovirus (CMV), Epstein-Barr virus (EBV), herpes simplex virus, and varicella zoster virus. CMV infections may occur as either primary or reactive infections and have a peak incidence at about 6 weeks after transplant. The classic signs include fever, malaise, myalgia, arthralgia, and leukopenia. CMV infection can affect several organ systems and result in pneumonitis; ulceration and hemorrhage in the stomach, duodenum, or colon; hepatitis; esophagitis; retinitis; encephalitis; or pancreatitis. The risk of developing posttransplant CMV depends on donor-recipient serology, with the greatest risk in seronegative patients who receive organs from seropositive donors. Pyelonephritis, cholecystitis, intra-abdominal abscesses, and parotitis are caused by bacterial infections or GI perforation and not primarily by CMV infection.

203. The answer is b. (*Townsend, pp 707-708.*) The MELD score is a statistical model employed for adult patients that has been shown to have a high predictive capacity in identifying patients with end-stage liver disease at greatest risk of mortality within 3 months. The MELD score was part of a new system put into place by the United Network for Organ Sharing for liver allocation which did not suffer from emphasis on waiting time and subjective clinical parameters (degree of ascites or encephalopathy). The MELD score enables liver allocation to be based on objective variables: total bilirubin, international normalized ratio, and creatinine.

204. The answer is d. (*Greenfield, p 557.*) Donor-type lymphoid cells transplanted within a graft may recognize the host's tissue as foreign and mount an immune response against the host. This response, termed GVHD, is common in bone marrow transplantation and is an important source of morbidity and mortality. Treatment requires more aggressive immunosuppression. Current clinical practice includes depletion of lymphocytes from the marrow graft in order to prevent the development of GVHD. GVHD has been documented following liver transplantation, presumably because of the large amount of lymphoid tissue in the donor liver. GVHD has not been described following heart, lung, pancreas, or kidney transplantation.

205. The answer is d. (*Greenfield, pp 621-630.*) Many causes of end-stage lung disease have been appropriately treated with lung transplantation. Whether one lung or both lungs are replaced at the time of transplantation depends on recipient factors. Patients with restrictive processes such as primary pulmonary fibrosis do well with a single lung transplant. For patients with primary pulmonary hypertension, unloading of the right ventricle with single lung transplantation has been adequate, and replacement of both lungs has not been necessary in most cases. Cystic fibrosis patients do well after lung transplantation, but double lung transplant is frequently necessary because of chronic infections. Secondary pulmonary hypertension is due to left ventricular failure with concomitant increases in pulmonary pressures secondary to increases in left ventricular end-diastolic pressures. Reactive secondary pulmonary hypertension is best treated with heart transplantation. Long-standing secondary pulmonary hypertension that is chiefly fixed is best treated with combined heart-lung transplantation.

206. The answer is a. (*Greenfield, pp 631-632.*) Whole-organ pancreas transplantation is the only therapy for type I insulin-dependent diabetes that maintains normal serum glucose levels and normal glucose tolerance tests. When the pancreas is transplanted along with a kidney, the tight glucose control generally prevents the recurrence of diabetic nephropathy. No series has shown the reversal of diabetic retinopathy or reduction in the rate of diabetic ulcers or of amputations, although some parameters of diabetic retinopathy may improve after pancreas transplantation.

207. The answer is a. (*Brunicardi, pp 316-318.*) Specific exclusion criteria for liver transplantation are not formally established. Some of the more common contraindications to liver transplantation are ongoing or recent substance abuse, presence of active sepsis, current extrahepatic malignancy, poor cardiac or pulmonary function, and patients with hepatocellular carcinoma with metastatic disease, obvious vascular invasion, or significant tumor burden. Patients with hepatocellular carcinoma who would not tolerate resection because of portal hypertension and uncompensated liver disease can be successfully treated with liver transplantation. The best candidates are patients with a single lesion less than 5 cm in size or no more than three lesions, none of which are greater than 3 cm in size. The presence of hepatorenal syndrome is an indication, not a contraindication, to liver transplantation. Presence of an extrahepatic malignancy should defer transplantation for 2 years after curative therapy for their malignancy.

208. The answer is d. (*Brunicardi, p 302.*) OKT3 is a monoclonal antibody against the CD3 antigen complex on mature T cells. In addition to minor side effects such as fevers and headaches that result from cytokine release after OKT3 administration, severe complications may occur such as noncardiogenic pulmonary edema, encephalopathy, aseptic meningitis, and nephrotoxicity. OKT3 administration results in clearance of T cells from the circulation, and thus drug efficacy can be measured by assessing the percentage of CD3 positive cells in the blood. OKT3 can be used as the primary treatment or second-line therapy for acute rejection, rejection prophylaxis, and induction therapy.

209. The answer is b. (*Brunicardi, p 1538.*) In following patients with nonseminomatous testicular tumors, elevated serum levels of the β subunit of human chorionic gonadotropin (hCG), alpha fetoprotein (AFP), and lactate dehydrogenase have been found to be useful indicators of tumor activity or recurrence. PSA has been utilized in screening for prostate cancer, although its role is controversial. CA125 has been used to follow ovarian cancers; it is fairly nonspecific but can alert the physician to the need for a more aggressive search for persistent disease when relative increases are noted in a patient after therapy. The p53 oncogenes have been found in soft tissue sarcomas, osteogenic sarcomas, and colon cancers; they have no role in the detection of recurrence.

210. The answer is a. (*Brunicardi, pp 530-531.*) Isolated enlarged cervical lymph nodes in adults are malignant nearly 80% of the time (excluding benign tumors of the thyroid gland). They are usually metastatic squamous cell carcinomas arising from primary sources above the clavicles in the aerodigestive tract. Fine-needle aspiration cytology is commonly used to obtain histologic confirmation of suspected cancer. Aspiration cytology can usually diagnose carcinoma accurately, but lymphoma may be difficult to identify by this method, and open biopsy is often necessary. Bone marrow biopsy is not indicated prior to lymph node biopsy. It is done as part of the staging process after a diagnosis of lymphoma has been made. Endoscopy and scanning of the oropharynx and nasopharynx are part of the diagnostic workup of a suspected malignant cervical lymph node, but do not provide histologic proof of cancer.

211. The answer is e. (*Brunicardi, pp 269-271.*) The management of malignant tumors may be guided by knowledge obtained by grading and staging the tumors. Histologic grading reflects the degree of anaplasia of tumor cells. Tumors in which histologic grading seems to have prognostic value include soft tissue sarcoma, transitional cell cancers of the bladder, astrocytoma, and chondrosarcoma. Grading has been of little predictive value in melanoma, hepatocellular carcinoma, or osteosarcoma. Staging is based on the extent of spread rather than histologic appearance and is more relevant in predicting the course of lung and colorectal cancers.

212. The answer is e. (*Brunicardi, pp 1508-1510.*) Wilms tumor is the most common abdominal malignancy of childhood, but represents only about 10% of childhood malignant tumors. This is a nephroblastoma (Wilms tumor) adherent to the left kidney. These tumors are associated with aniridia (rarely) and with hemihypertrophy, cryptorchidism, or hypospadias in about 10% of cases. Most patients present with an asymptomatic mass found by a parent. Less than one-third of patients experience hematuria. As would be expected in over half such cases, this child is hypertensive, probably due to compression of the renal artery by the mass. Surgical treatment consists of resection of the kidney and ureter. Chemotherapy is indicated in patients with malignancy confined to one kidney, and chemoradiation is indicated after surgical excision for more advanced disease. Cure rates exceeding 80% are achieved in patients with hematogenous metastases. CT scan is used to assess the tumor characteristics and evaluate for metastases. Ultrasonography is utilized to assess for vascular invasion into the renal vein or vena cava.

213. The answer is a. (*Brunicardi, pp 1423-1425.*) Most medullary thyroid carcinomas (MTC) occur sporadically. However, approximately 25% occur in inherited syndromes such as familial medullary thyroid cancer and MEN type 2A and type 2B. These syndromes result secondary to germline mutations in the RET proto-oncogene. MEN 2A consists of medullary thyroid cancer, pheochromocytomas or adrenal medullary hyperplasia, and primary hyperparathyroidism. MEN 2B consists MTC, pheochromocytoma, mucosal neuromas, gangliomas, and a Marfanlike habitus. These patients may develop medullary carcinoma at a very young age, and any patient with MEN 2A or MEN 2B should be assumed to have medullary cancer until proved otherwise. Patients are followed carefully for pheochromocytoma with urine VMA, for hyperparathyroidism with serum calcium, and for medullary carcinoma with serum calcitonin. However, as some patients have a normal basal calcitonin, a pentagastrin or provocative calcium infusion test should be performed in these high-risk patients. Patients thought to have MEN 1 syndrome (pituitary, parathyroid, and pancreatic tumors) or Zollinger-Ellison syndrome should be assayed for serum gastrin, insulin, glucagon, and somatostatin. These assays may prove to be inappropriately high in MEN 1 syndrome due to pancreatic islet cell tumors.

214. The answer is c. (*Brunicardi, pp 1671-1673.*) Benign soft tissue tumors far outnumber their malignant counterparts. Because of this, prolonged delays are common before definitive treatment of soft tissue sarcomas is instituted. Risk for malignancy is increased for tumors greater than 5 cm in largest diameter, as well as for those lesions that are symptomatic or that have enlarged rapidly over a short period of time. Properly performed biopsy is critical in the initial treatment of any soft tissue mass. Improperly performed biopsies can complicate the care of the sarcoma patient and, in rare circumstances, even eliminate certain surgical options. Excisional biopsies should be reserved for small masses for which complete excision would not jeopardize subsequent treatment should a sarcoma be found. For all other masses, incisional biopsy should be performed. The incision should be placed directly over the mass and should be oriented along the long axis of the extremity.

215. The answer is e. (*Gobbi, pp 2528-2536; Tondini, pp 831-837.*) The stomach is the most common site in the GI tract for non-Hodgkin lymphoma, followed by the small intestine and the colon. Lymphomas constitute 3% of all malignant gastric tumors. Ninety percent of these lymphomas are of the non-Hodgkin type. Surgery alone can be considered adequate treatment for patients with non-Hodgkin lymphoma that does not infiltrate beyond the submucosa. However, gastric resection is not considered mandatory, and there are no substantial differences in response to therapy and survival when resection is compared with combined chemotherapy and radiation therapy, including in advanced cases. Moreover, chemotherapy and radiation therapy have been shown to be effective even in unresected bulky cases, and provide minimal risk of hemorrhage and perforation even in this setting.

216. The answer is d. (*Greenfield, pp 651-653.*) Acinar, adenoid cystic, and low grades of mucoepidermoid carcinomas exhibit moderately malignant behavior. Undifferentiated, squamous, and high grades of mucoepidermoid carcinomas are considered highly malignant tumors. Regional node dissection is indicated for malignant tumors because of the high (up to 50%) incidence of occult regional metastases. Facial nerve preservation should be attempted when the margins are adequate and the tumor is well localized. The minimal appropriate procedure for parotid carcinoma is a superficial parotidectomy with nerve preservation. The nerve must be partially or totally sacrificed if the tumor directly involves the nerve trunk or its branches.

217. The answer is b. (*Brunicardi, pp 276-281.*) A surgeon is frequently asked to evaluate patients who are receiving systemic chemotherapy. Most complications of chemotherapy do not require surgical therapy. Perirectal abscesses are more common in these immunosuppressed patients. GI bleeding occurs secondary to mucosal irritation and thrombocytopenia. Pancreatitis is uncommon, but is associated with L-asparaginase use. Up to 20% of patients treated with floxuridine by continuous hepatic artery infusion develop some degree of inflammation and obstruction of the bile duct. Systemic chemotherapy does not increase the likelihood of acute cholecystitis, appendicitis, incarcerated femoral hernia, or diverticulitis.

218. The answer is e. (*Greenfield, pp 2091-2093.*) After radical orchiectomy, lymph node dissection is indicated in embryonal carcinoma, teratocarcinoma, and adult teratoma if there is no supradiaphragmatic spread. This dissection increases the 5-year survival and helps in staging. Seminoma is extremely radiosensitive, and lymph node dissection is unnecessary. Choriocarcinoma are frequently associated with pulmonary metastases and are treated with chemotherapy. Orchiectomy for a testicular mass is approached via an inguinal incision in order to perform a high ligation of the cord and to eliminate spread of the tumor. Cryptorchidism (undescended testicle) is associated with decreased spermatogenesis and carries a lifelong risk of malignant degeneration even after being surgically corrected.

219. The answer is e. (*Brunicardi, p 306.*) Kidney transplant is the treatment of choice for patients with end-stage renal disease. It offers the patients a chance to lead healthy, normal lives. Compared with dialysis, it is associated with better patient survival, improved quality of life, and decreased longterm costs. Dialysis is less expensive than renal transplantation if the graft functions for less than 2 years. Renal transplantation requires lifelong immunosuppression which has its associated risks.

220. The answer is e. (*Brunicardi, p 1460.*) Pheochromocytoma is associated with MEN IIA, MEN IIB, von Hippel-Lindau disease, and neurofibromatosis I. Hereditary pheochromocytomas are more likely to be multiple and bilateral.

221. The answer is e. (*Brunicardi, pp 1088-1089.*) In an average-risk patient, colorectal cancer screening according to the American Cancer Society should begin at age 50 and then an annual fecal occult blood test *or* flexible sigmoidoscopy every 5 years *or* air contrast barium enema (which has a sensitivity of 90% for polyps >1 cm in size) every 5 years or colonoscopy every 10 years is recommended. If an adenomatous polyp is detected, then colonoscopy is recommended every 3 years. If no polyps are detected subsequently, colonoscopy can be performed every 5 years. If more than five polyps are detected, colonoscopy should occur annually. For patients with HNPCC, screening should begin either between the ages of 20 and 25 or 10 years earlier than the youngest family member with colorectal cancer, whichever comes earlier.

222. The answer is b. *(Brunicardi, pp 285-286.)* Only about 30% of the biologic damage from x-rays is due to the direct effects on the target molecule. The remainder is due to an indirect action mediated by free radicals and can be modified by free radical scavengers such as sulfhydryl. The percentage of cells killed by a given dose of x-rays or gamma rays is greatly increased by molecular oxygen; cells deficient in oxygen are resistant to radiation. Among the basic principles of radiation biology is the observation that the sensitivity of mammalian cells to radiation varies with their position in the cell division cycle. M-phase (mitotic phase) cells are the most radiosensitive. Radiation is frequently employed for local control of disease. Overall and disease-free survival rates for breast lumpectomy and radiation are equivalent to those for mastectomy, in patients with Stage I and II breast cancers. Rapidly dividing cells of the GI mucosa and bone marrow are particularly sensitive to the effects of radiation.

223. The answer is c. *(Heys, pp 614-623.)* Malignant tumors require energy substrates to grow and ordinarily claim these substrates from the host. In animal studies, withholding dietary proteins diminishes the rate of tumor growth. There is no evidence in the human to suggest acceleration of tumor growth when nutritional support is provided. There is also no evidence that nutritional therapy improves the response of the tumor to therapy. For nearly a century, the association of stomach cancer and diet has been recognized. Among the wide variety of substances incriminated are nitrates and nitrosamides in food and drinking water. There is evidence that regular ingestion of vitamin C from childhood may reduce the forma-tion of carcinogens, though reduction in the incidence of cancer has not been demonstrated. Excess amounts of dietary fat and deficiency of fiber have been clearly associated with colon cancer. Animal fats have also been associated with cancer of the exocrine pancreas, the prostate, and the endometrium. Alcohol consumption, especially when combined with cigarette smoking, increases the incidence of esophageal cancer. Con-sumption of alcohol also increases the incidence of pancreatitis, but not pancreatic cancer.

224. The answer is d. (*Greenfield, pp 581-586, 610-620.*) Cardiac allograft has become an accepted treatment for end-stage heart disease. One-year cardiac allograft survival exceeds 80%, which is comparable to renal allograft survival. Cardiac allografts have a cold ischemia preservation time of 4 to 5 hours, and therefore tissue typing is not practical. Cardiac donors are matched to recipients only by size and ABO blood type. Tissue typing remains an important component of cadaveric kidney allograft matching. The mainstay of immunosuppression for both cardiac and renal allografts continues to include calcineurin inhibitors (FK506, cyclosporine), steroids, and antimitotic agents (azathioprine, mycophenolate mofetil).

225. The answer is b. (*Greenfield, pp 971-972, 1386-1391, 2052.*) Resection of metastases of lung, liver, and brain can result in occasional 5-year cures. In general, surgery should be undertaken only when the primary tumor is controlled, diffuse metastatic disease has been ruled out, and the affected patient's condition and the location of the metastasis permit safe resection. The best results have come from resection of pulmonary metastases, in which 5-year survival rates exceed those for resection for primary bronchogenic carcinoma. For example, resection of pulmonary metastases in patients with osteogenic sarcoma can have survival rates up to 25% to 35%.

226. The answer is c. (*Rhame, pp 141-152; Wilson, pp 193-201.*) The risk of contracting HIV is much less than the risk of contracting hepatitis B from a patient. Although the risk of transmission of HIV in the health care setting is very low, there are reported cases of seroconversion after parenteral exposure. Particular precautions should be taken in operating on patients who are known to be seropositive for HIV or who have known risk factors. Recommendations include elimination of inexperienced personnel or personnel with open lesions on body surfaces from the operating room. Disposable gowns, drapes, masks, and eye shields should be used. Contaminated clothing should be soaked in a dilute solution (1:10) of chlorine bleach prior to washing. Double gloving does not reduce the major intraoperative risk of needle puncture, which is the primary source of risk to the operating team. Needles should never be capped; an uncapped needle is less dangerous than are the maneuvers to recap needles.

227. The answer is c. (*Brunicardi, pp 267-268.*) Risk factors for breast cancer include family history, breast cancer, and exposure to estrogen (nulliparity, previous, early menarche, and late menopause). A late age at first birth (after age 30) increases the risk of breast cancer compared with early parity (age 18 or earlier). Having one first-degree relative (mother, sister, or daughter) with breast cancer also increases the risk. Women of the upper social classes, as measured by either education or income, have been found to have the highest incidence of breast cancer. Neither cigarette smoking nor the use of hair dye has been correlated with breast cancer.

228. The answer is c. (*Brunicardi, pp 260-265.*) Li-Fraumeni syndrome is associated most commonly with a mutation in the p53 tumor suppressor gene. Li-Fraumeni syndrome in an individual is based on (1) bone or soft tissue sarcoma in that person before the age of 45, (2) a first-degree relative with cancer before the age of 45, and (3) a first- or second-degree relative with sarcoma at any age or any cancer before the age of 45. The APC gene is associated with familial adenomatous polyposis (FAP). The RET protooncogene is associated with MEN 2. The PTEN tumor suppressor gene is associated with Cowden disease, or multiple hamartoma syndrome. The p16 tumor suppressor gene is associated with hereditary malignant melanoma.

229. The answer is a. (*Brunicardi, pp 276-281.*) Doxorubicin, an antibiotic derived from *Streptomyces* species, has activity against sarcomas and carcinomas of the breast, liver, bladder, prostate, head and neck, esophagus, and lung. Its major side effect is production of a dilated cardiomyopathy. Patients receiving this agent should have an echocardiogram before and after treatment in order to monitor potential cardiac toxicity.

230. The answer is e. (*Brunicardi, pp 262-263.*) Both *BRCA1* and *BRCA2* are associated with an increased risk of ovarian cancer by age 70% to 44% and 27%, respectively. Approximately 10% of women under the age of 40 who develop breast cancer have a mutation in *BRCA1* or *2*. *BRCA1* is associated with an increased risk of colon cancer and prostate cancer in males. *BRCA2* is associated with an increased risk of gallbladder, bile duct, and pancreatic cancers as well as gastric cancer, malignant melanoma, and in men, prostate cancer. *BRCA1* breast cancers are more likely to be estrogen receptor–negative, and *BRCA2* breast cancers are more likely to be estrogen receptor–positive.

231. The answer is e. (*Brunicardi, pp 277-281.*) Cyclophosphamide is an alkylating agent used in the treatment of a variety of solid tumors. Its major side effect is hemorrhagic cystitis. Bleomycin can cause pulmonary fibrosis. Vincristine is an alkaloid that can cause peripheral and central neuropathies. Cisplatin is an alkylating agent that can lead to ototoxicity, neurotoxicity, and nephrotoxicity. 5-Fluorouracil is an antimetabolite that can cause mucositis, dermatitis, and cerebellar dysfunction.

232. The answer is d. *(Townsend, pp 675-676.)* Posttransplant lymphoproliferative disorders (PTLD) are associated with the EBV. PTLD has a range of clinical presentations, and treatment can include multiple modalities including withdrawal of immunosuppression, antiviral therapy with ganciclovir, chemotherapy, or immunotherapy with monoclonal antibodies. Other common posttransplantation malignancies include hepatocellular carcinomas, which are associated with hepatitis B and C; Kaposi sarcoma, which is associated with human herpesvirus 8; and cervical cancers, which are associated with human papillomavirus. Although CMV infection can occur when CMV-seronegative recipients receive an organ from a CMV-seropositive donor, CMV does not predispose transplantation patients to malignancy.

233. The answer is d. *(Brunicardi, pp 1447-1448.)* The patient has tertiary hyperparathyroidism, which is manifested by persistent hypercalcemia secondary to autonomous parathyroid function after renal transplantation. Treatment is total parathyroidectomy with autotransplantation or subtotal parathyroidectomy. The imaging modalities described would be more appropriate in the workup of primary hyperparathyroidism—24-hour urinary calcium levels are low in familial hypercalciuric hypercalcemia. Ultrasound, sestamibi scintigraphy, and CT scanning are all modalities that can be utilized to identify a parathyroid adenoma preoperatively.

234. The answer is e. *(Brunicardi, p 273.)* CEA is a glycoprotein that is present in early embryonic and fetal cells (an oncofetal antigen) and in colon cancer. It is not found in normal colon mucosa. It is not tumor-specific and may be elevated in a variety of benign and malignant conditions, including cirrhosis, ulcerative colitis, renal failure, pancreatitis, pancreatic cancer, stomach cancer, breast cancer, and lung cancer. However, the CEA assay is a sensitive serologic tool for identifying recurrent disease. In about two-thirds of patients with recurrent disease, an increased CEA level is the first indicator of tumor reappearance. A rising CEA following colon cancer surgery, in the absence of other conditions associated with an elevated CEA, predicts the appearance of liver metastases within 1 year with an accuracy approaching 70%. Although an elevated CEA level preoperatively predicts a higher risk of recurrence, the use of preoperative CEA levels as an indication for postoperative adjuvant chemotherapy is controversial and currently not supported by clinical practice guidelines.

235 to 237. The answers are 235-a, 236-g, 237-e. *(Brunicardi, pp 1090-1092.)* In order to resect the tumor with an adequate margin (traditionally 5 cm) on its proximal and distal ends and remove the draining lymph node basin, a left hemicolectomy should be performed. Patients with lymph node involvement are at significant risk for both local and distant recurrence, and adjuvant chemotherapy is routinely recommended in these patients. The liver is the most common site of bloodborne metastases from primary colorectal cancers. If the liver is the only site of metastasis and the lesion is able to be resected with clear margins then survival is improved with hepatic resection.

238 to 241. The answers are 238-f, 239-a, 240-d, 241-b *(Greenfield, pp 552-557, 587.)* Routine postoperative immunosuppression for a renal transplant recipient includes cyclosporine, azathioprine, and steroids. Cyclosporine is nephrotoxic and is frequently withheld in the postoperative period until the creatinine returns to normal following transplantation. Azathioprine has bone marrow toxicity as its major side effect, and both WBC and platelet counts need to be monitored in the immediate posttransplant period. The patient's decrease in WBCs is secondary to azathioprine toxicity, and the most appropriate step is to decrease the dose of azathioprine. Viral infections are a serious cause of morbidity following transplantation. A buffy coat is the supernatant of a centrifuged blood sample that contains the WBCs. Viral cultures from this supernatant as well as localization of inclusion bodies can identify transplant patients infected with CMV. This patient has CMV pneumonitis and needs to be treated with high-dose gancyclovir.

An elevation in creatinine at 3-month follow-up can be secondary to rejection, anastomotic problems, urologic complications, infection, or nephrotoxicity of various medications. With a normal ultrasound, no fever, and no graft tenderness, the most likely cause is cyclosporine-induced nephrotoxicity and the most appropriate step is a reduction in the cyclosporine dose. Finally, at 6 months with graft tenderness, fever, and an edematous kidney on ultrasound, rejection must be suspected. Negative cultures make infection unlikely, and a steroid boost is appropriate. Addition of monoclonal antibodies to CD3 (OKT3) or pooled antibodies against lymphocytes (ALGs) is also appropriate in the treatment of a first rejection.

Endocrine Problems and the Breast

Questions

242. A patient with mild skin pigmentation is admitted emergently to your service because of sudden abdominal pain, fever, and a rigid abdomen. Her blood work indicates a marked leukocytosis, a blood sugar of 55 mg/dL, a sodium value of 119 mEq/dL, and a potassium value of 6.2 mEq/dL. Her blood pressure is 88/58 mm Hg. She undergoes an exploratory laparotomy. Which of the following is the definitive treatment for her primary condition?

a. 10% dextrose infusion
b. Bicarbonate
c. Hypertonic saline
d. Corticosteroids
e. Vasopressors

243. A 45-year-old woman complains to her primary care physician of nervousness, sweating, tremulousness, and weight loss. The thyroid scan shown here exhibits a pattern that is most consistent with which of the following disorders?

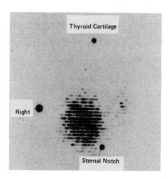

a. Hypersecreting adenoma
b. Graves disease
c. Lateral aberrant thyroid
d. Papillary carcinoma of thyroid
e. Medullary carcinoma of thyroid

244. A 35-year-old woman with a history of previous right thyroidectomy for a benign thyroid nodule now undergoes completion thyroidectomy for a suspicious thyroid mass. Several hours postoperatively, she develops progressive swelling under the incision, stridor, and difficulty breathing. Orotracheal intubation is successful. Which of the following is the most appropriate next step?

a. Fiberoptic laryngoscopy to rule out bilateral vocal cord paralysis
b. Administration of intravenous calcium
c. Administration of broad-spectrum antibiotics and debridement of the wound
d. Wound exploration
e. Administration of high-dose steroids and antihistamines

245. A 62-year-old woman presents with invasive ductal adenocarcinoma of the breast. Which of the following findings would still allow her to receive breast conservation therapy?

a. Diffuse suspicious microcalcifications throughout the breast
b. Multifocal disease in a single quadrant
c. Previous treatment of a breast cancer with lumpectomy and radiation
d. Two distinct tumors in two different quadrants of the breast
e. Persistently positive margins after multiple reexcisions of the breast cancer

246. A 29-year-old woman presents with a 6-month history of erythema and edema of the right breast with palpable axillary lymphadenopathy. A punch biopsy of the skin reveals neoplastic cells in the dermal lymphatics. Which of the following is the best next step in her management?

a. A course of nafcillin to treat the overlying cellulitis and then neoadjuvant chemotherapy for breast cancer
b. Modified radical mastectomy followed by adjuvant chemotherapy
c. Modified radical mastectomy followed by hormonal therapy
d. Combined modality chemotherapy and radiation therapy to the right breast with surgery reserved for residual disease
e. Combined modality therapy with chemotherapy, surgery, and radiation

247. A 15-year-old otherwise healthy female high school student begins to notice galactorrhea. A pregnancy test is negative. Which of the following is a frequently associated physical finding?

a. Gonadal atrophy
b. Bitemporal hemianopsia
c. Exophthalmos and lid lag
d. Episodic hypertension
e. Buffalo hump

248. A 52-year-old woman sees her physician with complaints of fatigue, headache, flank pain, hematuria, and abdominal pain. She undergoes a sestamibi scan that demonstrates persistent uptake in the right superior parathyroid gland at 2 hours. Which of the following laboratory values is most suggestive of her diagnosis?

a. Serum acid phosphatase above 120 IU/L
b. Serum alkaline phosphatase above 120 IU/L
c. Serum calcium above 11 mg/dL
d. Urinary calcium below 100 mg/day
e. Parathyroid hormone levels below 5 pmol/L

249. A 53-year-old woman with multiple endocrine neoplasia type I (MEN-1) syndrome presents with a dermatitic rash and is found to have an elevated fasting glucagon level. Which of the following statements is true regarding her need for further workup and treatment?

a. She should undergo visceral angiography as the initial test for localization of the lesion.
b. Localization of the lesion is typically difficult because of its small size.
c. Surgical treatment requires total pancreatectomy because there are usually multiple lesions.
d. Metastatic disease is rare.
e. Octreotide may be useful in the management of hyperglycemia in patients with unresectable disease.

250. A 49-year-old man has become irritable, his facies have changed to a round configuration, he is impotent, he has developed purplish lines on his flanks, and he is hypertensive. His workup includes a computed tomography (CT) scan that revealed a 3-cm right adrenal mass. Which of the following statements regarding his diagnosis and treatment is true?

a. Surgical intervention is indicated only for lesions greater than 6 cm in size.
b. Magnetic resonance imaging (MRI) and scintigraphic scans are not useful in distinguishing adenomas from carcinomas preoperatively.
c. Operative exploration of both adrenal glands is indicated.
d. Preoperative CT-guided biopsy of the adrenal lesion should be performed.
e. Steroid replacement therapy may be required for up to 6 to 12 months postoperatively.

251. A 40-year-old woman is found to have a 1- to 2-cm, slightly tender cystic mass in her breast; she has no perceptible axillary adenopathy. Which of the following represents the best management option?

a. Reassurance and reexamination in the immediate postmenstrual period
b. Immediate excisional biopsy
c. Aspiration of the mass with cytologic analysis
d. Fluoroscopically guided needle localization biopsy
e. Mammography and reevaluation of options with new information

252. A 62-year-old Polynesian woman, who grew up in the South Pacific in the 1950s, has a lump in her neck. Which of the following statements concerning radiation-induced thyroid cancer is true?

a. It usually follows high-dose radiation to the head and neck.
b. A patient with a history of radiation is safe if no cancer has been found 20 years after exposure.
c. Approximately 25% of patients with a thyroid nodule and a history of head and neck irradiation develop thyroid cancer.
d. Most radiation-induced thyroid cancers are follicular.
e. The treatment of choice is a near-total (or total) thyroidectomy.

253. A 55-year-old woman presents with a 6-cm right thyroid mass and palpable cervical lymphadenopathy. Fine-needle aspiration (FNA) of one of the lymph nodes demonstrates the presence of calcified clumps of sloughed cells. Which of the following best describes the management of this thyroid disorder?

a. The patient should be screened for pancreatic endocrine neoplasms and hypercalcemia.
b. The patient should undergo total thyroidectomy with modified radical neck dissection.
c. The patient should undergo total thyroidectomy with frozen section intraoperatively, with modified radical neck dissection reserved for patients with extracapsular invasion.
d. The patient should undergo right thyroid lobectomy followed by iodine 131 (^{131}I) therapy.
e. The patient should undergo right thyroid lobectomy.

254. A 45-year-old woman is found to have lobular carcinoma in situ (LCIS) on a breast biopsy. Regarding counseling for her risk for invasive breast cancer, which of the following statements is true?

a. The most common type of invasive carcinoma after a diagnosis of LCIS is lobular carcinoma.
b. Her risk of invasive carcinoma is greatest within 10 years after a diagnosis of LCIS, after which time the risk becomes minimal.
c. Her risk of invasive carcinoma is equivalent in both breasts.
d. Her risk of invasive carcinoma is significantly increased if a large focus of LCIS is present in the biopsy specimen.
e. Early menarche and late menopause are associated with increased relative risks for breast cancer when compared to LCIS.

255. A 14-year-old black girl has her right breast removed because of a large mass. The tumor weighs 1400 g and has a bulging, very firm, lobulated surface with a whorl-like pattern, as illustrated here. Which of the following is the most likely diagnosis?

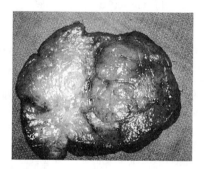

a. Cystosarcoma phyllodes
b. Intraductal carcinoma
c. Malignant lymphoma
d. Fibroadenoma
e. Juvenile hypertrophy

256. A 53-year-old woman presents with complaints of weakness, anorexia, malaise, constipation, and back pain. While being evaluated, she becomes somewhat lethargic. Laboratory studies include a normal chest x-ray, serum albumin 3.2 mg/dL, serum calcium 14 mg/dL, serum phosphorus 2.6 mg/dL, serum chloride 108 mg/dL, blood urea nitrogen (BUN) 32 mg/dL, and creatinine 2.0 mg/dL. Which of the following is the most appropriate initial management?

a. Intravenous normal saline infusion
b. Administration of thiazide diuretics
c. Administration of intravenous phosphorus
d. Use of mithramycin
e. Neck exploration and parathyroidectomy

257. Which of the following patients with primary hyperparathyroidism should undergo parathyroidectomy?

a. A 62-year-old asymptomatic woman
b. A 54-year-old woman with fatigue and depression
c. A 42-year-old woman with a history of kidney stones
d. A 59-year-old woman with mildly elevated 24-hour urinary calcium excretion
e. A 60-year-old woman with mildly decreased bone mineral density measured at the hip of less than 2 standard deviations below peak bone density.

258. A woman sustains an injury to her chest after striking the steering wheel of her automobile during a collision. Which of the following statements concerning fat necrosis of the breast is true?

a. Most patients report a history of trauma.
b. The lesion is usually nontender and diffuse.
c. It predisposes patients to the development of breast cancer.
d. It is difficult to distinguish from breast cancer.
e. Excision exacerbates the process.

259. A 45-year-old woman presents with hypertension, development of facial hair, and a 7-cm suprarenal mass. Which of the following is the most likely diagnosis?

a. Myelolipoma
b. Cushing disease
c. Adrenocortical carcinoma
d. Pheochromocytoma
e. Carcinoid

260. A 36-year-old woman presents with palpitations, anxiety, and hypertension. Workup reveals a pheochromocytoma. Which of the following is the best approach to optimizing the patient preoperatively?

a. Fluid restriction 24 hours preoperatively to prevent intraoperative congestive heart failure
b. Initiation of an α-blocker 24 hours prior to surgery
c. Initiation of an α-blocker at 1 to 3 weeks prior to surgery
d. Initiation of a β-blocker 1 to 3 weeks prior to surgery
e. Escalating antihypertensive drug therapy with β-blockade followed by α-blockade starting at least 1 week prior to surgery

261. A 31-year-old woman notices a breast lump during her second pregnancy. A biopsy confirms the presence of breast cancer. Which of the following statements is true?

a. Termination of a first-trimester pregnancy is mandatory.
b. Radiation therapy is safe in the third trimester provided appropriate shielding is provided.
c. Breast conservation is inappropriate for third-trimester pregnancies.
d. Modified radical mastectomy should be delayed until after delivery.
e. Administration of adjuvant chemotherapy is safe for the fetus during the second and third trimesters.

262. A 40-year-old woman notices a skin rash around her areola. There is an erosive area about the nipple. There is tenderness, itching, and intermittent bleeding. Which of the following statements is true regarding this entity?

a. It usually precedes development of Paget disease of bone.
b. It presents with nipple-areolar eczematous changes.
c. It does not involve axillary lymph nodes because it is a manifestation of intraductal carcinoma only.
d. It accounts for 10% to 15% of all newly diagnosed breast cancers.
e. It is adequately treated with wide excision when it presents as a mass.

263. A 40-year-old man who has a long history of peptic ulcer disease that has not responded to medical therapy is admitted to the hospital. His serum gastrin levels are markedly elevated; at celiotomy, a small, firm mass is palpated in the tail of the pancreas. Which of the following statements concerning this patient's condition is correct?

a. Histamine or a protein meal will markedly increase basal acid secretion.
b. Secretin administration will suppress acid secretion.
c. The pancreatic mass will probably be benign.
d. Distal pancreatectomy is the treatment of choice.
e. H_2-receptor antagonists have not been beneficial in the treatment of this condition.

264. A 29-year-old woman with a history of difficulty becoming pregnant presents to her primary care physician and is diagnosed with Grave disease on iodine uptake scan; her thyrotropin (TSH) level is markedly suppressed and her free thyroxine (T_4) level is elevated. She desires to conceive as soon as possible and elects to undergo thyroidectomy. After she is rendered euthyroid with medications preoperatively, which of the following management strategies should also be employed to reduce the risk of developing thyroid storm in the operating room?

a. Drops of Lugol iodine solution daily beginning 10 days preoperatively
b. Preoperative treatment with phenoxybenzamine for 3 weeks
c. Preoperative treatment with propranolol for 1 week
d. Twenty-four hours of corticosteroids preoperatively
e. No other preoperative medication is required

265. A 30-year-old woman presents with hypertension, weakness, bone pain, and a serum calcium level of 15.2 mg/dL. Hand films below show osteitis fibrosa cystica. Which of the following is the most likely cause of these findings?

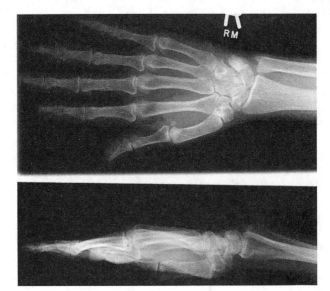

a. Sarcoidosis
b. Vitamin D intoxication
c. Paget disease
d. Metastatic carcinoma
e. Primary hyperparathyroidism

266. A 35-year-old woman presents with a serum calcium level of 15.2 mg/dL and an elevated parathyroid hormone level. Following correction of the patient's hypercalcemia with hydration and furosemide, which of the following is the best therapeutic approach?

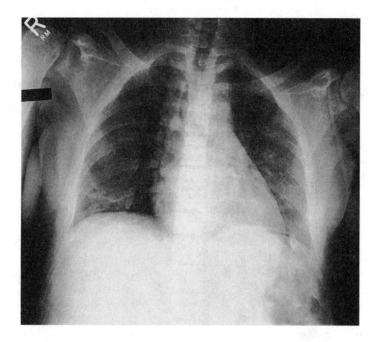

a. Administration of steroids
b. Radiation treatment to the neck
c. Neck exploration and resection of all four parathyroid glands
d. Neck exploration and resection of a parathyroid adenoma
e. Avoidance of sunlight, vitamin D, and calcium-containing dairy products

267. A 58-year-old man presents with tachycardia, fever, confusion, and vomiting. Work-up reveals markedly elevated (triiodothyronine) T$_3$ and (thyroxine) T$_4$ levels. He is diagnosed as having a thyroid storm. Which of the following is the most appropriate next step in the management of this patient?

a. Emergent subtotal thyroidectomy
b. Emergent total thyroidectomy
c. Emergent hemodialysis
d. Administration of fluid, antithyroid drugs, β-blockers, iodine solution, and steroids
e. Emergent radiation therapy to the neck

268. A 34-year-old woman presents with hypertension, generalized weakness, and polyuria. Her electrolyte panel is significant for hypokalemia. Which of the following is the best initial test given her presentation and laboratory findings?

a. Plasma renin activity and plasma aldosterone concentration
b. Urine electrolytes
c. Plasma cortisol level
d. Overnight low-dose dexamethasone suppression test
e. Twenty-four-hour urinary aldosterone level

269. Incisional biopsy of a breast mass in a 35-year-old woman demonstrates cystosarcoma phyllodes at the time of frozen section. Which of the following is the most appropriate management strategy for this lesion?

a. Wide local excision with a rim of normal tissue
b. Lumpectomy and axillary lymphadenectomy
c. Modified radical mastectomy
d. Excision and postoperative radiotherapy
e. Excision, postoperative radiotherapy, and systemic chemotherapy

270. A 36-year-old woman, 20 weeks pregnant, presents with a 1.5-cm right thyroid mass. FNA is consistent with a papillary neoplasm. The mass is cold on scan and solid on ultrasound. Which of the following methods of treatment is contraindicated?

a. Right thyroid lobectomy
b. Subtotal thyroidectomy
c. Total thyroidectomy
d. Total thyroidectomy with lymph node dissection
e. ^{131}I radioactive ablation of the thyroid gland

271. A 63-year-old woman notices lumps on both sides of her neck. A fine-needle aspirate is nondiagnostic, and she undergoes total thyroidectomy. On frozen section, pathology reveals Hürthle cell carcinoma. Correct statements concerning Hürthle cell carcinoma of the thyroid include which of the following?

a. It is a form of anaplastic thyroid cancer.
b. It can be diagnosed by FNA.
c. Treatment consists of a total thyroidectomy.
d. Microscopically, it consists of clusters of cells separated by areas of collagen and amyloid.
e. Once treated appropriately, it has a low rate of recurrence.

272. A 51-year-old man presents with a 2-cm left thyroid nodule. Thyroid scan shows a cold lesion. FNA cytology demonstrates follicular cells. Which of the following statements regarding this patient's condition is true?

a. Thyroid nodules in men are rarely malignant.
b. Increased age is associated with improved prognosis in patients with follicular carcinomas.
c. In the setting of abnormal cytology, an initial course of TSH suppression by thyroid hormone is recommended.
d. In the setting of a possible follicular neoplasm, prophylactic neck dissection is indicated.
e. Thyroid lobectomy is an acceptable treatment for this patient.

273. A 41-year-old woman has noted bilateral thin serous discharge from her breasts. There seems to be no mass associated with it. Which of the following statements would be appropriate to tell the patient?

a. Intermittent thin or milky discharge can be physiologic.
b. Expressible nipple discharge is an indication for open biopsy.
c. Absence of a mass on mammogram rules out malignancy.
d. Galactorrhea is indicative of an underlying malignancy.
e. Pathologic discharge is usually bilateral.

274. A 52-year-old woman is referred to you. She says that her doctor told her she had a condition called Cushing. She has hypertension, obesity, and new skin striae. True statements regarding Cushing disease and Cushing syndrome include which of the following?

a. Adrenocortical hyperplasia is the most common cause of Cushing disease.
b. Overproduction of adrenocorticotropic hormone (ACTH) is pathognomonic of Cushing syndrome.
c. Clinical manifestations of Cushing disease and Cushing syndrome are identical.
d. Cushing syndrome is caused only by neoplasms of either the pituitary or adrenal glands.
e. Cushing disease is incurable.

275. A 34-year-old woman has recurrent fainting spells induced by fasting. Her serum insulin levels during these episodes are markedly elevated. Correct statements regarding this patient's condition include which of the following?

a. The underlying lesion is more commonly located in the body or tail of the pancreas.
b. The underlying lesion is usually multifocal.
c. These lesions are usually malignant.
d. Serum calcium levels may be elevated.
e. She should be screened for a coexistent pheochromocytoma.

276. A 36-year-old woman whose mother has just undergone treatment for breast cancer is asking about how this affects her and what can be done to lessen her chances of having the disease. Which of the following has the lowest risk factor for breast cancer?

a. Dietary fat intake
b. Paternal relative with breast cancer 1 (*BRCA1*) mutation
c. Excessive estrogen exposure—early menarche, late menopause, nulliparity
d. Previous biopsy with atypical hyperplasia
e. Exposure to ionizing radiation

Questions 277 to 281

For each clinical description, select the appropriate stage of breast cancer. Each lettered option may be used once, more than once, or not at all.

a. Stage I
b. Stage II
c. Stage III
d. Stage IV
e. Inflammatory carcinoma

277. Tumor not palpable, clinically positive lymph nodes fixed to one another, no evidence of metastases.

278. Tumor 5.0 cm; clinically positive, movable ipsilateral lymph nodes; no evidence of metastases.

279. Tumor 2.1 cm, clinically negative lymph nodes, no evidence of metastases.

280. Tumor not palpable, but breast diffusely enlarged and erythematous, clinically positive supraclavicular nodes, and evidence of metastases.

281. Tumor 0.5 cm, clinically negative lymph nodes, pathological rib fracture.

Questions 282 to 286

A 43-year-old man presents with signs and symptoms of peritonitis in the right lower quadrant. The clinical impression and supportive data suggest acute appendicitis. At exploration, however, a tumor is found; frozen section suggests carcinoid features. For each tumor described, choose the most appropriate surgical procedure. Each lettered option may be used once, more than once, or not at all.

a. Appendectomy
b. Segmental ileal resection
c. Cecectomy
d. Right hemicolectomy
e. Hepatic wedge resection and appropriate bowel resection

282. A 2.5-cm tumor at the base of the appendix.

283. A 1.0-cm tumor at the tip of the appendix.

284. A 0.5-cm tumor with serosal umbilication in the ileum.

285. A 1.0-cm tumor of the midappendix; a 1-cm firm, pale lesion at the periphery of the right lobe of the liver.

286. A 3.5-cm tumor encroaching onto the cecum and extensive liver metastases.

Questions 287 to 291

For each clinical problem outlined, select acceptable treatment options. Each lettered option may be used once, more than once, or not at all.

a. No further surgical intervention
b. Wide local excision
c. Wide local excision with adjuvant radiation therapy
d. Wide local excision with axillary lymph node dissection and radiation therapy
e. Simple mastectomy (without axillary lymph node dissection)
f. Modified radical mastectomy (simple mastectomy with in-continuity axillary lymph node dissection)
g. Radical mastectomy
h. Bilateral prophylactic simple mastectomies

287. A 49-year-old woman undergoes biopsy of a 5.0-cm left breast mass; she has no palpable axillary lymph nodes. Biopsy of the mass shows cystosarcoma phyllodes.

288. A 42-year-old woman has a mammogram that demonstrates diffuse suspicious mammographic calcifications suggestive of multicentric disease. Biopsy of one of the lesions reveals ductal carcinoma in situ (DCIS).

289. A 51-year-old (premenopausal) woman undergoes needle localization biopsy for microcalcifications. Pathology reveals sclerosing adenosis.

290. A 49-year-old woman has a 6-cm palpable mass that is biopsy-proven ductal adenocarcinoma. She undergoes neoadjuvant chemotherapy which reduces the tumor to 3 cm in size. However, she has palpable axillary lymph nodes; FNA demonstrates adenocarcinoma. She desires breast conservation therapy if possible.

291. A neglected 82-year-old woman presents with a locally advanced breast cancer that is invading the pectoralis major muscle over a broad base. She is otherwise in good health.

Endocrine Problems and the Breast

Answers

242. The answer is d. *(Townsend, pp 1011-1016.)* Corticosteroids are the treatment of choice for adrenal insufficiency. Failure to recognize adrenal cortical insufficiency, particularly in the postoperative patient, may be a fatal error that is especially regrettable because therapy is effective and easy to administer. Adrenal insufficiency may occur in a host of settings including infections (eg, tuberculosis, [human immunodeficiency virus] HIV-associated infections), autoimmune states, adrenal hemorrhage (classically, during meningococcal septicemia), pituitary insufficiency, after burns, in the setting of coagulopathy, and after interruption of chronically administered exogenous steroids. Chronic adrenal insufficiency (classic Addison disease) should be recognizable preoperatively by the constellation of skin pigmentation, weakness, weight loss, hypotension, nausea, vomiting, abdominal pain, hypoglycemia, hyponatremia, and hyperkalemia. Adrenal insufficiency may also develop insidiously in the postoperative period, progressing over a course of several days. This insidious course is seen when adrenal injury occurs in the perioperative period, as would be the case with adrenal damage from hemorrhage into the gland in a patient receiving postoperative anticoagulant therapy. The other answers all address individual components of the patient's condition but not the underlying disease.

243. The answer is a. *(Brunicardi, pp 1405-1410.)* The thyroid scan shows a single focus of increased isotope uptake, often referred to as a hot nodule. Hyperfunctioning adenomas or hot nodules become independent of TSH control and secrete thyroid hormone autonomously, which results in clinical hyperthyroidism. The elevated thyroid hormone levels ultimately diminish TSH levels severely and thus depress function of the remaining normal thyroid gland. An isolated focus of increased uptake on a thyroid scan is virtually diagnostic of a hyperfunctioning adenoma. Grave disease demonstrate diffuse uptake of radioactive iodine by the thyroid gland. Carcinomas usually display diminished uptake and are called cold nodules. Multinodular goiter would display many nodules with varying activity.

244. The answer is d. (*Brunicardi, p 1429.*) The clinical presentation is consistent with a wound hematoma and necessitates exploration of the wound, drainage of the hematoma, and identification and control of any bleeding vessels. If airway control is unable to be obtained prior to the operating room, the wound should be opened at the bedside. Bilateral vocal cord dysfunction can be a cause of postoperative stridor and difficulty breathing, particularly after reoperative surgery; however, bilateral vocal cord dysfunction should manifest immediately after extubation. Hypocalcemia can occur in post-thyroidectomy due to ischemia or accidental removal of parathyroid tissue but is typically transient. Symptoms of hypocalcemia are usually neuromuscular and cardiac in nature.

245. The answer is b. (*Greenfield, pp 1275-1279.*) There is strong evidence from multiple randomized trials that there is no difference in survival in patients receiving modified radical mastectomy versus lumpectomy and axillary node dissection followed by radiation (breast conservation therapy) for stages I and II breast cancer. Absolute contraindications to breast conservation therapy include diffuse microcalcifications suspicious for malignancy, persistently positive margins in the face of multiple reexcisions, pregnancy (except in the third trimester with radiation therapy deferred until after delivery), multiple tumors in separate quadrants, and a previous history of therapeutic radiation to the breast. Relative contraindications include multifocal disease within a single quadrant and expected poor cosmetic results (eg, large tumor, small breast).

246. The answer is e. (*Townsend, p 885.*) Currently, treatment of inflammatory breast cancer consists of multimodality therapy with chemotherapy, surgery, and radiation, which results in a 50% 5-year survival rate. The clinical description of *peau d'orange* results from neoplastic invasion of dermal lymphatics with resultant edema of the breast; this clinical presentation and the skin biopsy findings are diagnostic for inflammatory breast cancer. Although the clinical picture may resemble that of a bacterial infection of the breast (mastitis), care must be taken to differentiate between the two pathologies.

247. The answer is b. (*Townsend, pp 2109-2110.*) Increased prolactin levels may be due to a variety of etiologies including but not limited to medications, pregnancy, cirrhosis, or tumors. Prolactin-secreting tumors in the pituitary gland may cause bitemporal hemianopsia because of compression of the optic chiasm. They are typically associated with amenorrhea and galactorrhea in women. In both sexes, lack of libido and impotence or infertility may be noted. Sexual vigor is usually restored after removal of the adenomas. Observation alone is recommended for asymptomatic patients. Symptomatic relief can be afforded by dopaminergic agonists (eg, bromocriptine), which usually cause tumor shrinkage. Surgery is reserved for those individuals with persistent symptoms despite adequate therapy or who do not desire long-term medical therapy.

248. The answer is c. (*Greenfield, pp 1321-1330.*) Elevated parathyroid hormone (PTH) levels in conjunction with elevated calcium levels are diagnostic for hyperparathyroidism. Primary hyperparathyroidism is a common disease, with approximately 50,000 new cases diagnosed each year in the United States. Essential to the diagnosis of hyperparathyroidism is the finding of hypercalcemia. Though there are many causes of hypercalcemia, hyperparathyroidism is by far the most prevalent. The majority of patients with primary hyperparathyroidism have a single parathyroid adenoma, which can be localized in 75% to 80% of patients with sestamibi scanning. Technetium 99m labeled sestamibi is taken up by the parathyroid and thyroid glands. Hyperfunctioning parathyroid glands take up the sestamibi to a greater extent than normal glands and therefore, sestamibi scanning can be used to identify parathyroid adenomas. Patients with primary hyperparathyroidism have either normal or elevated urinary calcium. As the name suggests, patients with familial hypocalciuric hypercalcemia (FHH) have hypercalcemia. They also usually have elevated PTH, but urine calcium excretion is low (as opposed to normal to high as with a parathyroid adenoma). Surgery is not indicated in this relatively rare setting of hypercalcemia.

249. The answer is e. (*Greenfield, pp 888-889*) Glucagonomas are usually solitary and large, and as such are easily identifiable on CT scanning of the abdomen. Usually located in the body or tail of the pancreas, resection requires distal pancreatectomy. Metastases are common and should be resected whenever feasible. Octreotide may be useful in the treatment of hyperglycemia in patients with unresectable disease.

250. The answer is e. (*Greenfield, pp 1339-1341.*) After adrenalectomy for a functioning adenoma, steroid replacement therapy may be required for up to 6 to 12 months postoperatively, even with a normally functioning contralateral adrenal gland. Primary adrenal pathology causes 10% to 20%

of all cases of Cushing syndrome. In 10% to 15% of cases, adenomas are bilateral. All functioning adenomas should be resected, while nonfunctioning adenomas should be resected if the lesion is greater than 6 cm in size or carcinoma is suspected. A hyperfunctioning adrenal adenoma can usually be lateralized by preoperative radiologic studies, eliminating the need to explore both adrenal glands—CT scanning is a sensitive, but not specific, initial study. MRI or scintigraphic studies (using radiolabeled norcholesterol, NP-59) are more specific and can be utilized to aid in distinguishing adrenal adenomas from carcinomas. Surgical approaches include transabdominal laparoscopy or a posterior unilateral flank route. The anterior transperitoneal approach is usually reserved for complicated cases such as large or obviously malignant lesions.

251. The answer is c. *(Brunicardi, pp 465-466, 476.)* Most clinicians would recommend aspiration and cytologic examination of the cyst fluid in this situation. Cysts are common lesions in the breasts of women in their thirties and forties; malignancies are relatively rare. All such lesions justify attention, however, and physicians must not underestimate the fear associated with the discovery of a mass in the breast, even in low-risk situations. If the lesion does not completely disappear after aspiration, excision is advised. In young women, the breast parenchyma is dense, which limits the diagnostic value of mammography. The National Cancer Center Network recommends a breast examination every 3 years for women of 20 years of age and older and a yearly mammogram and breast examination for women over the age of 40.

252. The answer is e. *(Brunicardi, pp 1413-1420.)* Treatment of radiation-induced thyroid cancer, which is usually of the papillary type, consists of a near-total (or total) thyroidectomy for multiple reasons: (1) a high incidence of bilaterality, (2) a greater incidence of complications if a second operation is necessary, (3) better detection of recurrent or persistent disease (using thyroglobulin levels), and (4) more effective use of radioactive iodine therapy postoperatively. The latent period for these tumors is 20 to 30 years or longer. Approximately 40% of patients with a history of radiation and a thyroid nodule are found to have thyroid cancer.

253. The answer is b. *(Brunicardi, pp 1417-1420.)* Treatment of high-risk papillary carcinomas consists of near-total (or total) thyroidectomy. If patients have lymph node metastases in the lateral neck, concomitant modified radical neck dissection should be performed with total thyroidectomy. Papillary carcinoma of the thyroid frequently metastasizes to cervical lymph nodes, but distant metastasis is uncommon. Overall, survival at 10 years is greater than 95%. Several scoring systems for determining prognosis have been developed; one of the more common systems takes into account age, grade, extrathyroidal invasion and metastases, and size (AGES). The surgical management of low-risk papillary thyroid cancers is controversial (lobectomy versus total thyroidectomy). Medullary, but not papillary, thyroid carcinoma is associated with multiple endocrine neoplasia syndrome.

254. The answer is c. (*Greenfield, p 1269.*) Lobular carcinoma in situ (LCIS) is considered to be a risk factor for invasive breast carcinoma, most commonly ductal carcinoma. The risk for breast cancer is equivalent in both breasts, lasts indefinitely, and is not correlated to the amount of LCIS in the biopsy specimen. The relative risk for invasive breast cancer is less than 2 for early menarche and late menopause, while the relative risk is greater than 5 for patients with a diagnosis of LCIS.

255. The answer is d. (*Brunicardi, p 466.*) Fibroadenomas occur infrequently before puberty but are the most common breast tumors between puberty and the early thirties. They usually are well-demarcated and firm. Although most fibroadenomas are no larger than 3 cm in diameter, giant or juvenile fibroadenomas are very large frequently. The bigger fibroadenomas (greater than 5 cm) occur predominantly in adolescent black girls. The average age at onset of juvenile mammary hypertrophy is 16 years. This disorder involves a diffuse change in the entire breast and does not usually manifest clinically as a discrete mass; it may be unilateral or bilateral and can cause an enormous and incapacitating increase in breast size. Regression may be spontaneous and sometimes coincides with puberty or pregnancy. Cystosarcoma phyllodes may also cause a large lesion. Together with intraductal carcinoma, it characteristically occurs in older women. Lymphomas are less firm than fibroadenomas and do not have a whorl-like pattern. They display a characteristic fish flesh texture.

256. The answer is a. (*Brunicardi, pp 1434-1440.*) Acute management of the hypercalcemic state includes vigorous hydration to restore intravascular volume, which is invariably diminished. This will establish renal perfusion and thus promote urinary calcium excretion. The patient described is exhibiting classic signs and symptoms of hyperparathyroidism. In addition, if a history is obtainable, frequently the patient will relate a history of renal calculi and bone pain—the syndrome characterized as "groans, stones, and bones." Thiazide diuretics are contraindicated because they frequently cause patients to become hypercalcemic. Instead, diuresis should be promoted with the use of loop diuretics such as furosemide (Lasix). The use of intravenous phosphorus infusion is no longer recommended because precipitation in the lungs, heart, or kidney can lead to serious morbidity. Mithramycin is an antineoplastic agent that in low doses inhibits bone resorption and thus diminishes serum calcium levels; it is used only when other maneuvers fail to decrease the calcium level. Calcitonin is useful at times. Bisphosphonates are used for lowering calcium levels in resistant cases, such as those associated with humoral malignancy. Emergency neck exploration is seldom warranted. In unprepared patients, the morbidity is unacceptably high.

257. The answer is c. *(Brunicardi, pp 1438-1439.)* Patients with symptomatic primary hyperparathyroidism as manifested by kidney stones, renal dysfunction, or osteoporosis should undergo parathyroidectomy. However, management of "asymptomatic" patients is controversial. Indications for surgical intervention for asymptomatic primary hyperparathyroidism include age less than 50 years, markedly elevated urine calcium excretion, kidney stones on radiography, decreased creatinine clearance, markedly elevated calcium or one episode of life-threatening hypercalcemia, and substantially decreased bone mass.

258. The answer is d. *(Townsend, p 868.)* Injury to breast tissue may cause necrosis of mammary adipose tissue and lead to the formation of a tender, localized, firm mass. A history of trauma is often elicited from affected patients, but less apparent factors, such as prolonged pressure, may also produce fat necrosis. Half the patients in whom the diagnosis is made do not recall a history of trauma. The pathophysiology of this lesion seems to involve early development of liquefaction of mammary fat with the formation of a cystic mass. Through a process of fibrosis, this lesion evolves into a firm, sometimes calcified lump that may be difficult to distinguish from carcinoma. There is, however, no relation between fat necrosis and the subsequent development of breast cancer. Excisional biopsy is usually required for definitive diagnosis; if the diagnosis of fat necrosis is confirmed, simple excision removes and terminates the process.

259. The answer is c. *(Brunicardi, pp 1458-1460.)* The constellation of symptoms in this patient is typical of a functional adrenocortical tumor (androgens).

Approximately 50% of adrenocortical tumors are functional and can secrete cortisol, androgens, estrogens, aldosterone, or multiple hormones. The single most important determinant of malignancy is the size of the tumor. Treatment consists of en bloc resection of the tumor and involved adjacent organs, such as the kidney or the tail of the pancreas. Symptoms related to hormone production can be minimized by complete resection despite the inability to cure advanced disease. Mitotane has been utilized as adjuvant therapy for unresectable or metastatic disease, but has not been proven to decrease mortality. Cushing disease refers to hypercortisolism due to a pituitary tumor and subsequent bilateral adrenal hyperplasia. Pheochromocytomas are characterized by hypertension and symptoms of excessive catecholamine production. Myelolipomas are benign adrenal lesions.

260. The answer is c. *(Brunicardi, pp 1461-1462.)* Patients with pheochromocytomas should be treated preoperatively with α-blockade using phenoxybenzamine 1 to 3 weeks before surgery. β-blockade may be necessary in addition to α-blockade for optimal blood pressure control, but should not be started in the absence of α-blockade because of the risk of cardiovascular collapse. With α-blockade, patients also require volume expansion.

261. The answer is e. *(Greenfield, pp 1282-1283.)* Chemotherapy can be administered to a pregnant patient but should be delayed until after the first trimester due to the increased risk of fetal abnormalities. Elective termination of pregnancy has not been demonstrated to improve survival. Since radiation exposure endangers the fetus and there is no evidence that general anesthesia and nonabdominal surgery increase premature labor, modified radical mastectomy is recommended for stage I or II carcinoma (tumor less than 4 cm in diameter). Patients in later stages of pregnancy, however, can start radiation therapy shortly after delivery, and some may be candidates for breast-conserving surgery and adjuvant radiotherapy. Radiation therapy is contraindicated in all trimesters of pregnancy. Chemotherapy does not appear to increase the risk of congenital malformation when given in the second or third trimester of pregnancy. Patients who require adjuvant chemotherapy during the first trimester may opt for a therapeutic abortion, however, since there is a slightly increased risk of fetal malformation in that circumstance.

262. The answer is b. *(Townsend, p 858)* Paget disease of the breast is unrelated to Paget disease of bone. It represents a small percentage (1%-3%) of all breast cancers and is thought to originate in the retroareolar lactiferous ducts. It progresses toward the nipple-areola complex in most patients, where it causes the typical clinical finding of nipple eczema and erosion. Up to 20% of patients with Paget disease have an associated breast mass, and these patients are more likely to have involvement of axillary nodes. Nipple-areolar disease alone usually represents in situ cancer; these patients have a 10-year survival rate of over 80%. In contrast, if Paget disease presents with a mass, the mass is likely to be an infiltrating ductal carcinoma. The generally recommended surgical procedure for Paget disease is currently a modified radical mastectomy. The validity of breast-saving surgery and adjuvant radiation therapy for patients without an associated mass is under investigation.

263. The answer is d. *(Brunicardi, pp 969-971.)* Zollinger-Ellison syndrome refers to hypergastrinemia resulting from an endocrine tumor of the pancreas. Over 50% of the tumors are malignant, and 40% have metastases at the time of surgery. Until recently, total gastrectomy was the primary operation for this tumor; however, it is now believed that operative exploration of the patient with resection of the tumor should be done if possible. H_2-receptor antagonists have also proved very promising in the management of these patients. Patients with Zollinger-Ellison tumors have very high basal levels of gastric acid (> 35 mEq/h) and serum gastrin (usually > 200 pg/mL). A protein meal or histamine usually does not increase acid and gastrin levels as it would in conventional duodenal ulcer patients. A paradoxical rise in serum gastrin after intravenous secretin is diagnostic of Zollinger-Ellison syndrome.

264. The answer is a. *(Brunicardi, p 1410.)* Drops of Lugol iodide solution daily beginning 10 days preoperatively should be prescribed to decrease the likelihood of postoperative thyroid storm, a manifestation of severe thyrotoxicosis. Propylthiouracil or methimazole can also be used preoperatively but are contraindicated in pregnant women. If thyroid storm occurs, treatment is β-blockade, for example, propranolol.

265. The answer is e. *(Brunicardi, pp 1436-1437.)* Osteitis fibrosa cystica is a condition associated with hyperparathyroidism that is characterized by severe demineralization with subperiosteal bone resorption (most prominent in the middle phalanx of the second and third fingers), bone cysts, and tufting of the distal phalanges on hand films. These specific bone findings would not be present in sarcoidosis, Paget disease, or metastatic carcinoma. Vitamin D deficiency can lead to osteitis fibrosa cystica but it would also be associated with hypocalcemia, not hypercalcemia.

266. The answer is d. *(Brunicardi, pp 1440-1444.)* Treatment for primary hyperparathyroidism in this setting is resection of the diseased parathyroid glands after initial correction of the severe hypercalcemia. Parathyroidectomy without preoperative localization studies have a high success rate and low complication rate. Neck exploration will yield a single parathyroid adenoma in about 85% of cases. Two adenomas are found less often (approximately 5% of cases) and hyperplasia of all four glands occurs in about 10% to 15% of patients. If hyperplasia is found, treatment includes resection of $3\frac{1}{2}$ glands. The remnant of the fourth gland can be identified with a metal clip in case reexploration becomes necessary. Alternatively, all four glands can be removed with autotransplantation of a small piece of parathyroid tissue into the forearm or sternocleidomastoid muscle. Subsequent hyperfunction, should it develop, can then be treated by removal of this tissue. Patients often need calcium supplementation postoperatively. Vitamin D supplementation may also be necessary if hypocalcemia develops and persists despite treatment with oral calcium. Steroids and radiation therapy have no role in the treatment of primary hyperparathyroidism.

267. The answer is d. *(Brunicardi, p 1410.)* Thyroid storm can be associated with high mortality rates if it is not appropriately managed in an intensive care unit setting. Treatment includes rapid fluid replacement, antithyroid medication such as propylthiouracil (PTU), β-blockers, iodine solutions, and steroids. β-Blockers are given to reduce peripheral conversion of T_4 to T_3 and decrease the hyperthyroid symptoms. Lugol iodine helps to decrease iodine uptake and thyroid hormone secretion. PTU therapy blocks formation of new thyroid hormone and reduces peripheral conversion of T_4 to T_3. Corticosteroids block hepatic thyroid hormone conversion. The thyroid storm needs to be treated before undergoing any surgery. Radiation therapy and hemodialysis have no role in the treatment of thyroid storm.

268. The answer is a. *(Brunicardi, pp1453-1455.)* The biochemical diagnosis of hyperaldosteronism requires demonstration of elevated plasma aldosterone concentration (PAC) with suppressed plasma renin activity (PAR). A PAC:PAR ratio of 25 to 30:1 is strongly suggestive of the diagnosis. Hyperaldosteronism must be suspected in any hypertensive patient who presents with hypokalemia. Hypokalemia occurs spontaneously in up to 90% of patients with this disorder. Other individuals who should be evaluated for hyperaldosteronism include those with severe hypertension, hypertension refractory to medication, and young age at onset of hypertension. Plasma cortisol level and overnight low-dose dexamethasone suppression test are laboratory studies used in diagnosing Cushing syndrome. Neither urine electrolytes nor 24-hour urinary aldosterone level is beneficial in diagnosing hyperaldosteronism.

269. The answer is a. *(Greenfield, pp 1284-1285.)* Cystosarcoma phyllodes is a tumor most often seen in younger women. It can grow to enormous size and at times ulcerate through the skin. Still, it is a lesion with low propensity toward metastasis. Local recurrence is common, especially if the initial resection was inadequate. Simple reexcision with adequate margins is curative. Very large lesions may necessitate simple mastectomy to achieve clear margins. Axillary lymphadenectomy, however, is seldom indicated without biopsy-positive demonstration of tumor in the nodes. The low incidence of metastatic disease suggests that adjunctive therapy is indicated only for known metastatic disease, even when the tumors are quite large and ulcerated.

270. The answer is e. *(Brunicardi, pp 1417-1420.)* This patient has cyto-logic evidence of a papillary lesion, possibly papillary carcinoma. Papillary carcinoma is a relatively nonaggressive lesion with 10-year survival of 95%. The lesion is frequently multicentric, which argues for more complete resection. Metastases, when they occur, are usually responsive to surgical resection or radioablation therapy. Removal of the involved lobe, and possibly the entire thyroid gland, is appropriate. Central and lateral lymph node dissection is performed for clinically suspect lymph nodes. Papillary carcinoma is frequently multifocal. Bilateral disease mandates total thyroidectomy. However, radioactive ^{131}I is contraindicated in pregnancy and should be used with caution in women of childbearing age.

271. The answer is c. *(Brunicardi, p 1421.)* Hürthle cell cancer is a type of follicular cancer, but differs from follicular neoplasms in that it is more often multifocal and bilateral, is more likely to spread to local nodes and distant sites, and has a higher mortality rate. Lobectomy can be performed for uni-lateral adenomas, but carcinomas (as evidenced by extracapsular or vascular invasion) should be treated with total thyroidectomy and central lymph node dissection. Because invasion cannot be determined by FNA, Hürthle cell cancer cannot be diagnosed on FNA. Amyloid deposits in the stroma of a thyroid tumor are diagnostic of medullary carcinoma.

272. The answer is e. *(Brunicardi, pp 1420-1421.)* Thyroid nodules are some-what less common in men and should always suggest malignancy. Follicular carcinomas cannot be diagnosed by FNA; capsular or vascular invasion on histology confirms a diagnosis of malignancy. For lesions less than 4 cm in size, thyroid lobectomy is adequate because at least 80% of follicular lesions are adenomas. For confirmed carcinomas or lesions greater than 4 cm in size, total thyroidectomy should be performed. There is no role for prophylactic neck dissection for follicular carcinomas. Age, tumor size, and tumor grade are all associated with increased mortality. Suppression with thyroid hormone (Synthroid) in the setting of abnormal cytology is not recommended.

273. The answer is a. *(Greenfield, pp 1260-1261.)* Nipple discharge from the breast may be classified as pathologic, physiologic, or galactorrhea. Galactorrhea may be caused by hormonal imbalance (hyperprolactinemia, hypothyroidism), drugs (oral contraceptives, phenothiazines, antihypertensives, tranquilizers), or trauma to the chest. Physiologic nipple discharge is intermittent, nonlactational (usually serous), and caused by stimulation of the nipple or to drugs (estrogens, tranquilizers). Both galactorrhea and physiologic discharge are frequently bilateral and arise from multiple ducts. Pathologic nipple discharge may be caused by benign lesions of the breast (duct ectasia, papilloma, fibrocystic disease) or by cancer. It may be bloody, serous, or gray-green. It is spontaneous and unilateral and can often be localized to a single nipple duct. When pathologic discharge is diagnosed, an effort should be made to identify the source. If an associated mass is present, it should be biopsied. If no mass is found, a terminal duct excision of the involved duct(s) should be performed.

274. The answer is c. *(Brunicardi, pp 1455-1456.)* Cushing disease is caused by hypersecretion of ACTH by the pituitary gland. This hypersecretion, in turn, is caused by either a pituitary adenoma (90% of cases) or diffuse pituitary corticotrope hyperplasia (10% of cases) because of hypersecretion of corticotropin-releasing hormone (CRH) by the hypothalamus. A high cure rate is achieved with surgery, occasionally followed by adjuvant radiotherapy for large pituitary adenomas. Cushing syndrome refers to the clinical manifestations of glucocorticoid excess due to any cause (Cushing disease, administration of exogenous glucocorticoids, adrenocortical hyperplasia, adrenal adenoma, adrenal carcinoma, ectopic ACTH-secreting tumors) and includes truncal obesity, hypertension, hirsutism, moon facies, proximal muscle wasting, ecchymoses, skin striae, osteoporosis, diabetes mellitus, amenorrhea, growth retardation, and immunosuppression. The most common cause of Cushing syndrome is iatrogenic, via administration of synthetic corticosteroids.

275. The answer is d. (*Greenfield, pp 884-885.*) Insulin-secreting endocrine tumors of the pancreas produce paroxysmal nervous system manifestations that may be a consequence of hypoglycemia, although the blood glucose level may bear little relation to the severity of the symptoms, even in the same patient from episode to episode. Most insulinomas are single discrete tumors (90%). They are evenly distributed between the head, body, and tail of the pancreas. Patients with insulinoma in the setting of the MEN-1 syndrome (synchronous islet cell tumors of the pancreas, pituitary hyperplasia or adenomas, and parathyroid chief cell hyperplasia) are more likely to have multiple tumors throughout the pancreas. If a careful examination of the pancreas reveals one or more specific adenomas, these can be enucleated. The finding of an elevated serum calcium level would raise the suspicion of MEN-1 and parathyroid hyperplasia. Insulinomas are not associated with MEN-2, which consists of coexistent medullary thyroid cancer, parathyroid hyperplasia, and pheochromocytoma. Approximately 10% of insulinomas are malignant. Streptozocin, a potent antibiotic that selectively destroys islet cells, can be useful in controlling symptoms from unresectable malignant tumors of the islet cells but probably has little to offer in the definitive management of the typical benign islet cell insulinoma.

276. The answer is a. (*Greenfield, pp 1266-1268.*) Studies have failed to demonstrate a correlation between diet and breast cancer risk. Age is the most common risk factor. Another important risk factor is family history in a first-degree relative or presence of a genetic mutation such as *BRCA 1* or *2*, which can be inherited through either the maternal or the paternal side of the family. Other risk factors include excessive estrogen exposure, obesity, alcohol use, hormone replacement, ionizing radiation, and a history of a prior breast cancer or abnormal breast biopsy (LCIS or atypical hyperplasia).

277 to 281. The answers are 277-c, 278-b, 279-b, 280-e, 281-d. (*Greenfield, p 1276.*) The TNM stage of breast cancer is assigned by measuring the greatest diameter of the tumor (T), assessing the axillary and clavicular lymph nodes for enlargement and fixation (N), and judging whether metastatic disease is present (M). In general, the worst of the three TNM parameters will determine the stage assignment. Tumors that are not palpable are classified as T0; tumors 2 cm or less as T1; tumors greater than 2 but not more than 5 cm as T2; tumors greater than 5 cm as T3; and tumors with extension into the chest wall or skin as T4. Clinically negative lymph nodes are classified as N0; positive, movable ipsilateral axillary nodes as N1; fixed ipsilateral axillary nodes as N2; and ipsilateral internal mammary nodes as N3. Absence of evidence of metastatic disease is classified as M0 and distant metastatic disease as M1. The patient in question 277 has a T0N2M0 lesion. This is stage III (fixed or matted nodes are a poor prognostic sign). The patient in question 278 has a T2N1M0 lesion. This is stage II. The patient in question 279 has a T2N0M0 lesion. Though smaller than the tumor in question 278 and without clinically involved nodes, this tumor is also stage II. The patient in question 280 has findings compatible with inflammatory breast cancer. A biopsy of the involved skin and a mammogram would confirm the diagnosis. The patient in question 281 has a T1N0M1 lesion. This is stage IV (stage IV is any T, any N, M1).

282 to 286. The answers are 282-d, 283-a, 284-b, 285-e, 286-c. (*Greenfield, pp 814-817.*) Carcinoid tumors are most commonly found in the appendix and small bowel, where they may be multiple. They have a tendency to metastasize, which varies with the size of the tumor. Tumors less than 1 cm uncommonly metastasize. Tumors greater than 2 cm are more often found to be metastatic. Metastasis to the liver and beyond may give rise to the carcinoid syndrome. The tumors cause an intense desmoplastic reaction. Spread into the serosal lymphatics does not imply metastatic disease; local resection is potentially curative. When metastatic lesions are found in the liver, they should be resected when technically feasible to limit the symptoms of the carcinoid syndrome. When extensive hepatic metastases are found, the disease is not curable. Resection of the appendix and cecum may be performed to prevent an early intestinal obstruction by locally encroaching tumor.

287 to 291. The answers are 287-b, 288-e, 289-a, 290-d, 291-g. (*Townsend, pp 871-896.*) Generally accepted treatment for stage I breast cancer in premenopausal women includes lumpectomy (wide excision, partial mastectomy, quadrantectomy), combined with axillary lymph node dissection (or sentinel lymph node biopsy) and adjuvant radiation therapy, or modified radical mastectomy. Both approaches offer equivalent chances of cure; there is a higher incidence of local recurrence with lumpectomy, axillary dissection, and radiation, but this observation has not been found to affect the overall cure rate in comparison with mastectomy. Patients with familial breast cancer (multiple first-degree relatives and penetrance of breast cancer through several familial generations) have extremely high risks of developing breast cancer in the course of their lifetimes. A subset of patients with familial breast cancer has been identified by a specific gene mutation (*BRCA1*); however, the genetic basis of most cases of familial breast cancer has yet to be elucidated. A patient with a history of familial breast cancer and multiple biopsies showing atypia may reasonably request bilateral prophylactic simple mastectomies. Alternatively, she may continue with routine surveillance. Lobular carcinoma in situ is a histologic marker that identifies patients at increased risk for the development of breast cancer. It is not a precancerous lesion in itself, and there is no benefit to widely excising it because the risk of subsequent cancer is equal for both breasts. As the risk for the future development of breast cancer is now estimated to be approximately 1% per year, prophylactic mastectomy is no longer recommended. Proper management consists of close surveillance for cancer by twice-yearly examinations and yearly mammography. Sclerosing adenosis is a benign lesion. DCIS is the precursor of invasive ductal carcinoma. It is described in four histologic variants (papillary, cribriform, solid, and comedo), of which the comedo subtype shows the greatest tendency to recur after wide excision alone. DCIS is treated with wide excision alone (for small noncomedo lesions) or wide excision plus radiation therapy. For multicentric DCIS, simple mastectomy is recommended. Cystosarcoma phyllodes is treated with wide local excision with at least 1-cm margins; axillary lymphadenectomy is not routinely recommended in the absence of clinically suspicious nodes. There are few indications for radical mastectomy, as it is both more traumatic and more disfiguring than any other method of local control of breast cancer and offers no greater survival benefit. However, one indication for radical mastectomy is locally advanced breast cancer with wide invasion of the pectoralis major in a patient who is physiologically able to tolerate general anesthesia.

Gastrointestinal Tract, Liver, and Pancreas

Questions

292. A 74-year-old woman is admitted with upper gastrointestinal (GI) bleeding. She is started on H$_2$ blockers, but experiences another bleeding episode. Endoscopy documents diffuse gastric ulcerations. Omeprazole is added to the H$_2$ antagonists as a therapeutic approach to the management of acute gastric and duodenal ulcers. Which of the following is the mechanism of action of omeprazole?

a. Blockage of the breakdown of mucosa-damaging metabolites of nonsteroidal antiinflammatory drugs (NSAIDs)
b. Provision of a direct cytoprotective effect
c. Buffering of gastric acids
d. Inhibition of parietal cell hydrogen potassium ATPase (adenosine triphosphatase)
e. Inhibition of gastrin release and parietal cell acid production

293. A 35-year-old woman presents with frequent and multiple areas of cutaneous ecchymosis. Workup demonstrates a platelet count of 15,000/µL, evaluation of the bone marrow reveals a normal number of megakaryocytes, and ultrasound examination demonstrates a normal-sized spleen. Based on the exclusion of other causes of thrombocytopenia, she is given a diagnosis of immune (idiopathic) thrombocytopenic purpura (ITP). Which of the following is the most appropriate treatment on diagnosis?

a. Expectant management with close follow-up of platelet counts
b. Immediate platelet transfusion to increase platelet counts to greater than 50,000/µL
c. Glucocorticoid therapy
d. Intravenous immunoglobulin (IVIG) therapy
e. Referral to surgery for laparoscopic splenectomy

294. A 59-year-old woman presents with right lower quadrant pain, nausea, and vomiting. She undergoes an uncomplicated laparoscopic appendectomy. Postoperatively, the pathology reveals a 2.5-cm mucinous adenocarcinoma with lymphatic invasion. Staging workup, including colonoscopy, chest x-ray, and computed tomography (CT) scan of the abdomen and pelvis, is negative. Which of the following is the best next step in her management?

a. No further intervention at this time; follow-up every 6 months for 2 years
b. Chemotherapy alone
c. Neoadjuvant chemotherapy followed by right hemicolectomy
d. Ileocecectomy
e. Right hemicolectomy

295. A 41-year-old man complains of regurgitation of saliva and of undigested food. An esophagram reveals a bird's-beak deformity. Which of the following statements is true about this condition?

a. Chest pain is common in the advanced stages of this disease.
b. More patients are improved by forceful dilatation than by surgical intervention.
c. Manometry can be expected to show high resting pressures of the lower esophageal sphincter (LES).
d. Surgical treatment consists primarily of resection of the distal esophagus with reanastomosis to the stomach above the diaphragm.
e. Patients with this disease are at no increased risk for the development of carcinoma.

296. A 32-year-old man with a 3-year history of ulcerative colitis (UC) presents for discussion for surgical intervention. Which of the following is true regarding total proctocolectomy for UC?

a. Patients with UC should consider surgery after 5 years because the risk of carcinoma increases to greater than 50%.
b. Symptoms relating to peripheral arthritis or ankylosing spondylitis will improve or resolve after proctocolectomy.
c. Early proctocolectomy can prevent the development of primary sclerosing cholangitis (PSC) in UC patients.
d. Proctocolectomy is not advised in younger patients because of the need for a permanent ileostomy.
e. Preservation of the rectum is a surgical option in the definitive management of UC.

297. A 39-year-old previously healthy male is hospitalized for 2 weeks with epigastric pain radiating to his back, nausea, and vomiting. Initial laboratory values revealed an elevated amylase level consistent with acute pancreatitis. Five weeks following discharge, he complains of early satiety, epigastric pain, and fevers. On presentation, his temperature is 38.9°C (102°F) and his heart rate is 120 beats per minute; his white blood cell (WBC) count is 24,000/mm³ and his amylase level is normal. He undergoes a CT scan demonstrating a 6-cm by 6-cm rim-enhancing fluid collection in the body of the pancreas. Which of the following would be the most definitive management of the fluid collection?

a. Antibiotic therapy alone
b. CT-guided aspiration with repeat imaging in 2 to 3 days
c. Antibiotics and CT-guided aspiration with repeat imaging in 2 to 3 days
d. Antibiotics and percutaneous catheter drainage
e. Surgical internal drainage of the fluid collection with a cyst-gastrostomy or Roux-en-Y cyst-jejunostomy

298. A previously healthy 79-year-old woman presents with early satiety and abdominal fullness. CT scan of the abdomen, pictured here, reveals a cystic lesion in the body and tail of the pancreas. CT-guided aspiration demonstrates an elevated carcinoembryonic antigen (CEA) level. Which of the following is the best treatment option for this patient?

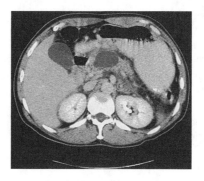

a. Distal pancreatectomy
b. Serial CT scans with resection if the lesion increases significantly in size
c. Internal drainage with Roux-en-Y cyst-jejunostomy
d. Percutaneous drainage of the fluid-filled lesion
e. Endoscopic retrograde cholangiopancreatography (ERCP) with pancreatic stent placement

299. A 56-year-old woman is referred to you about 3 months after a colostomy subsequent to a sigmoid resection for cancer. She complains that her stoma is not functioning properly. Which of the following is the most common serious complication of an end colostomy?

a. Bleeding
b. Skin breakdown
c. Parastomal hernia
d. Colonic perforation during irrigation
e. Stomal prolapse

300. A 56-year-old previously healthy physician notices that his eyes are yellow and he has pain in the right upper quadrant. Ultrasound and CT scan demonstrate a mass in the head of the pancreas. Endoscopic ultrasound suggests involvement of the superior mesenteric vein. Which of the following statements regarding his treatment and prognosis is true?

a. Total pancreatectomy is associated with improved survival.
b. Involvement of the superior mesenteric vein is a contraindication to pancreaticoduodenectomy.
c. Involvement of the superior mesenteric artery is a contraindication to pancreaticoduodenectomy.
d. Pylorus preservation is never indicated at the time of pancreaticoduodenectomy.
e. Preoperative biliary stenting is associated with improved survival after pancreaticoduodenectomy.

301. A 45-year-old woman with history of heavy nonsteroidal anti-inflammatory drug ingestion presents with acute abdominal pain. She undergoes exploratory laparotomy 24 hours after onset of symptoms and is found to have a perforated duodenal ulcer. Which of the following is the procedure of choice to treat her perforation?

a. Simple closure with omental patch
b. Truncal vagotomy and pyloroplasty
c. Truncal vagotomy and antrectomy
d. Highly selective vagotomy with omental patch
e. Hemigastrectomy

302. A 45-year-old man with a history of chronic peptic ulcer disease undergoes a truncal vagotomy and antrectomy with a Billroth II reconstruction for gastric outlet obstruction. Six weeks after surgery, he returns, complaining of postprandial weakness, sweating, lightheadedness, crampy abdominal pain, and diarrhea. Which of the following would be the best initial management strategy?

a. Treatment with a long-acting somatostatin analog
b. Dietary advice and counseling that symptoms will probably abate within 3 months of surgery
c. Dietary advice and counseling that symptoms will probably not abate but are not dangerous
d. Workup for neuroendocrine tumor (eg, carcinoid)
e. Preparation for revision to Roux-en-Y gastrojejunostomy

303. A 60-year-old male patient with hepatitis C with a previous history of variceal bleeding is admitted to the hospital with hematemesis. His blood pressure is 80/60 mm Hg, physical examination reveals splenomegaly and ascites, and initial hematocrit is 25%. Prior to endoscopy, which of the following is the best initial management of the patient?

a. Administration of intravenous octreotide
b. Administration of a β-blocker (eg, propranolol)
c. Measurement of prothrombin time and transfusion with cryoglobulin if elevated
d. Empiric transfusion of platelets given splenomegaly
e. Gastric and esophageal balloon tamponade (Sengstaken-Blakemore tube)

304. A 32-year-old alcoholic with end-stage liver disease has been admitted to the hospital three times for bleeding esophageal varices. He has undergone banding and sclerotherapy previously. He admits to currently drinking a six-pack of beer per day. On his abdominal examination, he has a fluid wave. Which of the following is the best option for long-term management of this patient's esophageal varices?

a. Orthotopic liver transplantation
b. Transection and reanastomosis of the distal esophagus
c. Distal splenorenal shunt
d. End-to-side portocaval shunt
e. Transjugular intrahepatic portosystemic shunt (TIPS)

305. A 55-year-old man complains of chronic intermittent epigastric pain. A gastroscopy demonstrates a 2-cm prepyloric ulcer. Biopsy of the ulcer yields no malignant tissue. After a 6-week trial of medical therapy, the ulcer is unchanged. Which of the following is the best next step in his management?

a. Repeat trial of medical therapy
b. Local excision of the ulcer
c. Highly selective vagotomy
d. Partial gastrectomy with vagotomy and Billroth I reconstruction
e. Vagotomy and pyloroplasty

306. A 45-year-old man was discovered to have a hepatic flexure colon cancer during a colonoscopy for anemia requiring transfusions. Upon exploration of his abdomen in the operating room, an unexpected discontinuous 3-cm metastasis is discovered in the edge of the right lobe of the liver. Preoperatively, the patient was counseled of this possibility and the surgical options. Which of the following statements is correct?

a. A diverting ileostomy should be performed and further imaging obtained.
b. Liver resection cannot be safely performed at the time of colon resection.
c. Five-year survival after complete resection of the primary lesion and liver metastasis is 25%.
d. Liver metastases are a contraindication to resection of the primary lesion.
e. Postoperative radiation therapy to the liver increases 5-year survival after resection of the primary lesion.

307. A 42-year-old man with no history of use of NSAIDs presents with recurrent gastritis. Infection with *Helicobacter pylori* is suspected. Which of the following statements is true?

a. Morphologically, the bacteria are a gram-positive, tennis-racket–shaped organism.
b. Diagnosis can be made by serologic testing or urea breath tests.
c. Diagnosis is most routinely achieved via culturing endoscopic scrapings.
d. The most effective way to treat and prevent recurrence of this patient's gastritis is through the use of single-drug therapy aimed at eradicating *H pylori*.
e. The organism is easily eradicated.

308. A 22-year-old college student notices a bulge in his right groin. It is accentuated with coughing, but is easily reducible. Which of the following hernias follows the path of the spermatic cord within the cremaster muscle?

a. Femoral
b. Direct inguinal
c. Indirect inguinal
d. Spigelian
e. Interparietal

309. An 80-year-old man with history of symptomatic cholelithiasis presents with signs and symptoms of a small-bowel obstruction. Which of the following findings would provide the most help in ascertaining the diagnosis?

a. Coffee-grounds aspirate from the stomach
b. Aerobilia
c. A leukocyte count of 40,000/µL
d. A pH of 7.5, P_{CO_2} of 50 kPa, and paradoxically acid urine
e. A palpable mass in the pelvis

310. A 42-year-old man has had bouts of intermittent crampy abdominal pain and diarrhea. Colonoscopy is performed. You must discuss the problem with the patient. Which of the following colonic pathologies is thought to have no malignant potential?

a. Ulcerative colitis
b. Villous adenomas
c. Familial polyposis
d. Peutz-Jeghers syndrome
e. Crohn colitis

311. A 70-year-old woman has nausea, vomiting, abdominal distention, and episodic crampy midabdominal pain. She has no history of previous surgery but has a long history of cholelithiasis for which she has refused surgery. Her abdominal radiograph reveals a spherical density in the right lower quadrant. Which of the following is the definitive treatment for this patient's bowel obstruction?

a. Ileocolectomy
b. Cholecystectomy
c. Ileotomy and extraction
d. Nasogastric (NG) tube decompression
e. Intravenous antibiotics

312. A 53-year-old man presents to the emergency room with left lower quadrant pain, fever, and vomiting. CT scan of the abdomen and pelvis reveals a thickened sigmoid colon with inflamed diverticula and a 7-cm by 8-cm rim-enhancing fluid collection in the pelvis. After percutaneous drainage and treatment with antibiotics, the pain and fluid collection resolve. He returns as an outpatient to clinic 1 month later. He undergoes a colonoscopy, which demonstrates only diverticula in the sigmoid colon. Which of the following is the most appropriate next step in this patient's management?

a. Expectant management with sigmoid resection if symptoms recur
b. Cystoscopy to evaluate for a fistula
c. Sigmoid resection with end colostomy and rectal pouch (Hartmann procedure)
d. Sigmoid resection with primary anastomosis
e. Long-term suppressive antibiotic therapy

313. A 29-year-old woman complains of postprandial right upper quadrant pain and fatty food intolerance. Ultrasound examination reveals no evidence of gallstones or sludge. Upper endoscopy is normal, and all of her liver function tests are within normal limits. She then undergoes a CCK-HIDA scan, which reveals that her gallbladder ejection fraction is 15% at 20 minutes. Which of the following is true regarding her treatment options?

a. Avoidance of fatty foods is the only therapeutic option.
b. Ultrasound examination should be repeated immediately, since the false-negative rate for ultrasound in detecting gallstones is 10% to 15%.
c. Treatment with ursodeoxycholic acid results in improvement in symptoms in 35% of patients.
d. Laparoscopic cholecystectomy results in improvement in symptoms in 85% of patients.
e. Surgical intervention should be reserved for patients whose symptoms do not resolve with conservative treatment.

314. A 47-year-old asymptomatic woman is incidentally found to have a 5-mm polyp and no stones in her gallbladder on ultrasound examination. Which of the following is the best management option?

a. Aspiration of the gallbladder with cytologic examination of the bile
b. Observation with repeat ultrasound examinations to evaluate for increase in polyp size
c. Laparoscopic cholecystectomy
d. Open cholecystectomy with frozen section
e. En bloc resection of the gallbladder, wedge resection of the liver, and portal lymphadenectomy

315. A 48-year-old woman develops pain in the right lower quadrant while playing tennis. The pain progresses and the patient presents to the emergency room later that day with a low-grade fever, a WBC count of 13,000/mm³ and complaints of anorexia and nausea as well as persistent, sharp pain of the right lower quadrant. On examination, she is tender in the right lower quadrant with muscular spasm, and there is a suggestion of a mass effect. An ultrasound is ordered and shows an apparent mass in the abdominal wall. Which of the following is the most likely diagnosis?

a. Acute appendicitis
b. Cecal carcinoma
c. Hematoma of the rectus sheath
d. Torsion of an ovarian cyst
e. Cholecystitis

316. A 32-year-old alcoholic man, recently emigrated from Mexico, presents with right upper quadrant pain and fevers for 2 weeks. CT scan of the abdomen demonstrates a non–rim-enhancing fluid collection in the periphery of the right lobe of the liver. The patient's serology is positive for antibodies to *Entamoeba histolytica*. Which of the following is the best initial management option for this patient?

a. Treatment with antiamebic drugs
b. Percutaneous drainage of the fluid collection
c. Marsupialization of the fluid collection
d. Surgical drainage of the fluid collection
e. Liver resection

317. A 45-year-old executive experiences increasingly painful retrosternal heartburn, especially at night. He has been chewing antacid tablets. An esophagogram shows a hiatal hernia. In determining the proper treatment for a sliding hiatal hernia, which of the following is the most useful modality?

a. Barium swallow with cinefluoroscopy during Valsalva maneuver
b. Flexible endoscopy
c. Twenty-four–hour monitoring of esophageal pH
d. Measurement of the size of the hernia on upper GI
e. Assessment of the patient's smoking and drinking history

318. A 22-year-old woman is seen in a surgery clinic for a bulge in the right groin. She denies pain and is able to make the bulge disappear by lying down and putting steady pressure on the bulge. She has never experienced nausea or vomiting. On examination she has a reducible hernia below the inguinal ligament. Which of the following is the most appropriate management of this patient?

a. Observation for now and follow up in surgery clinic in 6 months
b. Observation for now and follow up in surgery clinic if she develops further symptoms
c. Elective surgical repair of hernia
d. Emergent surgical repair of hernia
e. Emergent surgical repair of hernia with exploratory laparotomy to evaluate the small bowel

319. A 22-year-old woman presents with a painful fluctuant mass in the midline between the gluteal folds. She denies pain on rectal examination. Which of the following is the most likely diagnosis?

a. Pilonidal abscess
b. Perianal abscess
c. Perirectal abscess
d. Fistula-in-ano
e. Anal fissure

320. A 72-year-old man status post-coronary artery bypass graft (CABG) 5 years ago presents with hematochezia, abdominal pain, and fevers. Colonoscopy reveals patches of dusky-appearing mucosa at the splenic flexure without active bleeding. Which of the following is the most appropriate management of this patient?

a. Angiography with administration of intra-arterial papaverine
b. Emergent laparotomy with left hemicolectomy and transverse colostomy
c. Aortomesenteric bypass
d. Exploratory laparotomy with thrombectomy of the inferior mesenteric artery
e. Expectant management

321. A 62-year-old man has been diagnosed by endoscopic biopsy as having a sigmoid colon cancer. He is otherwise healthy and presents to your office for preoperative consultation. He asks a number of questions regarding removal of a portion of his colon. Which of the following statements is true regarding the effects of colon resection?

a. The majority (>50%) of normally formed feces is comprised of solid material.
b. Patients who undergo major colon resections suffer little long-term change in their bowel habits following operation.
c. Sodium, potassium, chloride, and bicarbonate are all absorbed by the colonic epithelium by a passive transport process.
d. The left colon absorbs more water than the right colon.
e. The colon absorbs long-chain fatty acids that result from bacterial breakdown of lipids.

322. A 39-year-old woman with no significant past medical history and whose only medication is oral contraceptive pills (OCP) presents to the emergency room with right upper quadrant pain. CT scan demonstrates a 6-cm hepatic adenoma in the right lobe of the liver. Which of the following describes the definitive treatment of this lesion?

a. Cessation of oral contraceptives and serial CT scans
b. Intra-arterial embolization of the hepatic adenoma
c. Embolization of the right portal vein
d. Resection of the hepatic adenoma
e. Systemic chemotherapy

323. A 43-year-old man without symptoms is incidentally noted on CT scan to have a 4-cm lesion in the periphery of the left lobe of the liver. The lesion enhances on the arterial phase of the CT scan and has a central scar suggestive of focal nodular hyperplasia (FNH). Which of the following is the recommended treatment of this lesion?

a. No further treatment is necessary
b. Wedge resection of the lesion
c. Formal left hepatectomy
d. Intra-arterial embolization of the lesion
e. Radiofrequency ablation of the liver lesion

324. A 57-year-old previously alcoholic man with a history of chronic pancreatitis presents with hematemesis. Endoscopy reveals isolated gastric varices in the absence of esophageal varices. His liver function tests are normal and he has no stigmata of end-stage liver disease. Ultrasound examination demonstrates normal portal flow but a thrombosed splenic vein. He undergoes banding, which is initially successful, but he subsequently rebleeds during the same hospitalization. Attempts to control the bleeding endoscopically are unsuccessful. Which of the following is the most appropriate next step in management?

a. Transjugular intrahepatic portosystemic shunt
b. Surgical portocaval shunt
c. Surgical mesocaval shunt
d. Splenectomy
e. Placement of a Sengstaken-Blakemore tube

325. A previously healthy 15-year-old boy is brought to the emergency room with complaints of about 12 hour of progressive anorexia, nausea, and pain of the right lower quadrant. On physical examination, he is found to have a rectal temperature of 38.18°C (100.72°F) and direct and rebound abdominal tenderness localizing to McBurney point as well as involuntary guarding in the right lower quadrant. At operation through a McBurney-type incision, the appendix and cecum are found to be normal, but the surgeon is impressed by the marked edema of the terminal ileum, which also has an overlying fibrinopurulent exudate. Which of the following is the most appropriate next step?

a. Close the abdomen after culturing the exudate.
b. Perform a standard appendectomy.
c. Resect the involved terminal ileum.
d. Perform an ileocolic resection.
e. Perform an ileocolostomy to bypass the involved terminal ileum.

326. A 32-year-old woman undergoes a cholecystectomy for acute chole-cystitis and is discharged home on the sixth postoperative day. She returns to the clinic 8 months after the operation for a routine visit and is noted by the surgeon to be jaundiced. Laboratory values on readmission show total biliru-bin 5.6 mg/dL, direct bilirubin 4.8 mg/dL, alkaline phosphatase 250 IU (nor-mal 21-91 IU), Serum glutamic oxaloacetic transaminase (SGOT) 52 kU (normal 10-40 kU), and Serum glutamic pyruvic transaminase (SGPT) 51 kU (normal 10-40 kU). An ultrasonogram shows dilated intrahepatic ducts. The patient undergoes the transhepatic cholangiogram seen here. Which of the following is the most appropriate next management step?

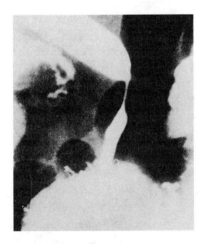

a. Choledochoplasty with insertion of a T tube
b. End-to-end choledochocholedochal anastomosis
c. Roux-en-Y hepaticojejunostomy
d. Percutaneous transhepatic dilatation
e. Choledochoduodenostomy

327. After complete removal of a sessile polyp of 2.0 cm by 1.5 cm found one finger length above the anal mucocutaneous margin, the pathologist reports it to have been a villous adenoma that contained carcinoma in situ. Which of the following is the most appropriate next step in management?

a. Reexcision of the biopsy site with wider margins
b. Abdominoperineal rectosigmoid resection
c. Anterior resection of the rectum
d. External radiation therapy to the rectum
e. No further therapy

328. A 62-year-old man has been noticing progressive difficulty swallowing, first solid food and now liquids as well. A barium study shows a ragged narrowing just below the carinal level. Endoscopic biopsy confirms squamous cell carcinoma. Which of the following statements concerning carcinoma of the esophagus is true?

a. Alcohol has not been implicated as a precipitating factor.
b. Squamous carcinoma is the most common type at the cardioesophageal junction.
c. It has a higher incidence in females.
d. It occurs more commonly in patients with corrosive esophagitis.
e. The standard of care is radiation therapy.

329. A 53-year-old woman with a history of a vagotomy and antrectomy with Billroth II reconstruction for peptic ulcer disease presents with recurrent abdominal pain. An esophagogastroduodenoscopy (EGD) demonstrates that ulcer and serum gastrin levels are greater than 1000 pg/mL on three separate determinations (normal is 40-150). Which of the following is the best test for confirming a diagnosis of gastrinoma?

a. A 24-hour urine gastrin level
b. A secretin stimulation test
c. A serum glucagon level
d. A 24-hour urine secretin level
e. A serum glucose to insulin ratio

330. A 52-year-old man with a family history of multiple endocrine neoplasia type I (MEN-1) has an elevated gastrin level and is suspected to have a gastrinoma. Which of the following is the most likely location for his tumor?

a. Fundus of the stomach
b. Antrum of the stomach
c. Within the triangle formed by the junction of the second and third portions of the duodenum, the junction of the neck and body of the pancreas, and the junction of the cystic and common bile duct
d. Tail of the pancreas
e. Within the triangle formed by the inferior edge of the liver, the cystic duct, and the common hepatic duct

331. A 73-year-old woman presents to the emergency room complaining of severe epigastric pain radiating to her back, nausea, and vomiting. CT scan of the abdomen demonstrates inflammation and edema of the pancreas. A right upper quadrant ultrasound demonstrates the presence of stones in the gallbladder. Which of the following is true regarding her prognosis?

a. An amylase level greater than 1000 mg/dL correlates with an increased risk for complications.
b. Her age is a negative prognostic factor.
c. A total bilirubin greater than 3.0 mg/dL is the most important predictor of outcome.
d. A low albumin is a positive prognostic factor.
e. A base deficit of more than 5 mEq/L is the most important predictor of outcome.

332. A 55-year-old man who is extremely obese reports weakness, sweating, tachycardia, confusion, and headache whenever he fasts for more than a few hours. He has prompt relief of symptoms when he eats. Which of the following statements is true regarding his diagnosis?

a. The tumor arises from the pancreatic α-cells.
b. Simple excision is curative in the majority of cases.
c. Symptoms arise from a rapidly rising glucose level.
d. The majority of tumors are malignant.
e. Standard of treatment is chemotherapy and radiation.

333. A 57-year-old woman sees blood on the toilet paper. Her doctor notes the presence of an excoriated bleeding 2.8-cm mass at the anus. Biopsy confirms the clinical suspicion of anal cancer. In planning the management of a 2.8-cm epidermoid carcinoma of the anus, which of the following is the best initial management strategy?

a. Abdominoperineal resection
b. Wide local resection with bilateral inguinal node dissection
c. Local radiation therapy
d. Systemic chemotherapy
e. Combined radiation therapy and chemotherapy

334. An 80-year-old man is admitted to the hospital complaining of nausea, abdominal pain, distention, and diarrhea. A cautiously performed transanal contrast study reveals an apple-core configuration in the rectosigmoid area. Which of the following is the most appropriate next step in his management?

a. Colonoscopic decompression and rectal tube placement
b. Saline enemas and digital disimpaction of fecal matter from the rectum
c. Colon resection and proximal colostomy
d. Oral administration of metronidazole and checking a *Clostridium difficile* titer
e. Evaluation of an electrocardiogram and obtaining an angiogram to evaluate for colonic mesenteric ischemia

335. Patients with Crohn disease are frequently seen in your office. A 46-year-old woman asks about the need for surgery, since she was recently diagnosed with the disease. Indications for operation in Crohn disease include all but which of the following?

a. Intestinal obstruction
b. Enterovesical fistula
c. Ileum–ascending colon fistula
d. Enterovaginal fistula
e. Free perforation

336. A 50-year-old man presents to the emergency room with a 6-hour history of excruciating abdominal pain and distention. The abdominal film shown here is obtained. Which of the following is the most appropriate next diagnostic maneuver?

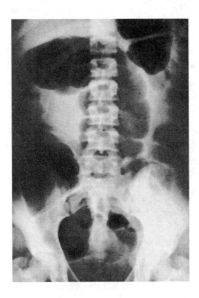

a. Emergency celiotomy
b. Upper GI series with small-bowel follow-through
c. CT scan of the abdomen
d. Barium enema
e. Sigmoidoscopy

337. A septuagenarian woman undergoes an uncomplicated resection of an abdominal aneurysm. Four days after surgery the patient presents with sudden onset of abdominal pain and distention. An abdominal radiograph demonstrates an air-filled, kidney-bean–shaped structure in the left upper quadrant. Which of the following is the most appropriate management at this time?

a. Decompression of the large bowel via colonoscopy
b. Placement of the NG tube and administration of low-dose cholinergic drugs
c. Administration of a gentle saline enema and encouragement of ambulation
d. Operative decompression with transverse colostomy
e. Right hemicolectomy

338. A visitor from abroad presents with abdominal pain and fever. CT scan shows a large, calcified cystic mass in the right lobe of the liver. Echinococcus is suggested by the CT findings. Which of the following is the most appropriate management of echinococcal liver cysts?

a. A large cyst should be treated by percutaneous aspiration of its contents.
b. Medical treatment with albendazole usually preempts the need for surgical drainage.
c. Negative serologic tests suggest that the cyst is chronic and inactive and that no treatment is indicated.
d. Leakage of cyst fluid puts the patient at risk for anaphylactic reaction.
e. Coexistent extrahepatic cysts are uncommon.

339. A 28-year-old woman who is 15 weeks pregnant has new onset of nausea, vomiting, and right-sided abdominal pain. She has been free of nausea since early in her first trimester. The pain has become worse over the past 6 hours. Which of the following statements regarding appendicitis during pregnancy is correct?

a. Appendicitis is the most prevalent extrauterine indication for celiotomy during pregnancy.
b. Appendicitis occurs more commonly in pregnant women than in nonpregnant women of comparable age.
c. Suspected appendicitis in a pregnant woman should be managed with a period of observation due to the risks of laparotomy to the fetus.
d. Noncomplicated appendicitis results in a 20% fetal mortality and premature labor rate.
e. The severity of appendicitis correlates with increased gestational age of the fetus.

340. A 56-year-old woman has nonspecific complaints that include an abnormal sensation when swallowing. An esophagram is obtained. Which of the following is most likely to require surgical correction?

a. Large sliding esophageal hiatal hernia
b. Paraesophageal hiatal hernia
c. Traction diverticulum of esophagus
d. Schatzki ring of distal esophagus
e. Esophageal web

341. A 65-year-old man who is hospitalized with pancreatic carcinoma develops abdominal distention and obstipation. The following abdominal radiograph is obtained. Which of the following is the most appropriate management of this patient?

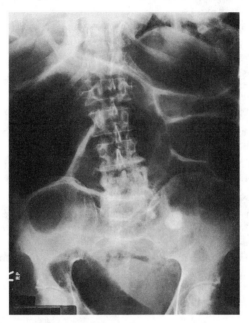

a. Urgent colostomy or cecostomy
b. Discontinuation of anticholinergic medications and narcotics and correction of metabolic disorders
c. Digital disimpaction of fecal mass in the rectum
d. Diagnostic and therapeutic colonoscopy
e. Detorsion of volvulus and colopexy or resection

342. A 48-year-old man presents with jaundice and right upper quadrant pain. Endoscopy shows blood coming from the ampulla of Vater. True statements regarding hemobilia include which of the following?

a. The classic presentation includes biliary colic, jaundice, and GI bleeding.
b. Spontaneous bleeding secondary to hematologic disorders is the major cause of this disorder.
c. Percutaneous transhepatic catheter placement of an absorbable gelatin sponge (Gelfoam) is the preferred treatment in cases of significant intrahepatic bleeding.
d. Angiography and endoscopy have no role in the treatment of intrahepatic bleeding.
e. Arterial embolization is advocated for hemobilia from the extrahepatic bile ducts.

343. A 30-year-old female patient who presents with bleeding per rectum is found at colonoscopy to have colitis confined to the transverse and descending colon. A biopsy is performed. Which of the following statements is true about this patient?

a. The inflammatory process is likely to be confined to the mucosa and submucosa.
b. The inflammatory reaction is likely to be continuous.
c. Superficial as opposed to linear ulcerations can be expected.
d. Noncaseating granulomas can be expected in up to 50% of patients with similar disease.
e. Microabscesses within crypts are common.

344. A 24-year-old man presents to the emergency room with abdominal pain and fever. CT scan of the abdomen reveals inflammation of the terminal ileum. He is referred to a gastroenterologist, where he is given the new diagnosis of Crohn disease. Regarding the risk of complications from this disease, which of the following statements is true?

a. The occurrence of toxic megacolon is common.
b. Perforation occurs in about 25% of patients with similar disease.
c. Fistulas between the colon and segments of intestine, bladder, vagina, urethra, and skin may develop.
d. Extraintestinal manifestations including uveitis and erythema nodosum would be exceedingly rare in this patient.
e. This patient would be at no increased risk for the development of cancer of the colon as compared with an age-matched population.

345. An upper GI series is performed on a 71-year-old woman who presented with several months of chest pain that occurs when she is eating. The film shown here is obtained. Investigation reveals a microcytic anemia and erosive gastritis on upper endoscopy. Which of the following statements about the patient's condition is true?

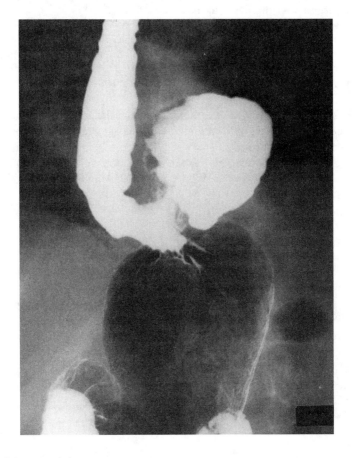

a. It is congenital.
b. The gastroesophageal junction is above the diaphragm.
c. Ulceration, gastritis, and anemia are common.
d. It usually is controlled by medical therapy.
e. Surgical treatment, if indicated, should be delayed up to 3 months to allow inflammation around the gastroesophageal junction to subside.

346. A 54-year-old man complains that his eyes are yellow. His bilirubin is elevated. His physical examination is unremarkable. A CT of the abdomen shows a mass in the head of the pancreas. Cytology from the ERCP is positive for cancer. Which of the following statements regarding adenocarcinoma of the pancreas is true?

a. It occurs most frequently in the body of the gland.
b. It carries a 1% to 2% 5-year survival rate.
c. It is nonresectable if it presents as painless jaundice.
d. It can usually be resected if it presents in the body or tail of the pancreas and does not involve the common bile duct.
e. It is associated with diabetes insipidus.

347. A 28-year-old woman presents with hematochezia. She is admitted to the hospital and undergoes upper endoscopy that is negative for any lesions. Colonoscopy is performed and no bleeding sources are identified, although the gastroenterologist notes blood in the right colon and old blood coming from above the ileocecal valve. Which of the following is the test of choice in this patient?

a. Angiography
b. Small-bowel enteroclysis
c. CT scan of the abdomen
d. Technetium 99m (^{99m}Tc) pertechnetate scan
e. Small-bowel endoscopy

348. A 32-year-old woman undergoes an uncomplicated appendectomy for acute appendicitis. The pathology report notes the presence of a 1-cm carcinoid tumor in the tip of the appendix. Which of the following is the most appropriate management of this patient?

a. Right hemicolectomy
b. Right hemicolectomy and chemotherapy
c. Chemotherapy only
d. Radiation only
e. No further treatment

349. A 58-year-old man presents with a bulge in his right groin associated with mild discomfort. On examination the bulge is easily reducible and descends into the scrotum. Which of the following statements regarding inguinal hernias is true?

a. They are more common in women.
b. Direct inguinal hernias protrude medially to the inferior epigastric vessels.
c. They should be immediately repaired if they descend into the scrotum.
d. Chronic incarceration is an indication for urgent surgical repair.
e. All incarcerated hernias eventually lead to strangulation.

350. A 35-year-old woman presents with pancreatitis. Subsequent ERCP reveals the congenital cystic anomaly of her biliary system illustrated in the film shown here. Which of the following statements regarding this problem is true?

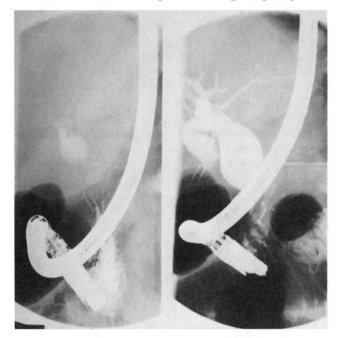

a. Treatment consists of internal drainage via choledochoduodenostomy.
b. Malignant changes may occur within this structure.
c. Most patients present with the classic triad of epigastric pain, an abdominal mass, and jaundice.
d. Cystic dilation of the intrahepatic biliary tree may coexist and is managed in a similar fashion.
e. Surgery should be reserved for symptomatic patients.

351. A 36-year-old man is in your intensive care unit following thoracotomy for a 24-hour-old esophageal perforation. His WBC is markedly elevated, and he is febrile and hypotensive. His NG tube fills with blood and continues to bleed. Emergency upper endoscopy documents diffuse gastric erosions. Which of the following statements regarding stress ulceration is true?

a. It is true ulceration, extending into and through the muscularis mucosa.
b. It classically involves the antrum.
c. Increased secretion of gastric acid has been shown to play a causative role.
d. It frequently involves multiple sites.
e. It is seen following shock or sepsis, but for some unknown reason does not occur following major surgery, trauma, or burns.

352. A patient with known gallstones presents with right upper quadrant pain, fever, jaundice, and shaking chills. He is febrile. Cholangitis is suspected. Which of the following statements concerning cholangitis is correct?

a. The most common infecting organism is *Staphylococcus aureus*.
b. The diagnosis is suggested by the Charcot triad.
c. The disease occurs primarily in young, immunocompromised patients.
d. Cholecystostomy is the procedure of choice in affected patients.
e. Surgery is indicated once the diagnosis of cholangitis is made.

353. An 88-year-old man with a history of end-stage renal failure, severe coronary artery disease, and brain metastases from lung cancer presents with acute cholecystitis. His family wants "everything done." Which of the following is the best management option in this patient?

a. Tube cholecystostomy
b. Open cholecystectomy
c. Laparoscopic cholecystectomy
d. Intravenous antibiotics followed by elective cholecystectomy
e. Lithotripsy followed by long-term bile acid therapy

354. After a weekend drinking binge, a 45-year-old alcoholic man presents to the hospital with abdominal pain, nausea, and vomiting. On physical examination, the patient is afebrile and is noted to have a palpable tender mass in the epigastrium. Laboratory tests reveal an amylase of 250 U/dL (normal <180 U/dL). A CT scan done on the second hospital day is pictured here. Which of the following statements concerning this patient's condition is true?

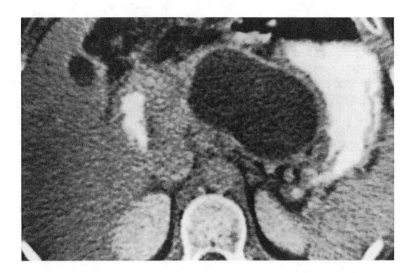

a. The mass may cause gastric outlet or extrahepatic biliary obstruction.
b. Spontaneous resolution almost never occurs.
c. The mass is seen only with acute pancreatitis.
d. The mass has an epithelial lining.
e. Malignant degeneration occurs in about 25% of cases if left untreated.

355. Upper endoscopy is performed on a patient with recurrent small upper GI bleeding episodes. A lesion is seen in the proximal stomach that is characterized as a bleeding vessel. Dieulafoy lesion of the stomach is suspected. Which of the following best characterizes this lesion?

a. A large mucosal defect with underlying friable vascular plexus
b. Frequent rebleeding after endoscopic treatment
c. Massive bleeding that requires subtotal gastrectomy
d. Location in the proximal stomach
e. Acid-peptic changes of the gastric mucosa

356. During an appendectomy for acute appendicitis, a 4-cm mass is found in the midportion of the appendix. Frozen section reveals this lesion to be a carcinoid tumor. Which of the following statements is true?

a. No further surgery is indicated.
b. A right hemicolectomy should be performed.
c. There is about a 50% chance that this patient will develop the carcinoid syndrome.
d. Carcinoid tumors arise from islet cells.
e. Carcinoid syndrome can occur only in the presence of liver metastases.

357. A 45-year-old man is examined for a yearly executive physical. A small mass is palpated in the rectum, and sigmoidoscopy demonstrates it to be a 2-cm mass covered by normal rectal mucosa. Biopsy suggests carcinoid. Which of the following is true regarding rectal carcinoid tumors?

a. Endoscopic resection is sufficient for tumors smaller than 2 cm.
b. Patients frequently present with the carcinoid syndrome.
c. They are rapidly growing tumors.
d. Local recurrence is rare with complete resection of the primary lesion.
e. Patients can develop the carcinoid syndrome even in the absence of liver metastases.

358. An ultrasound is performed on a patient with right upper quadrant pain. It demonstrates a large gallstone in the cystic duct but also a polypoid mass in the fundus. Which of the following is an indication for cholecystectomy for a polypoid gallbladder lesion?

a. Size greater than 0.5 cm
b. Presence of clinical symptoms
c. Patient age of older than 25 years
d. Presence of multiple small lesions
e. Absence of shadowing on ultrasound

359. An alcoholic man has been suffering excruciating pain recalcitrant to analgesics and splanchnic block. A surgeon recommends total pancreatectomy. A patient who has a total pancreatectomy might be expected to develop which of the following complications?

a. Diabetes mellitus
b. Hypercalcemia
c. Hyperphosphatemia
d. Constipation
e. Weight gain

360. Incidental finding of a liver mass that enhances with intravenous contrast prompts a surgical consultation. Magnetic resonance imaging (MRI) is suggestive of a hemangioma. Which of the following is true regarding hemangiomas of the liver in adults?

a. They are the most common benign tumor of the liver.
b. They may undergo malignant transformation.
c. They require hormonal stimulation for growth.
d. They should be resected to avoid spontaneous rupture and life-threatening hemorrhage.
e. Percutaneous biopsy is recommended prior to surgical resection.

361. A right hemicolectomy is performed on a 57-year-old woman with adenocarcinoma who had a preoperative elevation of CEA to 123 ng/mL. After falling to normal levels postoperatively, her most recent (24-month) follow-up level was 85 ng/mL. Correct statements regarding CEA and colorectal tumors include which of the following?

a. Elevated CEA is indicative of a tumor of GI origin.
b. A low CEA level after resection of a colon tumor is a poor marker of disease control.
c. Ninety percent of colorectal tumors produce CEA.
d. There is a high likelihood of liver involvement if the CEA level is high (greater than 100 ng/mL).
e. CEA levels are unusually low in cigarette smokers.

362. A 61-year-old woman with a history of unstable angina complains of hematemesis after retching and vomiting following a night of binge drinking. Endoscopy reveals a longitudinal mucosal tear at the gastroesophageal junction, which is not actively bleeding. Which of the following is the next recommended step in the management of this patient?

a. Angiography with embolization
b. Balloon tamponade
c. Exploratory laparotomy, gastrotomy, and oversewing of the tear
d. Systemic vasopressin infusion
e. Expectant management

Questions 363 to 366

Select the most appropriate diagnosis for each patient. Each lettered option may be used once, more than once, or not at all.

a. Symptomatic cholelithiasis
b. Acute cholecystitis
c. Gallstone pancreatitis
d. Choledocholithiasis
e. Cholangitis

363. A 62-year-old man presents with right upper quadrant abdominal pain and jaundice. He is afebrile with normal vital signs. On laboratory findings he has elevated bilirubin and alkaline phosphatase. Ultrasound demonstrates gallstones, normal gallbladder wall thickness, no pericholecystic fluid, and a common bile duct of 1.0 cm.

364. A 36-year-old woman presents with right upper quadrant abdominal pain and jaundice. She is febrile and tachycardic. On labs she has leukocytosis and elevated bilirubin and alkaline phosphatase. Ultrasound demonstrates gallstones, normal gallbladder wall thickness, no pericholecystic fluid, and a common bile duct of 1.0 cm.

365. A 55-year-old man presents with intermittent right upper quadrant abdominal pain. Each episode of pain lasts 1 to 2 hours. He is afebrile with normal vital signs. On labs he has no leukocytosis and normal bilirubin, alkaline phosphatase, amylase, and lipase. Ultrasound demonstrates gallstones, normal gallbladder wall thickness, no pericholecystic fluid, and a common bile duct of 3 mm.

366. A 23-year-old woman presents with epigastric abdominal pain and nausea. She is afebrile with normal vital signs. On labs she has no leukocytosis with normal bilirubin and alkaline phosphatase. The amylase and lipase are elevated. Ultrasound demonstrates gallstones, normal gallbladder wall thickness, no pericholecystic fluid, and a common bile duct of 3 mm.

Questions 367 to 370

Select the most appropriate surgical procedure for each patient. Each lettered option may be used once, more than once, or not at all.

a. Low anterior resection
b. Abdominoperineal resection
c. Subtotal colectomy with end ileostomy
d. Total proctocolectomy with ileoanal J-pouch
e. Sigmoid resection with end colostomy (Hartmann procedure)
f. Transanal excision
g. Diverting colostomy

367. A 37-year-old man with a 10-year history of UC who has a sessile polyp 10 cm from the anal verge with high-grade dysplasia.

368. A 60-year-old woman with recurrent squamous cell carcinoma of the anus after chemoradiation.

369. A 68-year-old woman with fecal incontinence who presents with a large fixed adenocarcinoma 3 cm from the anal verge.

370. A 33-year-old man with a history of Crohn disease presents with severe abdominal pain and fever. On examination, his heart rate is 130 beats per minute, blood pressure 105/62 mm Hg, and temperature 38.9°C (102°F). Workup reveals a leukocytosis of 32,000/mm^3. Plain films reveal a markedly dilated large colon.

Gastrointestinal Tract, Liver, and Pancreas

Answers

292. The answer is d. (*McQuaid, pp 285-316.*) Omeprazole (Prilosec) irreversibly inhibits the hydrogen-potassium-ATPase (proton pump) in the secretory canaliculus of the gastric parietal cell. This blocks the last step in the acid-secretory process. Omeprazole's duration of action exceeds 24 hours, and doses of 20 to 30 mg/day inhibit more than 90% of 24-hour acid secretion. Omeprazole provides excellent suppression of meal-stimulated and nocturnal acid secretion and seems very safe for short-term therapy. Prolonged administration in laboratory animals has been associated with significant hypergastrinemia, hyperplasia of enterochromaffin-like cells, and carcinoid tumors.

293. The answer is c. (*Townsend, pp 1628-1630.*) Patients with ITP who are asymptomatic and have a platelet count greater than 30,000/µL can be treated expectantly with follow-up. Of these patients, those with a platelet count between 30,000 and 50,000/µL have an increased risk for more severe thrombocytopenia. Patients with a platelet count lower than 30,000/µL or less than 50,000/µL with significant bleeding or risk factors for bleeding should be treated. Initial medical treatment with prednisone (1 mg/kg), and intravenous immunoglobulin is used in patients with severe bleeding or preoperatively prior to splenectomy. Platelet transfusions are reserved for patients with acute bleeding. Splenectomy is indicated in patients who have severe symptomatic thrombocytopenia, patients in whom remission is achieved only with toxic doses of steroids, patients with a relapse after initial steroid therapy, patients with persistent thrombocytopenia for more than 3 months and a platelet count less than 30,000/µL, and possibly in patients with a persistent platelet count of less than 10,000/µL after 6 weeks of therapy. The platelet count can be expected to rise shortly after splenectomy, and prolonged remissions are expected in approximately two-thirds of cases.

294. The answer is e. (*Townsend, p 1345.*) Patients with appendiceal adenocarcinoma, a rare neoplasm accounting for less than 0.5% of GI tumors, should undergo formal right hemicolectomy. Often affecting older patients, they may present with symptoms mimicking those of acute appendicitis. A thorough initial workup and follow-up are necessary because of the high rate of synchronous and metachronous tumors. Five-year survival is 55% but depends on the tumor stage.

295. The answer is c. (*Townsend, pp 1064-1069.*) Patients with achalasia, which is a functional disorder caused by failure of relaxation of the lower esophageal sphincter, typically present with dysphagia, chest pain, and regurgitation of saliva and undigested food. The characteristic appearance of the esophagram is the tapered bird's-beak deformity at the level of the esophagogastric junction; the esophagus is often dilated and may contain an air-fluid level. Manometry yields high resting pressures of the LES, which fails to relax or only partially relaxes. The absence of peristaltic deglutitory contractions in the body of the esophagus is also noted during manometry. Initial management of achalasia includes medications (calcium-channel blockers or long-acting nitrates), and other management options include endoscopic dilation or injection of botulinum toxin (Botox) into the LES. Surgery results in improvement in more than 90% of patients, compared with only 70% of patients treated by forceful dilatation. Surgical treatment is an esophagomyotomy. Patients with achalasia have seven times the risk of developing squamous cell carcinoma as the general population. This dreaded complication can occur even after successful treatment for the disease.

296. The answer is b. (*Townsend, pp 1373-1384.*) Although total procto-colectomy may relieve or resolve extraintestinal manifestations of UC such as peripheral arthritis or ankylosing spondylitis, surgery is not preventative or curative for primary sclerosing cholangitis. The risk of colon cancer in pancolitis is 0% to 3% at 5 and 10 years and increases to 50% after 30 years with the disease. In patients with both PSC and UC, the risk of cancer is increased fivefold from that for patients with UC alone. Indications for operative intervention in UC include acute management of toxic megacolon or fulminant colitis and definitive management for intractable disease or presence of high-grade dysplasia or carcinoma. Definitive surgical management options for UC include total proctocolectomy with end ileostomy (typically reserved for older or incontinent patients) and total proctocolectomy with ileoanal pouch anastomosis. In patients undergoing emergent colectomy for toxic megacolon, total abdominal colectomy without resection of the rectum can be performed initially. However, given that UC always involves the rectum, definitive management of UC requires resection of most of the rectal mucosa, although controversy exists regarding retention of the very distal rectal mucosa such as with a stapled ileoanal anastomosis.

297. The answer is d. *(Townsend, pp 1603-1606.)* The patient most likely has an infected pancreatic pseudocyst. Pseudocysts are nonepithelialized fluid collections that can present at earliest 4 to 6 weeks after an episode of acute pancreatitis. The treatment for infected pancreatic pseudocysts is similar to that for pancreatic abscesses—percutaneous catheter drainage with antibiotics. Aspiration of the fluid can be diagnostic but is not a definitive treatment, even with the addition of antibiotics. Internal drainage of pancreatic pseudocysts is contraindicated in the presence of infection but is the treatment of choice for mature, symptomatic, noninfected pseudocysts. Malignancy should be excluded if there is no preceding history of pancreatitis.

298. The answer is a. *(Townsend, pp 1610-1612.)* This woman has a cystadenocarcinoma arising from the pancreatic body and tail; the treatment is surgical resection. About 90% of primary malignant neoplasms of the exocrine pancreas are adenocarcinomas of duct cell origin. The remaining neoplasms include serous and mucinous cystadenomas/cystadenocarcinomas, solid pseudopapillary tumors, and intraductal mucinous papillary adenomas/tumors. Cystadenocarcinomas may be several times the size of typical ductal cancers and often arise in the body or tail of the pancreas. They may become very large without invading adjacent viscera and do not generally cause significant pain or weight loss. The clinical presentation is usually quite subtle, with symptoms related primarily to the enlarging mass. There are no diagnostic laboratory findings, and definitive preoperative diagnosis is rare. An elderly patient with no history of pancreatitis is unlikely to have a pseudocyst, and a benign neoplasm is also less likely in this age group. Endoscopic ultrasound and aspiration of the cyst fluid can assist with the diagnosis; a high CEA level and low amylase level in the cyst fluid can be suggestive of malignancy. Aggressive surgical resection is indicated for cystic neoplasms of the pancreas. Internal drainage is the treatment of choice for noninfected pancreatic pseudocysts (as opposed to external drainage which is the treatment of choice for infected pseudocysts) but is contraindicated if malignancy is suspected. ERCP with stent placement may be indicated in patients with pancreatic pseudocyst with fistula and proximal ductal stricture, but it has no role in the treatment of pancreatic malignancies. Percutaneous drainage is contraindicated in malignancies as well.

299. The answer is c. *(Townsend, pp 357-358.)* According to the United Ostomy Association Data Registry, the most frequent serious complication of end colostomies is parastomal herniation, which commonly occurs when the stoma is placed lateral to, rather than through, the rectus muscle. Symptomatic herniation requires operative relocation of the stoma or mesh herniorrhaphy. Minor problems are frequently encountered with colostomies. They include irregularity of function, irritation of the skin due to leakage of enteric contents, or bleeding from the exposed mucosa following trauma. Prolapse occurs most frequently with transverse loop colostomies and is likely due to the use of the transverse loop to decompress distal colon obstructions. As the intestine decompresses, it retracts from the edge of the surrounding fascia, which allows prolapse or herniation of the mobile transverse colon. Optimal treatment of stomal prolapse is restoration of intestinal continuity or conversion to an end colostomy. Perforation of a stoma is usually because of careless instrumentation with an irrigation catheter.

300. The answer is c. *(Blumgart, pp 1074, 1084.)* Involvement of the superior mesenteric artery by a pancreatic tumor precludes resection for cure and therefore is a contraindication to proceeding with a Whipple procedure of pancreaticoduodenectomy. Involvement of the superior mesenteric vein does not necessarily preclude resection for cure, as 2 to 3 cm of the portal vein/superior mesenteric vein can be resected and an end-to-end anastomosis or venous bypass can be performed. Pyloric preservation is a well-accepted modification of the Whipple procedure. Total pancreatectomy is reserved for patients with extensive low-grade or extensive intraductal papillary lesions involving most of the pancreas. Preoperative biliary stenting is controversial with regard to the risk of increased infectious complications postoperatively; preoperative stenting does not improve survival.

301. The answer is a. *(Greenfield, pp 725-727.)* In patients with no prior history of peptic ulcer disease, simple closure with an omental patch is recommended. Patients with long-standing ulcer disease require a definitive acid-reducing procedure, except in high-risk situations and if the perforation is more than 12 hours old secondary to extensive peritoneal soilage. The choice of procedure is made by weighing the risk of recurrence against the incidence of undesirable side effects of the procedure, and considerable controversy persists about this issue. Antrectomy and truncal vagotomy offers a recurrence rate of 1%, but carries a 15% to 25% incidence of sequelae such as diarrhea, dumping syndrome, bloating, and gastric stasis. Highly selective vagotomy, if technically feasible, offers a 1% to 5% incidence of side effects but carries a recurrence rate of 10% to 13% in some series, although results are better when gastric and prepyloric ulcers are excluded. Pyloroplasty and truncal vagotomy carries intermediate rates of recurrence and side effects, but has the advantage of speed in the setting of very ill patients with acute perforation.

302. The answer is b. (*Townsend, pp 1252-1253.*) Though reminiscent of the carcinoid syndrome, this patient's complaints in the context of recent gastric surgery are highly suggestive of the dumping syndrome, which is characterized by intestinal symptoms (bloating, cramping, diarrhea) and vasomotor symptoms (weakness, flushing, palpitations, diaphoresis, and dizziness) after ingestion of a meal following surgical removal of part of the stomach or alteration of the pyloric sphincter. Early dumping occurs within 20 to 30 minutes of eating and is attributed to the rapid influx of fluid with a high osmotic gradient into the small intestine from the gastric remnant. Late dumping syndrome occurs 2 to 3 hours after a meal; symptoms resemble those of hypoglycemic shock. Medical management consists of reassurance and dietary measures (avoidance of large amounts of sugars, frequent small meals, and separation of fluids and solids). The majority of cases will resolve within 3 months of operation on this regimen. Octreotide, a long-acting somatostatin analogue, can be used as well, but cost is a limiting factor. Surgery for intractable dumping consists of creation of an antiperistaltic limb of jejunum distal to the gastrojejunostomy.

303. The answer is a. (*Townsend, pp 1210-1213.*) Restoration of circulating blood volume is the first priority in patients with an acute variceal bleed. Initial resuscitation should be with isotonic crystalloids followed by transfusion of blood. Elevated prothrombin times should be corrected with fresh-frozen plasma, and although mild hypersplenism and thrombocytopenia are associated with portal hypertension, platelet transfusion is indicated only for platelet counts less than $50,000/\mu L$. Medical therapy consists of either octreotide or vasopressin to decrease splanchnic blood flow. Because of coronary vasoconstrictive effects, nitroglycerin is usually administered concomitantly with vasopressin. β-Blockade (eg, propranolol), with or without a long-acting nitrate, has been used to prevent recurrent variceal bleeding, but is not indicated in the acutely bleeding patients who are hemodynamically unstable. Balloon tamponade controls variceal hemorrhage immediately in more than 85% of patients. However, although balloon tamponade

(Sengstaken-Blakemore tube) has reduced the mortality and morbidity from variceal hemorrhage in good-risk patients, an increased awareness of the associated complications (aspiration, asphyxiation, and ulceration at the tamponade site), as well as a rebleeding rate of 40%, have reduced its use. Balloon tamponade is indicated as a temporary measure when vasopressin or octreotide and sclerotherapy fail and other therapies are not immediately available (such as endoscopy with banding).

304. The answer is e. (*Townsend, pp 1210-1213.*) Patients with poorly compensated liver disease who develop recurrent variceal bleeds should undergo transjugular intrahepatic portosystemic shunting. β-Blockade and endoscopic therapy are typically used as initial therapeutic options for patients with variceal bleeds. In patients with well-compensated liver disease, portosystemic shunts can be used to prevent recurrent variceal bleeds. Portocaval, mesocaval, and splenorenal shunts are considered nonselective shunts and are associated with the development or worsening of encephalopathy postoperatively. The distal splenorenal shunt is a selective shunt procedure and is associated with a lower rate of encephalopathy. However, in patients with Child C cirrhosis (poorly compensated liver disease), surgical shunting should be avoided because of increased operative mortality. Hepatic transplantation is contraindicated in a patient who is actively drinking. Esophageal transection and reanastomosis, or the Sugiura procedure, are typically reserved for patients with splanchnic venous thrombosis who are not shunt candidates.

305. The answer is d. (*Townsend, pp 1236-1256.*) This patient has a persistent gastric ulcer and should undergo surgical resection via either a distal gastrectomy with gastroduodenostomy (Billroth I reconstruction) or with gastrojejunostomy (Billroth II reconstruction) to definitively rule out a malignancy. The initial management of a gastric ulcer consists of antimicrobial therapy directed against *H pylori*. Indications for surgical intervention are hemorrhage, perforation, disease refractory to medical therapy, and inability to rule out a malignancy. Only ulcers associated with acid hypersecretion require a vagotomy as well (type II—body of stomach, with concomitant duodenal ulcer, or type III—prepyloric). Type I (in the body and along the lesser curvature) and type IV (near the gastroesophageal junction) ulcers do not require vagotomy.

306. The answer is c. (*Townsend, pp 1406-1415.*) Five-year survival rates of 25% have been reported after synchronous resection of primary colorectal cancers and liver metastases. Because approximately 5% of colorectal cancers are associated with resectable hepatic metastases, appropriate preoperative discussion should include obtaining permission for removal of synchronous peripheral hepatic lesions if they are found. Although concomitant colon and liver resections can be safely performed Adequate local resection, either by wedge or by limited partial hepatectomy, may be carried out whenever no extrahepatic disease is found and the hepatic lesion is technically removable. Any option that leaves the symptomatic colon cancer (bleeding) would be unacceptable. Radiation therapy has little to offer in colon cancer or its hepatic metastases.

307. The answer is b. (*Schwesinger, pp 411-416.*) Helicobacter pylori infections have become extremely common: nearly one-third of all American adults are now infected. Morphologically, the organism is a gram-negative, corkscrew-shaped, motile bacillus with three to seven flagella. Noninvasive approaches with simple, relatively inexpensive serologic and urea breath tests can establish the diagnosis of *H pylori* infection. Culturing endoscopic scrapings or biopsy specimens has proved to be impractical because of the need for special media and elaborate growth conditions. A rapid urease test is used when endoscopy provides a specimen for analysis. Therapy is problematic because the organism is not easily eradicated. Monotherapy is largely ineffective. Eradication of *H pylori* requires triple therapy with colloidal bismuth (Pepto-Bismol), an antibiotic (amoxicillin or ampicillin), and a nitroimidazole such as metronidazole. However, dual- and triple-drug therapy can achieve eradication in 80% to 90% of patients. Unfortunately, compliance rates with multidrug therapy are low.

308. The answer is c. (*Greenfield, pp 1187-1206.*) An indirect inguinal hernia leaves the abdominal cavity by entering the dilated internal inguinal ring and passing along the anteromedial aspect of the spermatic cord. The internal inguinal ring is an opening in the transversalis fascia for the passage of the spermatic cord; an indirect inguinal hernia, therefore, lies within the fibers of the cremaster muscle. A femoral hernia passes directly beneath the inguinal ligament at a point medial to the femoral vessels, and a direct inguinal hernia passes through a weakness in the floor of the inguinal canal medial to the inferior epigastric artery. Neither lies within the cremaster muscle fibers. Spigelian hernias, which are rare, protrude through an anatomic defect that can occur along the lateral border of the rectus muscle at its junction with the linea semilunaris. An interparietal hernia is one in which the hernia sac, instead of protruding in the usual fashion, makes its way between the fascial layers of the abdominal wall. These unusual hernias may be preperitoneal (between the peritoneum and transversalis fascia), interstitial (between muscle layers), or superficial (between the external oblique aponeurosis and the skin).

309. The answer is b. *(Greenfield, p 990.)* The finding of air in the biliary tract of a nonseptic patient is diagnostic of a biliary enteric fistula. When the clinical findings also include small-bowel obstruction in an elderly patient with history of gallstones and no prior abdominal surgery (a virgin abdomen), the diagnosis of gallstone ileus can be made with a high degree of certainty. In this condition, a large chronic gallstone mechanically erodes through the wall of the gallbladder into adjacent stomach or duodenum. A connection is formed between the biliary system and the GI tract which allows air into the biliary tract. When the gallstone arrives in the distal ileum, the caliber of the bowel no longer allows passage, and a small-bowel obstruction develops. Surgical removal of the gallstone is necessary. The diseases suggested by the other response items (bleeding ulcer, peritoneal infection, pyloric outlet obstruction, pelvic neoplasm) are common in elderly patients, but each would probably present with symptoms other than those of small-bowel obstruction.

310. The answer is d. *(Townsend, pp 1400-1414.)* Cancer of the colon in patients with chronic UC is 10 times more frequent than in the general population. Duration of disease is very important; the risk of developing cancer is low in the first 10 years but thereafter rises about 4% per year. The average age of cancer development in patients with chronic UC is 37 years; idiopathic carcinoma of the colon, however, develops at an average age of 65 years. Crohn colitis is currently felt to be a precancerous condition as well. The chance of development of carcinoma of the colon in patients with familial polyposis is essentially 100%. Treatment of the patient with familial polyposis generally consists of total proctocolectomy with ileoanal J-pouch. Villous adenomas have been demonstrated to contain malignant portions in about one-third of affected persons and invasive malignancy in another one-third of removed specimens. Anterior resection is performed for large lesions or those containing invasive carcinomas when the lesion is above the peritoneal reflection. Abdominal-perineal resection (APR) is indicated for low-lying rectal villous adenomas when they have demonstrated invasive carcinomas. Transrectal excision with regular follow-up examinations is sufficient for lesions without invasive carcinomas. Peutz-Jeghers syndrome is characterized by intestinal polyposis and melanin spots of the oral mucosa. Unlike the adenomatous polyps seen in familial polyposis, the lesions in this condition are hamartomas, which have no malignant potential.

311. The answer is c. (*Greenfield, p 990.*) Gallstone ileus is caused by erosion of a stone from the gallbladder into the GI tract (most commonly the duodenum). The stone becomes lodged in the small bowel (usually in the terminal ileum) and causes small-bowel obstruction. Plain films of the abdomen that demonstrate small-bowel obstruction and air in the biliary tract are diagnostic of the condition. Treatment consists of ileotomy, removal of the stone, and cholecystectomy if it is technically safe. If there is significant inflammation of the right upper quadrant, ileotomy for stone extraction followed by an interval cholecystectomy is often a safer alternative. Operating on the biliary fistula doubles the mortality rate compared with simple removal of the gallstone from the intestine.

312. The answer is d. (*Townsend, pp 1365-1369.*) The indications for surgical intervention for diverticular disease include hemorrhage secondary to diverticulosis, recurrent episodes of diverticulitis, intractability to medical therapy, and complicated diverticulitis. The latter includes perforated diverticulitis with or without abscess and fistulous disease. Diverticular abscesses are treated with percutaneous drainage initially followed by definitive resectional therapy. Initial percutaneous drainage allows for a one-stage procedure that consists of resection of the affected colon with primary anastomosis. Perforated diverticulitis is typically treated with either the Hartmann procedure (sigmoid resection with end colostomy and rectal stump) or sigmoid resection, anastomosis, and diverting loop ileostomy.

313. The answer is d. (*Townsend, p 1562.*) Cholecystectomy results in improvement in symptoms in 85% to 94% of patients with biliary dyskinesia. The diagnosis is confirmed by CCK-HIDA scan. Technetium labeled hydroxyiminodiacetic acid (HIDA) is injected intravenously, which is subsequently excreted into the biliary tract. After filling of the gallbladder, cholecystokinin (CCK), a hormone that is normally released by the duodenum after ingestion of a meal, is infused intravenously to stimulate gallbladder contraction. A gallbladder ejection fraction of less than 35% at 20 minutes is diagnostic of biliary dyskinesia. There is no role for oral dissolutional therapy with ursodeoxycholic acid in the treatment of biliary colic, since no gallstones are present.

314. The answer is b. (*Townsend, pp 1578-1579.*) Gallbladder polyps can be observed with serial ultrasounds if they are less than 1 cm in size. Patients with suspected gallbladder carcinoma should undergo cholecystectomy with intraoperative frozen section, and if there is invasion of the serosa and no evidence of metastatic or extensive local disease, they should undergo a radical cholecystectomy (portal lymphadenectomy and either wedge or formal resection of the liver surrounding the gallbladder fossa in addition to the cholecystectomy). Bile aspiration does not have a role in the workup of gallbladder polyps or gallbladder carcinoma.

315. The answer is c. (*Townsend, p 1136.*) Hematomas of the rectus sheath are more common in the elderly, and a history of trauma, sudden muscular exertion, or anticoagulation can usually be elicited. The pain is of sudden onset and is sharp in nature. The hematoma typically presents as an abdominal mass that does not change with contraction of the rectus muscles. The diagnosis can be established preoperatively with an ultrasound or CT scan showing a mass within the rectus sheath. Management is conservative unless symptoms are severe and bleeding persists, in which case surgical evacuation of the hematoma and ligation of bleeding vessels may be required.

316. The answer is a. (*Blumgart, pp 1147-1157.*) Amebic liver abscesses should be treated initially with metronidazole monotherapy, as opposed to pyogenic liver abscesses, which are treated initially with percutaneous catheter drainage and antibiotics against gram-negative and anaerobic organisms (eg, *Essherichia coli, Klebisella pneumoniae,* bacteroides, enterococcus, and anaerobic streptococci). If improvement fails to occur, then other antimicrobial agents can be added. Abscesses that are refractory to medical therapy may require laparotomy.

317. The answer is b. (*Brunicardi, pp 911-918.*) Surgical treatment for sliding esophageal hernias (type I paraesophageal hernias) should be considered only in symptomatic patients with objectively documented esophagitis or stenosis. The overwhelming majority of sliding hiatal hernias are totally asymptomatic, even many of those with demonstrable reflux. Even in the presence of reflux, esophageal inflammation rarely develops because the esophagus is so efficient at clearing the refluxed acid. Symptomatic hernias should be treated vigorously by the variety of medical measures that have been found helpful. Patients who do have symptoms of episodic reflux and who remain untreated can expect their disease to progress to intolerable esophagitis or fibrosis and stenosis. Neither the presence of the hernia nor its size is important in deciding on surgical therapy. Once esophagitis has been documented to persist under adequate medical therapy, manometric or pH studies may help determine the optimum surgical treatment.

318. The answer is c. (*Brunicardi, pp 1357-1358.*) The patient has a bulge identified below the inguinal ligament which is consistent with a femoral hernia. A femoral hernia occurs through the femoral canal bounded superiorly by the iliopubic tract, inferiorly by Cooper ligament, laterally by the femoral vein, and medially by the junction of the iliopubic tract and Cooper ligament. The incidence of strangulation in femoral hernias is high. Therefore, all femoral hernias, even asymptomatic ones, should be repaired. This patient has no evidence of an acute incarceration and does not need emergent repair of her hernia at this time.

319. The answer is a. (*Townsend, pp 1449-1450.*) The patient has a pilonidal abscess which develops from an infected pilonidal cyst. It typically presents as a painful fluctuant mass extending from the midline and is located between the gluteal clefts. Perianal and perirectal abscesses are usually much closer to the anus and are very painful on rectal examination. A fistula-in-ano is a chronically draining tract in the perianal region. It may become plugged and develop a perianal or perirectal abscess. An anal fissure is a linear ulcer along the anal canal and is not associated with an abscess.

320. The answer is e. (*Townsend, pp 1389-1392.*) Ischemic colitis presents as hematochezia, fever, and abdominal pain. Unlike acute mesenteric ischemia, which affects the small intestine and requires emergent intervention, ischemic colitis rarely requires surgical intervention unless full-thickness necrosis, perforation, or refractory bleeding is present. Expectant management with intravenous fluids, bowel rest, and supportive care is the treatment of choice.

321. The answer is b. (*Greenfield, pp 1035-1036.*) Patients may undergo resection of a large fraction of the colon and suffer little long-term change in bowel habits because the reserve capacity of the colon for water absorption greatly exceeds the normal requirements for maintaining stable bowel function. However, in diseases characterized by increased fluid secretion of the small bowel, the colon is more likely to be overwhelmed by the absorptive demand following partial colectomy than in the intact state. The colon absorbs electrolytes, water, short-chain fatty acids, and vitamins. The right colon absorbs more salt and water than the left colon. The majority of normal feces are comprised by water. Sodium is absorbed by colonic epithelium by active transport, and potassium is excreted into the colonic lumen passively. Chloride and bicarbonate are exchanged across the epithelium–chloride is absorbed and bicarbonate is excreted.

322. The answer is d. *(Brunicardi, pp 1160-1161.)* Hepatic adenomas are associated with oral contraceptive use, and cessation of OCPs may be adequate to allow regression of the lesion if smaller than 4 cm. However, for lesions greater than 4 cm in size, surgical resection is advocated. Other indications for resection include failure to regress with cessation of OCPs or inability to stop taking OCPs and desire to become pregnant. Lesions greater than 4 cm in size have an increased risk of rupture with hemorrhage, which may in fact be the initial clinical presentation.

323. The answer is a. *(Brunicardi, pp 1160-1161.)* Focal nodular hyperplasia is rarely symptomatic and unlike a hepatic adenoma does not carry an associated risk of malignant degeneration or rupture with hemorrhage. Therefore, surgical resection for FNH is indicated only if the lesion is symptomatic. If FNH cannot be distinguished from a hepatic adenoma on CT scan, a nuclear medicine scan can be obtained that may demonstrate a "hot" lesion in the setting of FNH and a "cold" lesion in the setting of hepatic adenoma.

324. The answer is d. *(Brunicardi, p 1260.)* Splenectomy is indicated for acute hemorrhage secondary to left-sided, or sinistral, portal hypertension, which is characterized by gastric varices in the setting of splenic or portal vein thrombosis in the absence of cirrhosis. Patients who have either had an episode of acute or have chronic pancreatitis can develop either splenic or portal venous thrombosis. In the absence of bleeding complications, surgery is indicated only if other surgical procedures are planned.

325. The answer is b. *(Brunicardi, pp 1076-1081, 1127.)* Patients with regional enteritis usually have a chronic and slowly progressive course with intermittent symptom-free periods. The usual symptoms are anorexia, abdominal pain, diarrhea, fever, and weight loss. Extraintestinal syndromes that may be seen include ankylosing spondylitis, polyarthritis, erythema nodosum, pyoderma gangrenosum, gallstones, hepatic fatty infiltration, and fibrosis of the biliary tract, pancreas, and retroperitoneum. However, in about 10% of patients, especially those who are young, the onset of the disease is abrupt and may be mistaken for acute appendicitis. Appendectomy is indicated in such patients as long as the cecum at the base of the appendix is not involved; otherwise, the risk of fecal fistula must be considered. Interestingly, about 90% of patients who present with the acute appendicitis-like form of regional enteritis will not progress to development of the full-blown chronic disease. Thus, resection or bypass of the involved areas is not indicated at this time.

326. The answer is c. *(Brunicardi, pp 1211-1213.)* This scenario is typical for a patient with iatrogenic injury of the common bile duct. These injuries commonly occur in the proximal portion of the extrahepatic biliary system. The transhepatic cholangiogram documents a biliary stricture, which in this clinical setting is best dealt with surgically. Choledochoduodenostomy generally cannot be performed because of the proximal location of the stricture. The best results are achieved with end-to-side choledochojejunostomy (Roux-en-Y) performed over a stent. Percutaneous transhepatic dilatation has been attempted in select cases, but follow-up is too short to make an adequate assessment of this technique. Primary repair of the common bile duct may result in recurrent stricture.

327. The answer is e. *(Greenfield, pp 1088-1090.)* The term *carcinoma in situ* refers to the presence of malignant cells in the mucosal layer only. Endoscopic polypectomy is adequate treatment when malignant cells are identified in a colonic polyp, even if an invasive component is identified, if: (1) no vascular or lymphatic invasion is present; (2) there is an adequate negative margin (2 mm), and the cancer is not poorly differentiated.

328. The answer is d. *(Greenfield, pp 700-707.)* A high incidence of esophageal carcinoma is reported in patients with corrosive esophagitis. Alcohol, tobacco, and dietary factors are also associated with a higher incidence of esophageal carcinoma. Carcinoma of the esophagus occurs primarily in the sixth and seventh decades of life in a male to female ratio of 3 to 1. Malignant tumors arising in the esophagus are usually squamous cell carcinomas except for those involving the esophagogastric junction. These are usually adenocarcinomas. The prognosis is poor for patients with esophageal carcinoma and multimodality therapy has been utilized in attempts to improve mortality. Neoadjuvant (preoperative) chemoradiation appears to result in improved local and regional control and to improve survival in patients with both squamous cell and adenocarcinoma. However, the standard of care is still esophageal resection. Radiation therapy alone has been used for palliation in patients with squamous cell carcinoma of the esophagus.

329. The answer is b. *(Townsend, pp 986-987.)* A secretin stimulation test is highly useful to confirm the diagnosis of Zollinger-Ellison syndrome (ZES) (gastrinoma). In this test a fasting gastrin level is measured before administration of intravenous secretin and further samples of serum gastrin are obtained at 2, 5, 10, and 20 minutes after secretin administration. A rise in serum gastrin levels greater than 200 pg/mL above baseline after secretin administration is found in patients with ZES. The rest of the tests do not confirm the diagnosis of a gastrinoma.

330. The answer is c. *(Greenfield, pp 1331-1332.)* Ninety percent of gastrinomas are located within the gastrinoma triangle—the three corners of the triangle are defined by the junction of the second and third portions of the duodenum, the junction of the neck and body of the pancreas, and the junction of the cystic and common bile duct.

331. The answer is b. *(Brunicardi, pp 1236-1237.)* The patient has acute gallstone pancreatitis. Ranson criteria consists of five criteria on admission and six during the first 48 hours that predict mortality: less than two criteria are associated with 0% mortality, three to five criteria with 10% to 20% mortality, and six or more with greater than 50% mortality. The criteria are slightly different for gallstone pancreatitis and non–gallstone pancreatitis. The first five criteria assess age, WBC count, low-density hormone (LDH), aspartate aminotransferase (AST), and glucose. The second set of criteria assesses hematocrit fall, blood urea nitrogen (BUN) elevation, serum calcium, base deficit, and estimated fluid sequestration. Amylase is not one of the criteria and does not correlate with the severity of disease.

332. The answer is b. *(Townsend, pp 983-986.)* The patient's presentation is classic for an insulinoma. These tumors are treated surgically, and simple excision of an adenoma is curative in the majority of cases. Seventy-five percent of these tumors are benign adenomas, and in 15% of affected patients the adenomas are multiple. Tumors arising from the pancreatic β cells give rise to hyperinsulinism. Symptoms relate to a rapidly falling blood glucose level and are caused by epinephrine release triggered by hypoglycemia (sweating, weakness, tachycardia). Cerebral symptoms of headache, confusion, visual disturbances, convulsions, and coma are caused by glucose deprivation of the brain. Whipple triad summarizes the clinical findings in patients with insulinomas: (1) attacks precipitated by fasting or exertion, (2) fasting blood glucose concentrations below 50 mg/dL, and (3) symptoms relieved by oral or intravenous glucose administration.

333. The answer is e. (*Greenfield, pp 1165-1171.*) Epidermoid cancers of the anal canal metastasize to inguinal nodes as well as to the perirectal and mesenteric nodes. The results of local radical surgery have been disappointing. Combined external radiation with synchronous chemotherapy (fluorouracil and mitomycin), also known as the Nigro protocol, has been used as the standard treatment of the disease, whereas radical surgical approaches are now generally reserved for treatment failures and recurrences.

334. The answer is c. (*Greenfield, pp 780-781.*) A markedly distended colon could have many causes in this 80-year-old man. The contrast study, however, reveals a classic apple-core lesion appropriate prior to relief of this large-bowel obstruction. After medical preparation (eg, hydration, normalization of electrolytes), this patient should undergo prompt surgical management of his mechanical obstruction; conservative management by resection and proximal colostomy would generally be preferred in this elderly patient with an obstructed, unprepared bowel.

335. The answer is c. (*Greenfield, pp 795-805.*) Surgical treatment of Crohn disease is aimed at correcting complications that are causing symptoms. Intestinal obstruction is usually partial and secondary to a fixed stricture that is not responsive to anti-inflammatory agents. When the obstruction causes symptoms that compromise nutritional status, surgery is warranted. Fistula formation in itself is not an indication for surgery. Fistulas between the intestine and the bladder and the intestine and the vagina, however, generally cause significant symptoms and warrant surgical intervention, while an ileum–ascending colon fistula is very common yet rarely symptomatic. Perforation of bowel into the free abdominal cavity is obviously a surgical emergency.

336. The answer is e. (*Brunicardi, pp 1097-1098.*) The film shows a markedly distended colon. The differential diagnosis includes tumor, foreign body, and colitis, but far more likely is either cecal or sigmoid volvulus. Sigmoid volvulus may be ruled out quickly by proctosigmoidoscopy, which is preferable to barium enema, since sigmoid volvulus may be treated successfully by rectal tube decompression via the sigmoidoscope. If sigmoidoscopy is negative, the working diagnosis, based on this classic film, must be cecal volvulus; barium enema would clinch the diagnosis, but the colon might rupture in the intervening 1 to 2 hours. Emergency celiotomy should be done.

337. The answer is e. *(Brunicardi, pp 1098-1099.)* The patient has a cecal volvulus and the procedure of choice is a right hemicolectomy. A cecal volvulus involves axial rotation of the terminal ileum, cecum, and ascending colon with concomitant twisting of the associated mesentery. Immediate operation is required to correct the volvulus and prevent ischemia. Colonoscopic decompression is usually unsuccessful and does not prevent recurrence of a cecal volvulus. A transverse colostomy "decompression" would not decompress the cecum, nor would it provide detorsion of the cecal mesentery to allow restoration of adequate blood supply to the right colon.

338. The answer is d. *(Greenfield, pp 912-913.)* Hydatid cysts secondary to echinococcal infection are most common in the liver in adults. Up to 20% to 30% of patients with hepatic cysts also have cysts in their lungs. In general, serologic tests are more likely to be positive the longer the lesion has been present, but false negativity occurs with sufficient frequency that results should not influence the decision to treat hepatic hydatid cysts. Spontaneous rupture of the cyst or leakage of cyst fluid during diagnostic or therapeutic aspiration may cause anaphylactic reactions or peritoneal dissemination of the disease. Classically, definitive treatment required surgical resection, enucleation, or evacuation of the cysts. As long as there is no evidence of biliary communication with the cyst, agents such as 0.5% silver nitrate or hypertonic saline are introduced into the cyst at the time of surgery, and efforts are made to avoid spillage and contamination of the peritoneal cavity. Treatment of patients with liver cysts with mebendazole or albendazole combined with percutaneous drainage has been demonstrated to have comparable outcomes to surgical cystectomy and should be considered in these patients.

339. The answer is a. *(Mahmoodian, pp 19-24.)* Appendicitis complicates approximately 1 in 1700 pregnancies at an incidence comparable with that in nonpregnant women matched for age. It is the most prevalent extrauterine indication for laparotomy in pregnancy. The duration of gestation does not influence the severity of the disease, but the diagnosis does become more difficult as the pregnancy progresses. By the twentieth week of gestation, the appendix often lies at the level of the umbilicus and more lateral than usual. Pregnancy should not delay surgery if appendicitis is suspected; appendiceal perforation greatly increases the chance of premature labor and fetal mortality (approximately 20% for each). In contrast, negative laparotomy under general anesthesia and nonperforated appendicitis are associated with very low risk to both the fetus and the mother (less than 1% and 5%, respectively).

340. The answer is b. (*Brunicardi, pp 911-918. Townsend, pp 1121-1123.*) Normal respiration creates negative pressure in the thoracic cavity. As a result of the pressure gradient, blood enters the chest via the vena cava and air via the trachea; both are life-sustaining results of this pressure gradient. The pathophysiologic consequence of a hole in the diaphragm is that eventually abdominal viscera will be aspirated into the thorax. The sliding hernia, contained in the lower mediastinum by intact pleura, may rarely cause symptoms of reflux that would justify surgical attention, but such patients are in no danger of vascular compromise or of obstructive displacement of hollow viscera. The paraesophageal hernia, on the other hand, leaves the patient at substantial risk for both strangulation and obstruction. Either result would be a surgical catastrophe; with rare exceptions, paraesophageal hernias should be surgically repaired whenever diagnosed. A traction diverticulum is usually caused by inflammatory contraction around mediastinal nodes, is rarely of any symptomatic consequence, and need not be repaired. Neither the Schatzki ring nor the esophageal web justifies esophageal surgery. They can be ignored or dilated as symptoms demand.

341. The answer is d. (*Greenfield, pp 784-785, 1038-1039.*) Ogilvie syndrome describes the condition in which massive cecal and colonic dilation is seen in the absence of mechanical obstruction. Other terms used to describe this condition are acute colonic pseudo-obstruction, colonic ileus, and functional colonic obstruction. It tends to occur in elderly patients in the setting of cardiopulmonary insufficiency, in other systemic disorders that require prolonged bed rest, and in the postoperative state. The diagnosis of Ogilvie syndrome cannot be confirmed until mechanical obstruction of the distal colon is excluded by colonoscopy or contrast enema. Anticholinergic agents and narcotics need to be discontinued, but any delay in decompressing the dilated cecum is inappropriate since colonic ischemia and perforation become a distinct hazard as the cecum reaches this degree of dilation (>10 cm to 12 cm). In patients with less than 10 cm of dilation and no evidence of ischemic bowel, management consists of bowel rest, NG suctioning if vomiting, correction of metabolic abnormalities, and discontinuation of medications that diminish GI motility. In patients with persistent distention or a dilated cecum greater than 10 cm, cautious endoscopic colonic decompression can be performed, or a sympatholytic agent such as neostigmine can be administered, with appropriate hemodynamic monitoring. Surgery is indicated in all patients in whom perforation or ischemic bowel is suspected.

342. The answer is a. *(Merrell, pp 621-625.)* The classic Quincke triad of abdominal pain in the right upper quadrant, jaundice, and GI bleeding is present in 30% to 40% of patients with hemobilia. With more frequent use of percutaneous liver procedures (eg, transhepatic cholangiogram, transhepatic catheter drainage), iatrogenic injury has replaced other trauma as the most common cause of bloody bile. Other causes include spontaneous bleeding during anticoagulation, gallstones, parasitic infections/abscesses, and neoplastic lesions. Angiography and endoscopy are useful diagnostic studies, and intrahepatic bleeding can be controlled by angiographic embolization in up to 95% of cases. Surgical treatment is advocated for bleeding from extrahepatic bile ducts or the gallbladder or in cases of penetrating trauma in which associated injuries might need attention.

343. The answer is d. *(Podolosky, pp 928-937.)* The patient depicted in this question has Crohn disease of the colon (Crohn colitis). Crohn colitis is characterized by linear mucosal ulcerations, discontinuous (skip) lesions, a transmural inflammatory process, and noncaseating granulomas in up to 50% of patients. Because their clinical features and management differ, Crohn colitis must be distinguished from UC. UC is usually found in the rectum, although in rare cases the rectum is spared involvement. The entire colon, from cecum to rectum, may be involved (pancolitis). UC typically presents as a grossly continuous inflammatory process (without skip lesions) that microscopically is confined to the mucosa and submucosa of the colon. In addition, crypt abscesses and superficial ulcerations are common in UC.

344. The answer is c. *(Podolosky, pp 928-937.)* Patients with Crohn disease can develop fistulas between the colon and other segments of intestine, the bladder, the urethra, the vagina, the skin, or the prostate. Intestinal perforation can occur in about 5% of patients. Toxic megacolon can occur in patients with Crohn disease, UC, or any severe inflammatory process of the large intestine. Extraintestinal manifestations are usually associated with active disease. Finally, patients with Crohn colitis have a 5.6-fold increased risk of colon cancer relative to an age-matched population.

345. The answer is c. *(Brunicardi, pp 911-918.)* The condition demonstrated is a paraesophageal hernia. It is encountered much less frequently (approximately 5%) than is the sliding hiatal hernia, and it has completely different therapeutic implications. Paraesophageal hernias are acquired, rarely present before middle age, and are most common in patients in their seventh decade. The position of the gastroesophageal junction distinguishes the different types of hernias, which occur near the esophageal hiatus of the diaphragm. In the more common sliding hernia, the gastroesophageal junction protrudes above the diaphragm (type I paraesophageal hernia). In the type II paraesophageal hernia, the anatomic junction between the esophagus and the stomach is anchored in its normal position below the diaphragm; the gastric cardia or fundus and occasionally other viscera herniate into the thorax within a true peritoneal sac alongside the gastroesophageal junction. In the type III paraesophageal hernia, the gastroesophageal junction and the gastric cardia or fundus are displaced above the level of the diaphragm. Surgical repair is indicated in patients with type II paraesophageal hernias as soon as the patient can be properly prepared for the procedure, as bleeding, ulceration, obstruction, necrosis of the stomach wall, and perforation are common.

346. The answer is b. *(Townsend, pp 1612-1619.)* The vast majority of pancreatic carcinomas are located in the head of the gland. Patients may present with painless jaundice by virtue of the carcinoma's obstruction of the intrapancreatic portion of the common bile duct. Approximately 10% to 15% of patients are candidates for resection. There is a very strong association with diabetes mellitus (but not diabetes insipidus), but the nature of this relationship is not known. Prognosis is poor; 5-year survival after pancreaticoduodenectomy is about 10% to 15%.

347. The answer is d. *(Townsend, pp 1321-1323.)* The patient most likely has bleeding from the small bowel, given the findings on endoscopy, and the most common cause of small intestinal bleeding in patients under the age of 30 is a Meckel diverticula. Because Meckel diverticula can contain ectopic gastric mucosa, acid secretion can cause small-bowel ulcerations. Small-bowel enteroclysis is a contrast study that can sometimes identify masses or lesions in the small bowel. While enteroclysis, small-bowel endoscopy, angiography, and CT scanning can all be useful adjuncts in the workup of GI bleeding, the patient in this scenario should have a ^{99m}Tc pertechnetate scan, which is diagnostic for a Meckel diverticula.

348. The answer is e. *(Brunicardi, p 1134.)* The most appropriate treatment for a 1-cm carcinoid tumor at the tip of the appendix is an appendectomy. Therapy for a carcinoid tumor of the appendix is based on tumor size and location. Simple appendectomy is adequate treatment for appendiceal carcinoid tumors less than 1 cm. Tumors larger than 2 cm should be treated with a right hemicolectomy to decrease locoregional recurrence. Treatment for tumors between 1cm and 2 cm is based on location. Tumors located at the base of the appendix or invading the mesentery are best treated with a right hemicolectomy. No further treatment is needed after an appendectomy for a 1- to 2-cm tumor located at the tip of the appendix.

349. The answer is b. *(Brunicardi, pp 1356-1357.)* Direct inguinal hernias occur medial to the inferior epigastric vessels while indirect inguinal hernias occur lateral to the inferior epigastric vessels. Immediate surgical repair of inguinal hernias are indicated in cases of acute incarceration. Chronically incarcerated hernias do not have an increased risk for strangulation. Descent of the hernia into the scrotum is not an indication for urgent surgical repair.

350. The answer is b. *(Cosentino, pp 740-748.)* Choledochal cysts are congenital cystic dilations of the extrahepatic biliary ducts. Intrahepatic cystic dilation can coexist (Caroli disease), but it represents a distinct problem and is managed differently. Patients may present with symptoms at any age, but the classic triad of epigastric pain, abdominal mass, and jaundice is not frequently seen. Rather, most patients present with other conditions such as cholecystitis, cholangitis, or pancreatitis. Ultrasonography or ERCP is helpful in demonstrating cysts. Nonsurgical treatment of these cysts results in high morbidity and mortality, and therefore surgery is advised in all cases. The present recommendation is for complete resection of the cyst and Roux-en-Y choledochojejunostomy. Since malignant changes in choledochal cysts have been frequently described, complete resection rather than the performance of an internal drainage procedure is preferred whenever the resection can be done safely.

351. The answer is d. *(Townsend, pp 1256-1258.)* Stress ulceration refers to acute gastric or duodenal erosive lesions that occur following shock, sepsis, major surgery, trauma, or burns. These lesions tend to be superficial and can involve multiple sites. McClelland and associates showed that patients subjected to trauma and subsequent hemorrhagic shock do not have increased gastric secretion, but rather show decreased splanchnic blood flow. Ischemic damage to the mucosa may therefore play a role. Unlike chronic benign gastric ulcers, which are generally found along the lesser curvature and in the antrum, acute erosive lesions usually involve the body and fundus and spare the antrum.

352. The answer is b. *(Brunicardi, p 1203.)* Cholangitis is suggested by the presence of the Charcot triad: fever, jaundice, and pain in the right upper quadrant. These symptoms are usually caused by choledocholithiasis, but they can also occur in association with obstructing neoplasms and choledochal cysts. The disease occurs primarily in the elderly. Therapy is aimed at decompression of the common bile duct. In patients with suppurative cholangitis who fail to respond to intravenous antibiotics and fluid resuscitation, the nonoperative approach is the preferred intervention via either percutaneous or endoscopic drainage of the obstructed common bile duct. If the nonoperative approach fails, surgery is indicated. This is usually best accomplished by surgical placement of a T tube into the duct. Percutaneous transhepatic catheter drainage is an acceptable alternative in select patients. This procedure can often provide effective decompression during the acute septic phase of the disease. Cholecystostomy will be effective only if there is free flow of bile into the gallbladder via the cystic duct and in general should not be depended on to secure drainage of the common bile duct.

353. The answer is a. *(Brunicardi, p 1200.)* High-risk, critically ill patients with multisystem disease and cholecystitis experience a significant increase in morbidity and mortality following operative intervention. Tube cholecystostomy can be performed under local anesthesia in the operating room or via a percutaneous approach in the radiology suite. Open or laparoscopic procedures would carry the same general anesthetic risk whether done urgently or in a delayed (elective) fashion. Lithotripsy has no role in the treatment of acute cholecystitis.

354. The answer is a. *(Townsend, pp 1603-1605.)* Pancreatic pseudocysts can develop in the setting of acute and chronic pancreatitis. They are cystic collections that do not have an epithelial lining and therefore have no malignant potential. Most pseudocysts spontaneously resolve. Therapy should not be considered for 6 weeks to allow for the possibility of spontaneous resolution as well as to allow for maturation of the cyst wall if the cyst persists. Complications of pseudocysts include gastric outlet and extrahepatic biliary obstructions as well as spontaneous rupture and hemorrhage. Pseudocysts can be excised, externally drained, or internally drained into the GI tract (most commonly the stomach or a Roux-en-Y limb of jejunum).

355. The answer is d. *(Reilly, pp 1702-1707.)* Recently, Dieulafoy lesion has been identified more frequently as a source of GI bleeding. It is characteristically located within 6 cm distal to the gastroesophageal junction. Dieulafoy lesion typically consists of an abnormally large submucosal artery that protrudes through a small, solitary mucosal defect. For unclear reasons, the lesions may bleed spontaneously and massively, in which case they require emergency intervention. Upper endoscopy is usually successful in localizing the lesion, and permanent hemostasis can be obtained endoscopically in most cases with injection sclerotherapy, electrocoagulation, or heater probe. If surgery is required, a gastrotomy and simple ligation or wedge resection of the lesion may be adequate. No large series have yet established the optimal surgical treatment for Dieulafoy lesion; however, acid-reducing procedures have not been successful in preventing further bleeding.

356. The answer is b. *(Brunicardi, p 1134.)* Carcinoid tumors arise from enterochromaffin cells in the crypts of Lieberkühn. When they are encountered in the appendix and are less than 2 cm in size, simple appendectomy is the procedure of choice. When the tumors are larger than 2 cm, a right hemicolectomy should be performed. Carcinoid syndrome (hepatomegaly, diarrhea, cutaneous flushing, right heart valvular disease, and asthma) usually occurs in the presence of liver metastases but can also be seen when there are metastases to sites drained by systemic (as opposed to portal) veins or from primary carcinoids outside the portal system. Carcinoid syndrome is rare in patients with carcinoid of the appendix because the tumors are usually discovered before metastases occur.

357. The answer is d. *(Brunicardi, pp 1094-1095.)* Rectal carcinoids are slowly growing tumors, but they can be locally invasive and metastasize in up to 15% of patients. Patients manifest systemic signs of the carcinoid syndrome only in the rare circumstance where hepatic metastases have occurred. The malignant potential is low in carcinoid tumors when they are less than 2 cm in diameter, as is typically the case when diagnosed. The tumors are curable by wide local transanal resection that includes the muscle layer. Endoscopic treatment leaves tumor cells near the margin of resection and is felt to increase the risk of recurrence. Whether more aggressive resection (abdominoperineal or low anterior resection [LAR]) improves the prognosis in larger tumors remains controversial. The prognosis is excellent for patients with local disease.

358. The answer is b. *(Reilly, pp 1702-1707.)* Polypoid lesions of the gall-bladder are found most often in the third through fifth decades of life and are increasingly being detected by ultrasonography. These are generally small lesions that typically do not show a shadow on ultrasound. Ninety percent are benign lesions, such as cholesterol polyps (pseudotumors). True adenomas, which constitute about 10% of these benign lesions, can undergo malignant transformation. The indications for operative intervention remain controversial. Recent reviews suggest that the vast majority of malignant polypoid lesions are solitary, larger than 1.0 cm, and much more common in patients older than 50 years of age. There is also an increased incidence of malignancy if the lesions are associated with gallstones. Symptomatic lesions should be removed regardless of their size. Asymptomatic small lesions can probably be safely followed by ultrasonography.

359. The answer is a. *(Blumgart, p 1085.)* The metabolic consequences of total pancreatectomy are manifold. They include weight loss, malabsorption attended by hypocalcemia and hypophosphatemia, diabetes mellitus, diarrhea, and both iron deficiency and pernicious anemia. Like pancreaticoduodenectomy, total pancreatectomy results in resection of the duodenum, distal common bile duct, and gallbladder. Because iron absorption occurs primarily in the duodenum, these patients will have iron deficiency anemia. Pernicious anemia results due to lack of pancreatic enzymes required for vitamin B_{12} absorption. In theory, total pancreatectomy should provide good surgical treatment for pancreatic carcinoma; in reality, the severe metabolic problems that result from total removal of the pancreas make partial pancreaticoduodenectomy a frequently preferred treatment for most cases of pancreatic carcinoma that are resectable.

360. The answer is a. *(Brunicardi, pp 1161-1162.)* Hepatic hemangiomas are the most common of all liver tumors. The diagnostic incidence of incidental hemangiomas in adults has increased in this era of noninvasive imaging of organs with MRI, ultrasonography, and CT. The mean age of presentation in adults is about 45 years, and the vast majority of these lesions are asymptomatic. There is no evidence that they undergo malignant transformation. The risk of rupture and severe hemorrhage into or from hemangiomas is extremely low; when it does occur, it is usually iatrogenic (following attempted biopsy). Given the typically benign and static nature of these lesions, management by angiographic embolization or resection should be reserved for the rare patient with symptomatic or complicated hemangioma.

361. The answer is d. (*Brunicardi, p 273.*) CEA is a nonspecific tumor marker that is elevated in only about one-half of patients with colorectal tumors and is often elevated in patients with lung, pancreatic, gastric, or gynecologic malignancies. CEA is also elevated in cigarette smokers. Patients in whom the primary colon tumor produced CEA and in whom the level falls below 2 to 3 ng/mL after resection have an excellent prognosis for disease control. In such patients, a subsequent rise in CEA has been demonstrated to be a very sensitive marker of the presence and extent of recurrent disease. Many surgeons follow CEA levels and perform second-look operations to resect local disease or possibly isolated metastatic disease if the levels become elevated postoperatively. Some surgeons recommend exploration in that circumstance even in the absence of other evidence (CT scan, colonoscopy) of recurrence. In some patients, the long-term survival seems to be improved following this aggressive approach. However, very high elevations of CEA suggest extensive liver disease or peritoneal spread, which is unresectable.

362. The answer is e. (*Brunicardi, p 985.*) Patients with Mallory-Weiss syndrome typically present with a massive, painless hematemesis after severe vomiting or retching. The majority of tears occur just below the gastroesophageal junction. These tears occur more commonly in cirrhotics than in the normal population. Most of the time (90%), bleeding will stop without any intervention. When bleeding persists, balloon tamponade, endoscopic control of the bleeding, and surgical intervention with gastrotomy and oversewing of the tear have all been successful. Both intravenous and intra-arterial infusion of vasopressin are also useful in controlling bleeding but are contraindicated in patients with coronary artery disease.

363 to 366. The answers are 363-d, 364-e, 365-a, 366-c. (*Townsend, pp 1556-1575.*) A patient with symptomatic cholelithiasis has pain from the gallbladder as it contracts against a gallstone lodged in the cystic duct. If the stone gets dislodged with the contractions then the pain resolves until another stone gets lodged in the cystic duct. If the gallstone remains stuck in the cystic duct, then the abdominal pain worsens as the gallbladder becomes more and more inflamed. The gallstones harbor bacteria and if the bile becomes static with an obstructed cystic duct, infection develops. At this point the patient has acute cholecystitis and needs antibiotics or urgent cholecystectomy. Eventually the pressure in the wall of the gallbladder exceeds the perfusion pressure of the vessels in the gallbladder and the gallbladder becomes ischemic. At this stage the gallbladder becomes necrotic and can perforate causing life-threatening peritonitis and sepsis. A gallstone remaining in the common bile duct is called choledocholithiasis. These patients may be asymptomatic, have abdominal pain, or progress to develop cholangitis depending on the status of the gallstone in the common bile duct. Stones that are not lodged in the sphincter of Oddi allow bile to empty out of the bile duct. Stones that become stuck in the common bile duct cause stasis of bile in the biliary system which can lead to cholangitis. The symptoms of cholangitis are right upper quadrant abdominal pain, fever, and jaundice (Charcot triad). Cholangitis is a life-threatening condition requiring emergent ERCP with stone extraction and common bile duct decompression. Sometimes patients develop acute pancreatitis with passage of the gallstone past the ampulla of Vater as it exits the common bile duct into the duodenum.

367 to 370. The answers are 367-d, 368-b, 369-b, 370-c. (*Brunicardi, pp 1076–1097. Townsend, pp 1454–1460.*) The definitive operation of choice for patients with UC is total proctocolectomy with either end ileostomy or ileoanal J-pouch anastomosis. Indications for operation in UC include high-grade dysplasia or carcinoma, toxic megacolon, and intractability to medical therapy. Patients with either UC or Crohn can develop toxic megacolon, which is manifested by fever, abdominal pain, and marked dilation of the large bowel. Treatment consists of a subtotal colectomy with end ileostomy. For patients with UC and toxic megacolon, completion proctectomy can be performed at a later date.

For squamous cell carcinoma of the anus, the mainstay of therapy is chemoradiation with the Nigro protocol. However, recurrent or persistent disease after chemoradiation requires surgery—abdominal-perineal resection involves removing the rectum and anus with formation of a permanent end colostomy. APR is also the procedure of choice for distal rectal cancers that involve the sphincters or are too close to obtain an adequate margin (2 cm) and in patients for whom sphincter-sparing surgery is contraindicated because of fecal incontinence. Preoperative or neoadjuvant chemoradiation can sometimes cause distal rectal tumors to shrink in size such that a sphincter-sparing operation can be performed. For proximal and midrectal cancers, low anterior resection (LAR) is the procedure of choice. LAR involves the removal of the rectum to below the peritoneal reflection through an abdominal approach.

Cardiothoracic Problems

Questions

371. A 75-year-old woman with history of angina is admitted to the hospital for syncope. Examination of the patient reveals a systolic murmur best heard at the base of the heart that radiates into the carotid arteries. Electrocardiogram (ECG) is notable for left ventricular hypertrophy with evidence of left atrial enlargement. ECG reveals an aortic valve area of 0.7 cm^2. Which of the following statements regarding the patient's diagnosis is true?

a. It is most often caused by rheumatic fever.
b. Congestive heart failure is the presenting symptom in one-third of the patients.
c. Patients do not develop symptoms until the aortic valve area is less than 0.8 cm^2.
d. There is no long-term treatment for this condition.
e. Percutaneous aortic balloon valvuloplasty is reserved for patients with mild disease.

372. A 68-year-old man is diagnosed with lung cancer. In preparation for pulmonary resection he undergoes pulmonary function tests. Which of the following results indicate a favorable prognosis?

a. Elevated P_{CO_2}
b. Forced expiratory volume in 1 second (FEV$_1$) more than 60% of predicted
c. Carbon monoxide diffusing capacity (DLCO) less than 40%
d. Low FEV$_1$/FVC (forced vital capacity)
e. Normal FEV$_1$/FVC

373. A 71-year-old woman is diagnosed with small-cell lung cancer. Which of the following statements regarding small-cell lung carcinoma is true?

a. It represents about 80% of all lung cancers.
b. Most are located peripherally.
c. It rarely spreads to mediastinal lymph nodes.
d. It is slow growing and rarely metastasizes.
e. Most are treated with chemotherapy and radiation instead of surgery.

374. A 42-year-old homeless man presents with a 3-week history of shortness of breath, fevers, and pleuritic chest pain. Chest x-ray (CXR) reveals a large left pleural effusion. Thoracentesis reveals thick, purulent-appearing fluid, which is found to have glucose less than 40 mg/dL and a pH of 6.5. A chest tube is placed, but the pleural effusion persists. Which of the following is the most appropriate management of this patient?

a. Placement of a second chest tube at the bedside and antibiotic therapy
b. Infusion of antibiotics via the chest tube
c. Intravenous antibiotics for 6 weeks
d. Thoracotomy with instillation of antibiotics into the pleural space
e. Thoracotomy with decortication and antibiotic therapy

375. A 63-year-old man is seen because of facial swelling and cyanosis, especially when he bends over. There are large, dilated subcutaneous veins on his upper chest. His jugular veins are prominent even while he is upright. Which of the following conditions is the most likely cause of these findings?

a. Histoplasmosis (sclerosing mediastinitis)
b. Substernal thyroid
c. Thoracic aortic aneurysm
d. Constrictive pericarditis
e. Bronchogenic carcinoma

376. During endoscopic biopsy of a distal esophageal cancer, perforation of the esophagus is suspected when the patient complains of significant new substernal pain. An immediate chest film reveals air in the mediastinum. Which of the following is the most appropriate management of this patient?

a. Placement of a nasogastric tube to the level of perforation, antibiotics, and close observation
b. Spit fistula (cervical pharyngostomy) and gastrostomy
c. Left thoracotomy, pleural patch oversewing of the perforation, and drainage of the mediastinum
d. Left thoracotomy with esophagectomy
e. Thoracotomy with chest tube drainage and esophageal exclusion

377. A 63-year-old woman with chronic obstructive pulmonary disease (COPD) presents with a several-week history of fever, night sweats, weight loss, and cough. Her CXR is noted to have a density in the left upper lobe with a relatively thin-walled cavity. Bronchoscopy and computed tomographic (CT) scan are suggestive of a lung abscess rather than a malignant process. Which of the following is the most appropriate initial management of this patient?

a. Percutaneous drainage of the lung abscess
b. Systemic antibiotics directed against the causative agent
c. Tube thoracostomy
d. Left upper lobectomy
e. Surgical drainage of the abscess

378. A 45-year-old man with poorly controlled hypertension presents with severe chest pain radiating to his back. An ECG demonstrates no significant abnormalities. A CT scan of the chest and abdomen is obtained, which demonstrates a descending thoracic aortic dissection extending from distal to the left subclavian takeoff down to above the iliac bifurcation. A Foley catheter is placed, and urine output is 30 to 40 cc/h. His feet are warm, with less than 2-second capillary refill. Which of the following is the most appropriate initial management?

a. Emergent operation for repair of the aortic dissection
b. Angiography to confirm the diagnosis of aortic dissection
c. Echocardiography to rule out cardiac complications
d. Initiation of a β-blocker
e. Initiation of a vasodilator such as nitroprusside

379. A stockbroker in his mid-40s presents with complaints of episodes of severe, often incapacitating chest pain on swallowing. Diagnostic studies on the esophagus yield the following results: endoscopic examination and biopsy—mild inflammation distally; manometry—prolonged high-amplitude contractions from the arch of the aorta distally, lower esophageal sphincter (LES) pressure 20 mm Hg with relaxation on swallowing; barium swallow—2-cm epiphrenic diverticulum. Which of the following is the best management option for this patient?

a. Myotomy along the length of the manometric abnormality
b. Diverticulectomy, myotomy from the level of the aortic arch to the fundus, fundoplication
c. Diverticulectomy, cardiomyotomy of the distal 3 cm of esophagus and proximal 2 cm of stomach with antireflux fundoplication
d. A trial of calcium-channel blockers
e. Pneumatic dilatation of the LES

380. A 4-year-old boy is seen 1 hour after ingestion of a lye drain cleaner. No oropharyngeal burns are noted. The CXR is normal, but the patient continues to complain of significant chest pain. Which of the following is the most appropriate next step in his management?

a. Parenteral steroids and antibiotics
b. Esophagogram with water-soluble contrast
c. Administration of an oral neutralizing agent
d. Induction of vomiting
e. Rapid administration of a quart of water to clear remaining lye from the esophagus and dilute material in the stomach

381. A previously healthy 20-year-old male is admitted to the hospital with acute onset of left-sided chest pain. Electrocardiographic findings are normal, but CXR shows a 40% left pneumothorax. Appropriate treatment consists of which of the following procedures?

a. Observation
b. Barium swallow
c. Thoracotomy
d. Tube thoracostomy
e. Thoracostomy and intubation

382. A 50-year-old salesman is on a yacht with a client when he has a severe vomiting and retching spell punctuated by a sharp substernal pain. He arrives in your emergency room 4 hours later and has a chest film in which the left descending aorta is outlined by air density. Which of the following is the most appropriate next step in his workup?

a. Contrast esophagram
b. Echocardiogram
c. Flexible bronchoscopy
d. Flexible esophagogastroscopy
e. Aortography

383. A 26-year-old man is brought to the emergency room after being extricated from the driver's seat of a car involved in a head-on collision, in which the patient was not wearing his seat belt. An echocardiogram (shown here) demonstrates wall motion abnormalities suggestive of a myocardial contusion. Which of the following is true regarding the diagnosis of and outcome after a traumatic myocardial contusion?

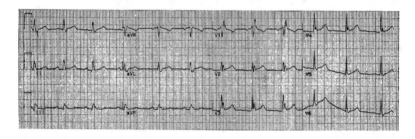

a. Significant pump failure occurs in less than 5% of patients with major chest trauma.
b. ST- and T-wave abnormalities on ECG are diagnostic.
c. An elevation in the creatine kinase, myocardial bound (CKMB) fraction of greater than 5% of total is predictive of increased mortality.
d. Cardiac enzymes are the most sensitive test for diagnosing myocardial contusion.
e. Patients should be placed on antiarrhythmics regardless of ECG findings for at least 24 hours postinjury.

384. A 63-year-old man underwent a three-vessel coronary artery bypass graft (CABG) 5 hours ago. Initially, his mediastinal chest tube output was 300 mL blood/h, but an hour ago, there was no further evidence of bleeding from the tube. His mean arterial pressure has fallen, and several fluid boluses were administered. His central venous pressure (CVP) is elevated to 20 mm Hg, and he has required the addition of inotropes. Which of the following is the best management strategy?

a. Addition of vasopressors along with the inotropes
b. Transfusion of packed red blood cells
c. Return to the operating room for exploration of the mediastinum
d. Placement of an intraaortic balloon pump
e. Infusion of streptokinase into the mediastinal chest tube

385. Several days following esophagectomy, a patient complains of dyspnea and chest tightness. A large pleural effusion is noted on chest radiograph, and thoracentesis yields milky fluid consistent with chyle. Which of the following is the most appropriate initial management of this patient?

a. Immediate operation to repair the thoracic duct
b. Immediate operation to ligate the thoracic duct
c. Tube thoracostomy and low-fat diet
d. Observation and low-fat diet
e. Observation and antibiotics

386. A 56-year-old woman presents for evaluation of a murmur suggestive of mitral stenosis and is noted on echocardiography to have a lesion attached to the fossa ovalis of the left atrial septum. The mass is causing obstruction of the mitral valve. Which of the following is the most likely diagnosis?

a. Endocarditis
b. Lymphoma
c. Cardiac sarcoma
d. Cardiac myxoma
e. Metastatic cancer to the heart

387. A 56-year-old woman has been treated for 3 years for wheezing on exertion, which was diagnosed as asthma. Chest radiograph, shown here, reveals a midline mass compressing the trachea. Which of the following is the most likely diagnosis?

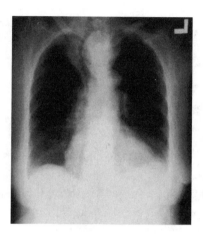

a. Lymphoma
b. Neurogenic tumor
c. Lung carcinoma
d. Goiter
e. Pericardial cyst

388. A 59-year-old man is found to have a 6-cm thoracic aortic aneurysm for which he desires repair, but he is concerned about the risk of paralysis postoperatively. Which of the following maneuvers has not been demonstrated to decrease the risk of paraplegia after repair?

a. Infusion of a bolus of steroids immediately postoperatively with a continuous infusion for 24 hours
b. Minimization of cross-clamping time
c. Reattachment of segmental intercostal and lumbar arteries
d. Cerebrospinal fluid (CSF) drainage
e. Left heart bypass

389. An 89-year-old man has lost 30 lb over the past 2 years. He reports that food frequently sticks when he swallows. He also complains of a chronic cough. Barium swallow is shown here. Which of the following statements is true?

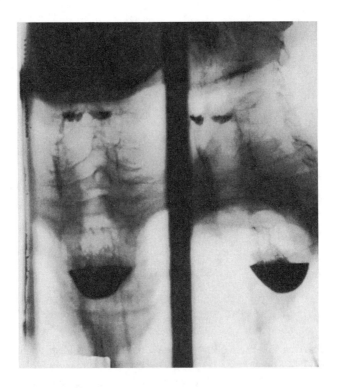

a. Radiation therapy and stenting can be expected to produce the same long-term survival as would surgery.
b. Esophagoscopy and biopsy should be performed to confirm the x-ray findings.
c. This patient is atypical in that the lesion usually appears in the second or third decade of life.
d. The patient should be administered a trial of a promotility agent prior to surgical intervention.
e. The origin of the lesion is at the cricopharyngeus muscle.

390. A 70-year-old woman undergoes a cardiac catheterization for exertional chest pain. Her pain continues to worsen and she is interested in having surgical treatment. Which of the following statements is true concerning CABG?

a. It is indicated for chronic and unstable angina.
b. It is indicated for congestive heart failure.
c. It is not indicated in patients with diabetes.
d. It is associated with a 10% operative mortality in low-risk patients.
e. It is indicated only if significant triple vessel disease is documented angiographically.

391. A 27-year-old woman seeks your advice regarding pain and numbness in the right arm and hand. She reports that it is exacerbated by raising her arm over her head. A provisional diagnosis is made. Which of the following statements is true regarding this condition?

a. It is associated with cervical spine disk disease.
b. It is reliably diagnosed by positional obliteration of the radial pulse.
c. If conservative measures fail, it is best treated by surgical decompression of the brachial plexus.
d. It most commonly affects the median nerve.
e. It can be reliably ruled out by angiography.

392. A 35-year-old man presents with a history of 4 days of severe substernal pain and fever of 38.89°C (102°F). He has a past medical history of peptic ulcer disease that resulted in a Billroth II procedure 5 years earlier. On admission, the chest film shown here is obtained. A true statement regarding this patient's case is which of the following?

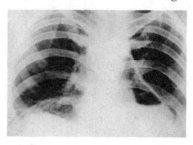

a. Pericardial effusion is present.
b. The condition may be managed with antibiotics and close observation if the patient remains hemodynamically stable.
c. The condition could have resulted from recurrent peptic ulcer disease.
d. The condition could have resulted from a myocardial infarction.
e. The previous Billroth II procedure effectively rules out peptic ulcer as the cause of the condition.

393. A 65-year-old woman has had pain in her right shoulder and has been treated with analgesics without relief. The CXR reveals a mass in the apex of the right chest. A transthoracic needle biopsy documents carcinoma. Superior pulmonary sulcus carcinomas (Pancoast tumors) are bronchogenic carcinomas that typically produce which of the following clinical features?

a. Atelectasis of the involved apical segment
b. Horner syndrome
c. Pain in the T4 and T5 dermatomes
d. Nonproductive cough
e. Hemoptysis

394. A 63-year-old man has a chylothorax that after 2 weeks of conservative therapy appears to be persistent. The chest tube output is approximately 600 mL/day. Appropriate management at this time includes which of the following procedures?

a. Neck exploration and ligation of the thoracic duct
b. Subdiaphragmatic ligation of the thoracic duct
c. Thoracotomy and repair of the thoracic duct
d. Thoracotomy and ligation of the thoracic duct
e. Thoracotomy and abrasion of the pleural space

395. A 32-year-old woman has a CXR screening, and a 1.5-cm mass is noted in the right lower lobe. She is a nonsmoker. Bronchoscopy shows a mass in the right lower lobe orifice, covered with mucosa. Biopsy indicates this is compatible with a carcinoid tumor. Which of the following statements is true regarding carcinoids in the lung?

a. They frequently metastasize.
b. They most commonly arise in peripheral terminal bronchioles.
c. They rarely produce the carcinoid syndrome.
d. They are radiosensitive.
e. Five-year survival rate is less than 50%.

396. Six months ago at the time of lumpectomy for breast cancer, a 60-year-old female attorney quit a 30-year smoking habit of two packs per day. She had the chest radiograph shown here as part of her routine follow-up examination. True statements about the lesion visualized on the film include which of the following?

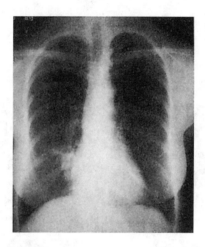

a. It is more apt to be metastatic breast carcinoma than primary lung carcinoma.
b. There is a 90% chance that this mass is malignant.
c. Since the diagnosis can be established with certainty only by a tissue diagnosis, the mass should be biopsied.
d. If the mass is malignant, the possibility for cure with excision is remote.
e. The mass is most likely benign.

397. A 42-year-old man presents with a solitary lung lesion. At the time of operation on this patient, a firm, rubbery lesion in the periphery of the lung is discovered. It is sectioned in the operating room to reveal tissue that looks like cartilage and smooth muscle. Which of the following is the most likely diagnosis?

a. Fibroma
b. Chondroma
c. Osteochondroma
d. Hamartoma
e. Aspergilloma

398. A 45-year-old woman presents with dysphagia, regurgitation of undigested food, and weight loss. She had x-rays shown here as part of her workup. Which of the following statements regarding her condition is true?

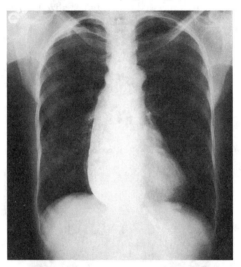

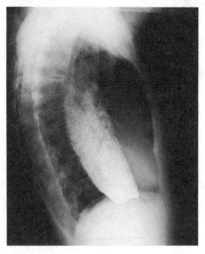

a. Difficulty swallowing solids but not liquids
b. Higher than normal incidence of esophageal carcinoma
c. Failure of the upper esophageal sphincter to relax in response to swallowing
d. Normal pressure in the body of the esophagus
e. Normal esophageal motility

Questions 399 to 403

For each physical finding or group of findings, select the cardiovascular disorder with which it is most likely to be associated. Each lettered option may be used once, more than once, or not at all.

a. Massive tricuspid regurgitation
b. Aortic regurgitation
c. Coarctation of the aorta
d. Thoracic aortic aneurysm
e. Myocarditis

399. An elderly man with abnormal pupillary responses (Argyll Robertson pupil).

400. A 24-year-old drug addict with jugular venous distention and exophthalmos.

401. A patient with flushing and paling of the nail beds (Quincke pulse) and a bounding radial pulse.

402. A patient with conjunctivitis, urethral discharge, and arthralgia.

403. A patient with short stature, webbed neck, low-set ears, and epicanthal folds.

Questions 404 to 408

For each clinical scenario, select the mediastinal tumor with which it is most likely to be associated. Each lettered option may be used once, more than once, or not at all.

a. Thymoma
b. Hodgkin disease
c. Pheochromocytoma
d. Parathyroid adenoma
e. Cystic teratoma

404. A 23-year-old patient with hypertension and increased urinary catecholamine levels.

405. A 21-year-old woman presents with generalized weakness and double vision. During her workup, she is noted to have a widened mediastinum on her CXR prompting a CT scan, which demonstrates an anterior mediastinal mass.

406. A 63-year-old woman with vague symptoms of fatigue and depression presents with hematuria. CT scan of the abdomen and pelvis reveals a stone at the ureteropelvic junction.

407. A 35-year-old woman with fever and weight loss. CT scan revealed a mediastinal mass, which was biopsied and revealed Reed-Sternberg cells.

408. A 33-year-old woman presents with cough and chest pain for 2 months. More recently, she complains of coughing up hair. The CXR reveals a mediastinal mass.

Questions 409 to 413

For each clinical scenario, select the most appropriate pharmacologic agent for the patient. Each lettered option may be used once, more than once, or not at all.

a. Epinephrine
b. Norepinephrine
c. Phenylephrine
d. Dopamine
e. Dobutamine
f. Nitroprusside
g. Nitroglycerin

409. A 56-year-old man presents with a blood pressure of 220/110 mm Hg, chest pain, and ST-elevations on an ECG.

410. A 65-year-old man presents with cardiogenic shock following a myocardial infarction.

411. A 30-year-old man presents with perforated appendicitis and heart rate of 120 beats per minute, blood pressure of 80/40 mm Hg, and central venous pressure of 17 mm Hg. The patient remains hypotensive after a continuous infusion of dopamine.

412. A 21-year-old man undergoes major abdominal surgery after a motor vehicle collision. He has a cardiac arrest in the intensive care unit shortly after returning from surgery.

413. A 45-year-old woman presents with a blood pressure of 220/130 mm Hg and a headache. After several hours of an intravenous drip of medication to control her hypertension she becomes acidotic.

Cardiothoracic Problems

Answers

371. The answer is b. *(Townsend, pp 1841-1844.)* The patient's history, physical examination, and findings on heart studies is classic for aortic stenosis. Nearly one-third of patients will have congestive heart failure as the presenting symptom. Patients with aortic stenosis and congestive heart failure have worse prognosis. Aortic stenosis is most often thought to result from calcification of the aortic valve associated with advanced age. The process is mostly idiopathic, with only a small percentage associated with rheumatic fever. Patients may not develop symptoms until the aortic valve area is about 1 cm^2. The only effective therapy with good long-term results is aortic valve replacement. Symptoms are relieved in nearly all the patients after surgery. Percutaneous aortic balloon valvuloplasty involves passing balloon catheters through the aortic orifice and inflating them in an effort to break the calcium that is retarding leaflet motion. Immediate results show an increase in the aortic valve area of 50%, but the long-term results are disappointing with a third of the patients having recurrent symptoms by 6 months. For this reason balloon valvuloplasty is reserved for patients who are not candidates for aortic valve replacement or whose long-term survival is poor.

372. The answer is b. *(Townsend, pp 1700-1703.)* The predicted postoperative forced expiratory volume in 1 second is the most commonly used predictor of postoperative pulmonary reserve. Usually FEV$_1$ may be expressed as an actual value of liter per second or as a percentage. The percent predicted value takes into account the body habitus. Most patients will tolerate a lobectomy with an FEV$_1$ greater than 60% of predicted. An elevated PCO$_2$ greater than 45 mm Hg suggests severe pulmonary disease with nearly 50% functional loss of the lung. Carbon monoxide diffusing capacity measures the rate at which carbon monoxide moves from the alveolar space to combine with hemoglobin in the red blood cells. It is determined by calculating the difference between inspired and expired samples of gas.

DLCO levels less than 40% to 50% are associated with increased perioperative risk. FEV$_1$/FVC is useful in determining obstructive versus restrictive lung disease. The ratio is low (FEV$_1$ is reduced and FVC is high) in obstructive disease. In restrictive disease the ratio is normal because both FEV$_1$ and FVC are reduced.

373. The answer is e. *(Townsend, p 1711.)* Small cell lung cancers are treated primarily with chemotherapy and radiation; they are rarely amenable to surgical resection because of extensive disease at presentation. Small cell lung cancer accounts for about 20% of primary lung cancers. Most are centrally located and characterized by an aggressive tendency to metastasize. They spread early to mediastinal lymph nodes and distant sites, most commonly to the bone marrow and the brain.

374. The answer is e. *(Way, pp 360-366.)* The patient has an empyema or the accumulation of pus in the pleural cavity. Based on the history (3 weeks of symptoms) and the fluid analysis demonstrating a glucose level less than 40 mg/dL and a pH less than 7.0 and its thick consistency, the patient's empyema is in the most advanced stage or the chronic organizing phase. In this phase, the fluid collection is loculated and depositions of fibrin create a thick pleural rind, which prevents apposition of the lung to the parietal pleura. Reexpansion of the lung requires thoracotomy with decortication to remove the purulent fluid and the pleural rind. Antibiotic therapy tailored to the organism(s) identified is necessary but not sufficient to treat an empyema.

375. The answer is e. *(Greenfield, pp 1423-1424.)* Superior vena cava obstruction (SVC syndrome) is almost always due to malignancy (90% of cases) and in three out of four cases, results from invasion of the vena cava by bronchogenic carcinoma. Lymphomas are the second most common cause of the SVC syndrome. Fibrosing mediastinitis as a complication of histoplasmosis or ingestion of methysergide may occur, but is rare. Rarely, a substernal thyroid or thoracic aortic aneurysm may be responsible for the obstruction. SVC syndrome can be caused iatrogenically secondary to indwelling catheters. Although constrictive pericarditis may decrease venous return to the heart, it does not produce obstruction of the superior vena cava. Whatever the cause of the superior vena cava syndrome, the resultant increased venous pressure produces edema of the upper body, cyanosis, dilated subcutaneous collateral vessels in the chest, and headache.

Cervical lymphadenopathy may also be present as a result of either stasis or metastatic involvement. Initial management of superior vena cava syndrome consists of diuresis, and for malignancies, the treatment consists of radiation and chemotherapy if applicable. Occasionally, surgical intervention or thrombolysis may be indicated for severe life-threatening complications.

376. The answer is d. (*Greenfield, pp 692-696.*) Perforation of the esophagus in the chest is a surgical catastrophe that requires aggressive intervention in virtually all circumstances. In a patient with no underlying esophageal disorder, surgical intervention is directed at primary repair of the perforation and drainage of the mediastinum. In patients with an underlying motility disorder, stricture, or malignancy, surgical intervention must address both the perforation and the esophageal abnormality. For patients with a distal esophageal carcinoma, treatment usually requires esophagectomy. Esophageal exclusion or proximal diversion (with a cervical esophagostomy or "spit fistula") are typically reserved for patients in whom a late diagnosis of esophageal perforation was made.

377. The answer is b. (*Brunicardi, pp 573-575.*) Initial treatment of a lung abscess, once the diagnosis has been made, is systemic antibiotics directed against the causative agent. The duration of therapy is dependent on the severity of the underlying pneumonia that resulted in the abscess and can last up to 12 weeks. Often, the abscess drains spontaneously via the tracheobronchial tree, but if it fails to resolve with medical therapy, intervention may be required, ranging from percutaneous to surgical drainage of the abscess or resectional therapy.

378. The answer is d. (*Brunicardi, pp 707-709.*) The initial treatment for a descending aortic dissection is reduction in the change in blood pressure over the change in time (*dP/dT*), which is achieved with β-blockade. Nitroprusside may be added after β-blockade has been achieved. Indications for operative intervention for a descending aortic dissection are end-organ failure (renal failure, lower extremity ischemia, intestinal ischemia), inadequate pain relief despite optimal medical therapy, and rupture or signs of impending rupture (increasing diameter or periaortic fluid).

379. The answer is a. (*Brunicardi, pp 878-880.*) The finding of prolonged high-amplitude contractions in the body of the esophagus in a highly symptomatic patient is diagnostic of diffuse esophageal spasm (DES). None of the findings revealed by the diagnostic studies listed (minimal reflux esophagitis, normal LES relaxation and pressure, and an incidental small epiphrenic diverticulum) justifies treatment and none explains the patient's symptoms. The cause of the hypermotility disorder known as DES is unknown, but its symptoms can be disabling. The recommended treatment for this relatively rare disorder is a long myotomy guided by the manometric evidence. More than 90% of patients treated in this fashion will experience acceptable relief of symptoms if the myotomy is performed correctly.

380. The answer is b. (*Greenfield, pp 696-697.*) Corrosive injuries of the esophagus most frequently occur in young children because of accidental ingestion of strong alkaline cleaning agents. Signs of airway injury or imminent obstruction warrant close observation and possibly tracheostomy. An initial esophagogram with water-soluble contrast (Gastrografin) is performed if a perforation is suspected or for localization of a perforation prior to surgical intervention. Vomiting should be avoided, if possible, to prevent further corrosive injury and possible aspiration. Administration of oral antidotes is ineffective unless given within moments of ingestion; even then, the additional damage potentially caused by the chemical reactions of neutralization often makes use of them unwise. Attempted dilution of the caustic agent is not recommended, given that most of the damage has already occurred, and increasing the gastric volume may induce nausea and vomiting. Based on lack of evidence of efficacy in preventing strictures and potential deleterious side effects, steroids are not recommended. Parenteral antibiotics are indicated in cases with significant esophageal injury. It is probably wise to avoid all oral intake until the full extent of injury is ascertained.

381. The answer is d. (*Greenfield, pp 1412-1414.*) Spontaneous pneumothorax usually results from the rupture of subpleural blebs in young men (age 20-40 years), which is often signaled by a sudden onset of chest and shoulder pain. Large pneumothoraxes require placement of a chest tube; thoracotomy with bleb excision and pleural abrasion is generally recommended if spontaneous pneumothorax is recurrent. Small pneumothoraxes in patients with minimal symptoms usually resolve and therefore can simply be observed. A spontaneous perforation of the esophagus (Boerhaave syndrome) can result in hydropneumothorax as well as the more usual pneumomediastinum, but would not present with an isolated 40% pneumothorax. Gastrografin swallow followed by a barium study are appropriate diagnostic tests for evaluation of a suspected leaking esophagus.

382. The answer is a. *(Townsend, pp 1082-1086)* The presence of air in the mediastinum after an episode of vomiting and retching is virtually pathognomonic of spontaneous rupture of the esophagus (Boerhaave syndrome). A contrast esophagram is the initial test of choice and is indicated with barium for a suspected thoracic perforation and water-soluble contrast (Gastrografin) for an abdominal perforation. Barium is inert in the chest but causes peritonitis in the abdomen, whereas aspirated Gastrografin can cause severe pneumonitis. CT scanning may be useful if a small, contained leak is suspected. A surgical endoscopy needs to be performed if the imaging studies are negative with a high degree of suspicion for an esophageal injury. If the leak is contained and the patient does not have any evidence of sepsis, then the leak can be managed with antibiotics and expectant management. For leaks associated with systemic signs, patients should undergo prompt surgical therapy. The operation of choice is dependent on the time to diagnosis. Leaks that are less than 24 hours old in patients without an underlying esophageal disorder may be managed with thoracotomy, repair, and drainage. Leaks older than 24 hours typically require more extensive surgery.

383. The answer is a. *(Brunicardi, p 134. Greenfield, pp 411-412.)* Significant pump failure occurs in less than 5% of patients with major chest trauma. There are no universally accepted criteria for the diagnosis of myocardial contusion, but an ECG may demonstrate ST- or T-wave changes (which are not specific for a myocardial contusion), arrhythmias, or bundle branch blocks. Similarly, cardiac enzymes may be elevated, including the CKMB fraction, but are neither sensitive nor specific for a myocardial contusion. Echocardiography may demonstrate wall motion abnormalities, valvular disruption, or a pericardial effusion with or without tamponade. Antiarrhythmics are not indicated prophylactically in a patient with a myocardial contusion, but should be used to treat any rhythm disturbances. Supportive therapy for myocardial contusion is directed at inotropic support of the ventricle; the coronary arteries are usually intact after the injury, so there is little role for coronary vasodilators and less for CABG.

384. The answer is c. *(Townsend, pp 1819-1820.)* Cardiac tamponade is a life-threatening complication that can occur after CABG. If the patient has bleeding postoperatively, the patient's coagulopathy should be corrected. Clotting of the mediastinal chest tube followed by hemodynamic decompensation with decreased mean arterial pressures (MAPs) and cardiac output with increasing filling pressures is suggestive of tamponade. Equalization of pressures across the four chambers on Swan-Ganz catheter monitoring or collapse of the right atrium on echocardiography are diagnostic of tamponade. The patient should return to the operating room for exploration and drainage of the mediastinal hematoma.

385. The answer is c. *(Greenfield, pp 1411-1412.)* A low-fat, medium-chain triglyceride diet often reduces the flow of chyle. Chylothorax may occur after intrathoracic surgery, or it may follow malignant invasion or compression of the thoracic duct. Intraoperative recognition of a thoracic duct injury is managed by ligation of the duct. Direct repair is impractical owing to the extreme friability of the thoracic duct. Injuries not recognized until several days after intrathoracic surgery frequently heal following the institution of a low-fat diet and either repeated thoracentesis or tube thoracostomy drainage.

386. The answer is d. *(Brunicardi, pp 679-680.)* The most common benign cardiac tumor is a myxoma. Symptoms can include valvular obstruction (mitral or tricuspid valve) or embolization systemically. They are often attached by a pedicle to the fossa ovalis of the left atrial septum. Treatment is resection.

387. The answer is d. *(Greenfield, pp 1416-1423.)* The boundaries of the mediastinum are the thoracic inlet, the diaphragm, the sternum, the vertebral column, and the pleura bilaterally. The mediastinum itself is divided into three portions delineated by the pericardial sac: the anterosuperior and posterosuperior regions are in front of and behind the sac, respectively, while the middle region designates the contents of the pericardium. In adults, mediastinal masses occur most frequently in the anterosuperior region and less often in the posterosuperior and middle regions. Cysts (pericardial, bronchogenic, or enteric) are the most common tumors of the middle region; neurogenic tumors are the most common of the primary tumors of the posterior mediastinum. The primary neoplasms of the mediastinum in the anteroposterior region (in order of descending frequency) are thymomas, lymphomas, and germ cell tumors. More commonly, though, a mass in this area represents the substernal extension of a benign substernal goiter. Diagnosis may be made by visualization of an enhancing structure on CT; radioactive iodine scanning is useful in management because it may make the diagnosis if the mediastinal tissue is functional and will also document the presence of functioning cervical thyroid tissue to prevent removal of all functional thyroid tissue during mediastinal excision.

388. The answer is a. (*Brunicardi, pp 696-701.*) Operative intervention is usually recommended for thoracic aortic aneurysms greater than 5 or 6 cm in diameter or those that are increasing in size. Spinal cord ischemia can result in paraplegia with a risk of 5% to 15%, depending on the extent of the repair. Various strategies that have been employed to prevent spinal cord ischemia include minimizing cross-clamp time, hypothermia, moderate systemic heparinization, left heart bypass, and cerebrospinal fluid drainage (using a lumbar drain). The rationale for cerebrospinal fluid drainage is that it decreases the pressure on the blood supply to the spinal cord and therefore improves perfusion. Postoperative steroids do not reduce the risk of paraplegia.

389. The answer is e. (*Greenfield, pp 697-698.*) Pharyngoesophageal (Zenker) diverticulum is an outpouching of mucosa between the lower pharyngeal constrictor and the cricopharyngeus muscles. It is thought to result from an incoordination of cricopharyngeal relaxation with swallowing. These diverticula occur in elderly patients and more commonly on the left. The typical patient presents with complaints of dysphagia, weight loss, and choking. Other patients present symptoms such as repeated aspiration, pneumonia, or chronic cough. A mass is sometimes palpable, and a gurgle may be heard. Surgical treatment is excision of the diverticulum and division of the cricopharyngeus muscle (cricopharyngeal myotomy), which can be done under local anesthesia in a cooperative patient. Diagnosis is made with a barium swallow; endoscopy is indicated if there is concern for malignancy (which is rarely associated with Zenker diverticulum). Esophagoscopy should be performed cautiously because the blind pouch is easily perforated. Even though the pouch may extend down into the mediastinum, the origin of the diverticulum is at the cricopharyngeus muscle near the level of the bifurcation of the carotid artery.

390. The answer is a. (*Townsend, pp 1802-1812.*) CABG is indicated in patients with angina (chronic, unstable, or postinfarction) and in asymptomatic patients with ischemia on cardiac stress tests. Operative mortality depends on the presence of risk factors such as age, other comorbidities, and preoperative ventricular function. Mortality in low risk, younger patients is approximately 3%. CABG offers a long-term survival benefit in patients with multivessel disease, left main coronary artery disease, and one-vessel and two-vessel disease with proximal left anterior descending coronary artery obstruction. CABG is the treatment of choice in diabetic patients. CABG is not indicated for patients with congestive heart failure unless this condition is ischemic in origin and angiography identifies disease amenable to surgical revascularization.

391. The answer is c. *(Greenfield, pp 1406-1407.)* The thoracic outlet syndrome designates a symptom complex whose precise cause is unknown. It is felt to result from compression of the brachial plexus or subclavian vessels, or both, in the anatomic space bounded by the first rib, the clavicle, and the scalene muscles. Carpal tunnel syndrome (compression of the median nerve as it passes through the carpal tunnel of the wrist) and cervical disk disease are the two entities most commonly confused with the thoracic outlet syndrome, whose symptoms and signs include pain, paresthesias, edema, venous congestion, and digital vasospastic changes. Positional dampening or obliteration of the radial pulse is an unreliable finding, since it is present in up to 70% of the normal population. Plain films may diagnose bony abnormalities, and MRI can be useful in detecting cervical disease. Neurologic abnormalities may be documented by nerve conduction studies. Angiographic studies are often negative. Conservative management, which generally should precede surgery, consists of an exercise program to strengthen shoulder girdle muscles and decrease shoulder droop. Operative treatment includes division of the scalenus anticus and medius muscles, first rib resection, cervical rib resection, or a combination of all three.

392. The answer is c. *(Cummings, pp 511-518.)* This x-ray demonstrates an air-fluid level in the pericardium. Pneumopericardium can result from penetrating or blunt chest trauma, spontaneous formation of gas from anaerobic bacteria, iatrogenic causes, or direct extension into the pericardium by diseased adjacent organs. In this case, a patient with a high gastrojejunostomy developed a recurrent ulcer that eroded through the diaphragm and into the pericardium and thus caused a pneumopyopericardium. Often these patients have an unrecognized gastrinoma (Zollinger-Ellison syndrome) and therefore continue to have peptic ulcer disease despite aggressive surgical therapy. The presence of pneumopyopericardium as seen in this chest film should be treated as a surgical emergency in this setting. Inability to demonstrate a fistula on radiographic investigation should not preclude the diagnosis of this entity. If the cause of the pericardial fluid is not clearly diagnosed by available means, then a pericardial window should be performed for diagnostic as well as therapeutic reasons. The pericardial sac should be irrigated, and adequate continuing drainage should be ensured. Although myocardial infarction may result in pericardial effusion or (rarely) tamponade, it does not cause pneumopericardium.

393. The answer is b. (*Greenfield, p 1382.*) Pancoast tumors are peripheral bronchogenic carcinomas that produce symptoms by involvement of extrapulmonary structures adjacent to the cupula. These structures include the nerve roots of C8 and T1, as well as the sympathetic trunk. Interruption of the cervical sympathetic trunk leads to miosis, ptosis, and anhidrosis, the triad of signs that constitutes Horner syndrome. Involvement of the nerve roots causes pain along the corresponding dermatomes. The peripheral location of the neoplasm makes pulmonary signs, such as atelectasis, cough, and hemoptysis, unlikely.

394. The answer is d. (*Brunicardi, pp 602-603.*) The initial treatment for a chylothorax consists of nonoperative therapy: drainage of the chest cavity, bowel rest, and total parenteral nutrition. However, if chyle drainage continues to be greater than 500 mL/day, then operative ligation of the thoracic duct should be performed. The best approach if the site of the leak cannot be identified is from a right thoracotomy—the thoracic duct is ligated from the diaphragm to T6. The thoracic duct enters the chest from the abdomen through the aortic hiatus of the diaphragm, courses on the right side of the chest, and then curves to the left at the level of the fifth thoracic vertebra.

395. The answer is c. (*Greenfield, pp 1382-1383.*) Bronchial carcinoid tumors rarely produce the carcinoid syndrome. They are slow-growing, infrequently metastatic tumors that histologically resemble carcinoid tumors of the small intestine. More than 80% arise in the major proximal bronchi, and their intraluminal growth is responsible for the frequent presentation of bronchial obstruction. The only therapy for this lesion is operative resection, because neither the primary tumor nor the infrequent lymph node metastasis is radiosensitive. The low malignant potential for this lesion is reflected by a long-term survival rate that approaches 90%.

396. The answer is c. (*Brunicardi, pp 556-557.*) Coin lesions have been defined as densities within the lung field of up to 3 cm, usually round, and free of signs of infections such as cavitation or surrounding infiltrates.

Malignant solitary lesions may contain flecks of calcification, but heavy calcification or concentric rings of calcium generally suggest a benign etiology. The differential diagnosis for coin lesions includes primary pulmonary carcinomas, metastatic carcinomas to the lung, benign lung neoplasms such as chondromas, other benign lung processes such as granulomas, or vascular abnormalities such as arteriovenous malformations. Coin lesions should be biopsied to rule out malignancy. Transthoracic fine-needle aspiration (FNA) can be used for diagnosis, with an accuracy of 95% for peripheral pulmonary lesions, but is associated with a high rate of complications. Thoracoscopic resection can be used for peripheral nodules not amenable to FNA. If the patient has had a previous malignancy of tissue other than lung, the likelihood that the lesion represents a metastatic lesion depends on the tissue of origin of the previous malignancy. If all patients with a history of prior cancer are considered together, a lung nodule will be a new lung primary in 60%, a metastatic lesion in 25%, and a benign process in 15% of cases. However, 80% of solitary lesions in patients with melanoma represent metastatic disease, while only 40% of lesions in patients with breast cancer represent metastasis, and solitary lesions in patients with colon carcinoma are equally likely to be metastatic or primary lung cancers.

397. The answer is d. *(Greenfield, pp 1391-1392.)* The term *hamartoma* denotes a tumor that arises from the disorganized arrangement of tissues normally found in an organ. Pulmonary hamartomas are solitary lesions of the pulmonary parenchyma and generally appear as asymptomatic peripheral nodules; they represent the most common benign epithelial and mesodermal elements. Pulmonary chondromas consist of mesodermal elements alone and arise centrally in major bronchi, where they produce signs and symptoms of bronchial obstruction. Fibromas are the most common benign mesodermal tumors found in the lung; they may occur either within the lung parenchyma or, more commonly, within the tracheobronchial tree. Osteochondromas are lesions of bone and are not found in the lung. Aspergillomas are caused by infection with the fungus *Aspergillus* and most commonly appear in the upper lobes as oval, friable, necrotic gray, or yellow masses often surrounded by evidence of preexisting parenchymal lung disease.

398. The answer is b. *(Brunicardi, pp 877-878.)* The x-rays are consistent with a diagnosis of achalasia, a motility disorder of the esophagus that usually affects persons between 30 and 50 years of age. The x-rays show a classic beak-like narrowing of the distal esophagus and a large, dilated esophagus proximal to the narrowing. The diagnosis of achalasia is generally suspected on the basis of barium studies, but, because other esophageal disorders may mimic the condition, an esophageal motility study is usually required to confirm the diagnosis. The characteristic findings on a motility study are small-amplitude, repetitive, simultaneous postdeglutition contractions in the body of the esophagus, failure of the lower esophageal sphincter to relax after deglutition, and a higher than normal pressure in the body of the esophagus. Carcinoma of the esophagus is approximately seven times more frequent in persons who have achalasia than in the general population. Patients usually describe difficulty in swallowing solids and liquids.

399 to 403. The answers are 399-d, 400-a, 401-b, 402-e, 403-c. (*Greenfield, pp 1466-1468.*) The Argyll Robertson pupil (a pupil that constricts with accommodation but not in response to light) is characteristic of central nervous system syphilis and is associated with vascular system manifestations of that disease. *Treponema pallidum* invades the vasa vasorum and causes an obliterative endarteritis and necrosis. The resulting aortitis gradually weakens the aortic wall and predisposes it to aneurysm formation. Once an aneurysm has formed, the prognosis is grave. Massive isolated tricuspid regurgitation produces a markedly elevated venous pressure, usually manifested by a severely engorged (often pulsating) liver. If the venous pressure is sufficiently elevated, exophthalmos may result. Tricuspid regurgitation of rheumatic origin is almost never an isolated lesion, and the major symptoms of patients who have rheumatic heart disease are usually attributable to concurrent left heart lesions. Bacterial endocarditis from intravenous drug abuse is becoming an increasingly important cause of isolated tricuspid regurgitation. A Quincke pulse, which consists of alternate flushing and paling of the skin or nail beds, is associated with aortic regurgitation. Other characteristic features of the peripheral pulse in aortic regurgitation include the waterhammer pulse (Corrigan pulse, caused by a rapid systolic upstroke) and pulsus bisferiens, which describes a double systolic hump in the pulse contour. The finding of a wide pulse pressure provides an additional diagnostic clue to aortic regurgitation. Myocarditis, aortitis, and pericarditis have all been described in association with Reiter syndrome; the original description included conjunctivitis, urethritis, and arthralgias. Although its cause is unknown, Reiter syndrome is associated with HLA-B27 antigen, as are aortic regurgitation, pericarditis, and ankylosing spondylitis. Short stature, webbed neck, low-set ears, and epicanthal folds are the classic features of patients who have Turner syndrome. Persons affected by the syndrome, which is commonly linked with aortic coarctation, are genotypically XO. However, females and males have been described with normal sex chromosome constitutions (XX, XY) but with the phenotypic abnormalities of Turner syndrome. Additional cardiac lesions associated with Turner syndrome include septal defects, valvular stenosis, and anomalies of the great vessels.

404 to 408. The answers are 404-c, 405-a, 406-d, 407-b, 408-e. (*Greenfield, pp 1416-1423.*) Mediastinal pheochromocytomas comprise less than 2% of all pheochromocytomas. Their presentation is consistent with overproduction of catecholamines resulting in paroxysmal or sustained hypertension. Diagnosis is by measurement of urinary catecholamines and their metabolites. Thymomas are associated with myasthenia gravis, agammaglobulinemia, and red blood cell aplasia. These tumors are typically cystic and occur in the anterior mediastinum. Most thymic lesions associated with myasthenia gravis are hyperplastic rather than neoplastic. Renal stones occur in about half the cases of hyperparathyroidism. Other disorders sometimes associated with hyperparathyroidism include peptic ulcers, pancreatitis, and bone disease; central nervous system symptoms may also arise in connection with hyperparathyroidism. Occasionally, parathyroid adenomas occur in conjunction with neoplasms of other endocrine organs, a condition known as multiple endocrine adenomatosis. Persons afflicted with Hodgkin disease have impaired cell-mediated immunity and are particularly susceptible to mycotic infections and tuberculosis. The severity of the immune deficiency correlates with the extent of the disease. The nodular sclerosing variant of primary mediastinal Hodgkin disease is the most common type. Histology reveals Reed-Sternberg cells. Cystic teratomas, or dermoid cysts, include endodermal, ectodermal, and mesodermal elements. They are characteristically cystic and contain poorly pigmented hair, sebaceous material, and, occasionally, teeth. If there is a connection between the teratoma and the tracheobronchial tree, the patient may present with symptoms of coughing up hair or sebaceous material. Dermoid cysts occur in the gonads and central nervous system, as well as in the mediastinum. With rare exceptions, these lesions are benign.

409 to 413. The answers are 409-g, 410-e, 411-b, 412-a, 413-f. (*Greenfield, pp 187-189.*) Epinephrine is a circulating endogenous catecholamine, released mainly from the adrenal medulla, whose effects are mediated by binding of free circulating hormone to β_1 and β_2 receptors, with lesser effects on α adrenoreceptors. At low infusion rates the β_1-adrenergic effects predominate causing increased heart rate, stroke volume, and contractility. At higher infusion rates, α-adrenergic receptors are stimulated resulting in an increase in blood pressure and systemic vascular resistance. Prolonged use of high-dose epinephrine is limited by renal and splanchnic vasoconstriction, cardiac dysrhythmias, and increased myocardial oxygen demand. Epinephrine is typically used as a short-term agent given in intravenous boluses during cardiac arrests. Norepinephrine is also endogenously produced, but acts locally through release at nerve synapses. It acts on α-adrenergic and β-adrenergic receptors resulting in an increase in afterload and glomerular perfusion pressure with preservation of cardiac output. Norepinephrine is associated with increase in urine output in hypotensive, septic patients. Dopamine is an endogenous catecholamine that is released into the circulation and acts by binding to α_1 receptors as well as to specific dopamine receptors in the renal, mesenteric, coronary, and intracerebral vascular beds, causing vasodilation. It has effects that change with increasing doses by binding to different receptors. At low serum concentrations, dopamine binds to dopaminergic receptors in the renal and splanchnic beds leading to increased urine output and natriuresis. At modest concentrations, dopamine binds to cardiac β_1-adrenergic receptors leading to increased myocardial contractility and increased heart rate. At high doses, dopamine binds to α-adrenergic receptors and causes an increase in blood pressure and peripheral vascular resistance. Dopamine is an effective agent in increasing blood pressure in hypotensive patients with adequate fluid resuscitation. Dobutamine is a synthetic catecholamine that predominately binds to β-adrenergic receptors and enhances myocardial contractility with minimal changes in heart rate. It is often used in treatment of cardiogenic shock following myocardial infarction to support myocardial contractility while reducing peripheral resistance. Phenylephrine is a pure α-agonist and its use results in increased peripheral vascular resistance and blood pressure. The increase in afterload increases left ventricular work and oxygen demand and may cause a decrease in stroke volume and cardiac output. Nitroprusside is an arterial and venous smooth muscle vasodilator. Continuous infusions of nitroprusside require monitoring of serum thiocyanate levels and arterial pH for cyanide toxicity. Nitroglycerin is primarily a venous smooth muscle vasodilator. It is an effective treatment for myocardial ischemia because it diminishes myocardial oxygen demand by reducing excessive preload and ventricular end-diastolic pressure.

Peripheral Vascular Problems

Questions

414. A 64-year-old woman complains of calf pain and swelling following an uncomplicated left hemicolectomy for diverticular disease. An ultrasound confirms the presence of deep vein thrombosis (DVT) of the calf. Which of the following statements is true?

a. The patient will not have long-term complications from the DVT if treated promptly with anticoagulants.
b. This condition may be effectively treated with low-dose heparin.
c. This condition may be effectively treated with pneumatic compression stockings.
d. This condition may be effectively treated with acetylsalicylic acid.
e. The patient is still at risk for pulmonary embolism.

415. For the first 6 hours following a long and difficult surgical repair of a 7-cm abdominal aortic aneurysm, a 70-year-old man has a total urinary output of 25 mL since the operation. Which of the following is the most appropriate diagnostic test to evaluate the cause of his oliguria?

a. Renal scan
b. Aortogram
c. Left heart preload pressures
d. Urinary sodium concentration
e. Creatinine clearance

416. A 72-year-old man undergoes an aortobifemoral graft for symptomatic aortoiliac occlusive disease. The inferior mesenteric artery (IMA) is ligated at its aortic attachment. Twenty-four hours after surgery the patient has abdominal distention, fever, and bloody diarrhea. Which of the following is the most appropriate diagnostic study for this patient?

a. Aortogram
b. Magnetic resonance imaging (MRI)
c. Computed tomographic (CT) scan
d. Sigmoidoscopy
e. Barium enema

417. A 25-year-old woman presents to the emergency room complaining of redness and pain in her right foot up to the level of the midcalf. She reports that her right lower extremity has been swollen for at least 15 years, but her left leg has been normal. On physical examination, she has a temperature of 39°C (102.2°F) and the right lower extremity is nontender with nonpitting edema from the groin down to the foot. There is cellulitis of the right foot without ulcers or skin discoloration. The left leg is normal. Which of the following is the most likely underlying problem?

a. Congenital lymphedema
b. Lymphedema praecox
c. Venous insufficiency
d. Deep venous thrombosis
e. Acute arterial insufficiency

418. A 76-year-old woman presents with acute onset of persistent back pain and hypotension. A CT scan is obtained (shown below), and the patient is taken emergently to the operating room. Three days after surgery she complains of abdominal pain and bloody mucus per rectum. Which of the following is the most likely diagnosis?

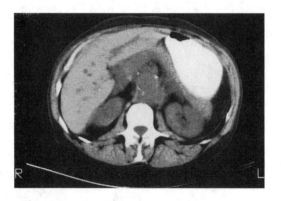

a. Staphylococcal enterocolitis
b. Diverticulitis
c. Bleeding arteriovenous (AV) malformation
d. Ischemia of the left colon
e. Bleeding colonic carcinoma

419. An 80-year-old man is found to have an asymptomatic pulsatile abdominal mass. An arteriogram is obtained (shown below). Which of the following statements concerning this patient's condition is correct?

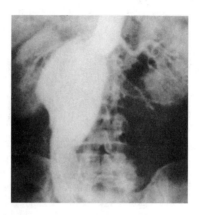

a. There is a 20% chance of mortality with surgical repair.
b. Surgery should be performed only after the patient becomes symptomatic.
c. Surgery will improve his chance of 5-year survival.
d. Surgery should not be performed in a patient of his age.
e. Surgery should be performed only if follow-up ultrasound demonstrates increasing size.

420. A 75-year-old man is found by his internist to have an asymptomatic carotid bruit. Which of the following is the most appropriate next test?

a. Transcranial Doppler studies
b. Doppler ultrasonography (duplex)
c. Spiral CT angiography
d. Arch aortogram with selective carotid artery injections
e. Magnetic resonance arteriogram (MRA)

421. A 69-year-old man with mild hypertension and chronic obstructive pulmonary disease (COPD) presents with transient ischemic attacks and the angiogram shown here. Which of the following is the most appropriate treatment recommendation?

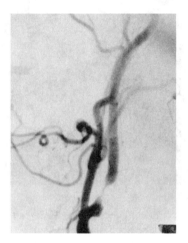

a. Medical therapy with aspirin 325 mg/day and medical risk factor management
b. Medical therapy with warfarin
c. Angioplasty of the carotid lesion followed by carotid endarterectomy if the angioplasty is unsuccessful
d. Carotid endarterectomy
e. Medical risk factor management and carotid endarterectomy if neurologic symptoms develop

422. A 55-year-old man with recent onset of atrial fibrillation presents with a cold, numb, pulseless left lower extremity. He is immediately taken to the operating room for an embolectomy of the left popliteal artery. Which additional procedure should be performed along with the embolectomy?

a. Electromyography (EMG) of the leg
b. Measurement of anterior compartment pressure in the leg
c. Fasciotomy of the anterior compartment in the leg
d. Fasciotomy of all the compartments in the leg
e. Application of a posterior splint to the leg

423. A 58-year-old man presents with pain in the left leg after walking more than one block that is relieved with rest. On physical examination distal pulses are not palpable in the left foot and there is dry gangrene on the tip of his left fifth toe. An ankle-brachial index on the same side is 0.5. Which of the patient's symptoms or signs of arterial insufficiency qualifies him for reconstructive arterial surgery of the left lower extremity?

a. Ankle-brachial index less than 0.7
b. Rest pain
c. Claudication
d. Absent palpable pulses
e. Toe gangrene

424. A 64-year-old man presents with a history of a triple coronary artery bypass 2 years ago. His only medication is a thiazide diuretic. You are considering administration of antiplatelet therapy. Which of the following statements concerning antiplatelet therapy is correct?

a. Aspirin has been shown to be an effective antiplatelet agent.
b. Most antiplatelet agents work by enhancing prostaglandin synthesis.
c. Antiplatelet agents have not been shown to increase patency rates of coronary artery bypass grafts.
d. Aspirin can be used to treat deep venous thrombophlebitis.
e. The antiplatelet effect of aspirin will last for the life of the platelet, which is generally 20 to 25 days.

425. A patient who has had angina as well as claudication reports feeling light-headed on exertion, especially when lifting and working with his arms. The subclavian steal syndrome is associated with which of the following hemodynamic abnormalities?

a. Antegrade flow through a vertebral artery
b. Venous congestion of the upper extremities
c. Occlusion of the carotid artery
d. Occlusion of the vertebral artery
e. Occlusion of the subclavian artery

426. An angiogram of a patient to be referred to you for a surgical opinion shows almost total occlusion of the aorta at the aortoiliac bifurcation. Which of the following is most consistent with the findings on the angiogram?

a. Claudication of the hips, buttocks, and thighs
b. Causalgia of the lower leg
c. Retrograde ejaculation
d. Gangrene of the feet
e. Dependent rubor of the feet

427. A 66-year-old woman with a history of smoking has a slowly enlarging abdominal aortic aneurysm. Surgery is considered, but her hypertension, smoking, and diabetes puts her at risk for associated coronary heart disease. What test is most predictive of postoperative ischemic cardiac events following peripheral vascular surgery?

a. Exercise stress testing
b. Gated blood pool studies that demonstrate an ejection fraction of 50% or less
c. Coronary angiography
d. Dipyridamole-thallium imaging
e. Transesophageal echocardiography

428. Fourteen months after a femoropopliteal bypass graft procedure, a 64-year-old man is admitted with a cold foot and no graft pulse. Urokinase infusion is begun. Which of the following statements regarding management is true?

a. Clot lysis is accomplished in 25% of patients.
b. After successful clot lysis, surgical revision of the opened graft should be considered only if early reocclusion occurs.
c. With optimal treatment, a 20% reocclusion rate is expected within 1 year.
d. Urokinase is less successful in lysing acute thromboses of prosthetic grafts than those of vein grafts.
e. Streptokinase is the preferred thrombolytic agent when treating graft occlusions.

429. A 60-year-old man is admitted to the coronary care unit with a large anterior wall myocardial infarction. On his second hospital day, he begins to complain of the sudden onset of numbness in his right foot and an inability to move his right foot. On physical examination, the right femoral, popliteal, and pedal pulses are no longer palpable. Which of the following statements concerning this condition is true?

a. Appropriate management is embolectomy of the right femoral artery.
b. Duplex imaging of the right lower extremity arteries is the appropriate next step.
c. Prophylactic exploration of the contralateral femoral artery should be done despite the presence of a normal pulse.
d. The source of the embolus is most likely the right ventricle.
e. Arteriography is mandatory prior to operative intervention.

430. A 60-year-old man is found on a routine physical examination to have a large pulsatile mass in the right popliteal fossa. X-ray of the right of the right lower extremity is shown below. Which of the following statements about this condition is true?

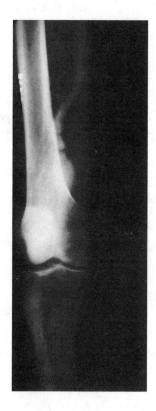

a. Surgery is reserved for symptomatic patients.
b. Limb loss is a definite risk in the untreated patient.
c. The contralateral limb is affected in a similar fashion in over 85% of cases.
d. Embolic complications are unlikely.
e. Rupture is the most common presentation.

431. A 65-year-old male cigarette smoker reports onset of claudication of his right lower extremity approximately 3 weeks previously. He can walk three blocks before the onset of claudication. Physical examination reveals palpable pulses in the entire left lower extremity, but no pulses are palpable below the right groin level. Noninvasive flow studies are obtained and are pictured here. Which of the following statements regarding this patient's condition is true?

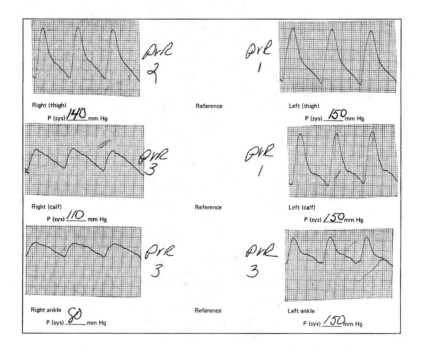

a. Femoropopliteal bypass is indicated on a relatively urgent basis in order to salvage the right leg.
b. The occlusive process is in the right superficial femoral artery, with flow to the right foot supplied by the profunda femoris artery.
c. About half of patients with similar symptoms will ultimately require amputation.
d. The occlusive process is most likely caused by embolic disease.
e. The noninvasive studies suggest iliac as well as superficial femoral occlusive disease on the right side.

432. A 56-year-old woman presents to her primary care physician for a routine check up. She states that she was recently hospitalized for surgery and was told she had some metal placed in a large blood vessel to prevent blood clots from moving to her lungs. An abdominal x-ray is shown here. Which of the following is the most appropriate indication for placement of this device?

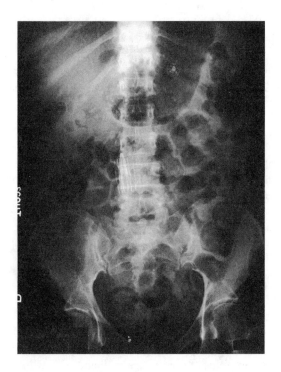

a. Recurrent pulmonary embolus despite adequate anticoagulation therapy
b. Axillary vein thrombosis
c. Pulmonary embolus due to DVT of the lower extremity that occurs 2 weeks post-operatively
d. DVT in a patient with patient with metastatic carcinoma
e. Pulmonary embolus in a patient with metastatic carcinoma

433. Two days after admission to the hospital for a myocardial infarction, a 65-year-old man complains of severe, unremitting midabdominal pain. His cardiac index is 1.6. Physical examination is remarkable for an absence of peritoneal irritation or distention despite the patient's persistent complaint of severe pain. Serum lactate is 9 mmol/L (normal is less than 3 mmol/L). Which of the following is the most appropriate next step in this patient's management?

a. Perform computed tomography
b. Perform mesenteric angiography
c. Perform laparoscopy
d. Perform flexible sigmoidoscopy to assess the distal colon and rectum
e. Defer decision to explore the abdomen until the arterial lactate is greater than 10 mmol/L

434. A postoperative patient with swelling and pain in his right calf is suspected of having a deep venous thrombosis. Prior to initiating treatment with anticoagulants, he requires a confirmatory examination. Which of the following statements regarding duplex imaging of the lower extremity is true?

a. It is not very sensitive for detecting calf thrombi in symptomatic patients.
b. A negative venous duplex examination is sufficient to withhold treatment with anticoagulation.
c. It cannot differentiate between acute and chronic venous thrombi.
d. The presence of enlarged collaterals confirms the diagnosis of an acute venous thrombosis.
e. The lack of compressibility of the vein is the hallmark of a chronic venous thrombosis.

435. A 52-year-old man with human immunodeficiency virus (HIV) and a history of intravenous drug use presents with a new heart murmur and fever. He also complains of severe back pain and on further evaluation is found to have an enlarged, saccular-appearing abdominal aorta below the renal arteries. Which of the following statements is correct regarding his diagnosis and treatment options?

a. The most likely organisms involved are *Staphylococcus* and *Salmonella*.
b. The mainstay of therapy should consist of antifungal antibiotics for 3 to 6 months.
c. Surgical intervention is indicated only if he remains febrile after 6 weeks of intravenous antibiotics.
d. The treatment of choice is aortic replacement with a synthetic graft and perioperative antibiotics only.
e. The treatment of choice is 6 weeks of intravenous antibiotics followed by aortic replacement with a synthetic graft.

436. A 72-year-old woman with severe COPD who requires home oxygen is unable to ambulate inside her home without experiencing severe left hip pain. She was hospitalized 1 year ago for a viral pneumonia and was ventilator-dependent at that time for 6 weeks. On examination, her blood pressure is 165/80 mm Hg. She has weakly palpable bilateral femoral pulses. An angiogram demonstrates severe aortoiliac disease involving bilateral iliac vessels. Which of the following is the most appropriate vascular procedure for this patient?

a. Femorofemoral bypass
b. Axillofemoral bypass
c. Femoropopliteal bypass
d. Aortobifemoral bypass
e. Common femoral and profunda femoral endarterectomies

Peripheral Vascular Problems

Answers

414. The answer is e. (*Greenfield, pp 1783-1786.*) The initial treatment for DVT is therapeutic heparinization with either with intravenous heparin or low-molecular-weight heparin administered subcutaneously. Even following prompt, aggressive treatment of DVT of the calf, as many as half of affected patients will develop symptoms of chronic venous hypertension, and a larger number will have abnormal venous hemodynamic findings. Both low-dose heparin and pneumatic compression stockings are acceptable prophylactic measures in patients at moderate risk for DVT; however, they are not effective against established thrombosis. Salicylates have not been shown to have either a prophylactic or a therapeutic role in the treatment of DVT. A small percentage of patients undergoing appropriate treatment of DVT can still develop a pulmonary embolus. These patients would then be candidates for an inferior vena cava filter. Long-term anticoagulation for patients with DVT is achieved with warfarin; the appropriate duration of therapy is based upon the risk factors (reversible or time-limited versus ongoing), the number of previous episodes, and the location (isolated calf versus femoral).

415. The answer is c. (*Greenfield, pp 183-187.*) By far the most likely cause of the oliguria observed in this patient is hypovolemia. Volume status would be best assessed by placing a Swan-Ganz catheter to measure the preload pressures in the left atrium (by inference from the pulmonary capillary wedge pressures). Patients who undergo long, difficult operations in large surgical fields collect third-space fluids and become intravascularly depleted despite large volumes of intravenous fluid and blood replacement. The proper management usually involves titrating the cardiac output by providing as much fluid as necessary to keep the wedge pressures near 15 mm Hg. The other studies listed might become useful if urinary flow remains depressed after optimal cardiac output has been achieved, but in view of the probability of hypovolemia, they are not indicated as first diagnostic studies.

416. The answer is d. (*Townsend, pp 1923-1924.*) The patient has ischemia of the left colon and rectum. Intestinal ischemia develops when a patent inferior mesenteric artery is ligated in the setting of superior mesenteric artery (SMA) or bilateral hypogastric artery occlusion. Ligation of the IMA too far from the aorta can also interfere with the collateral blood supply to the rectosigmoid and lead to ischemia. Abdominal distention, fever, elevation of white blood cell count, and/or bloody diarrhea in the postoperative period should raise suspicion for colon ischemia. The best study to evaluate the sigmoid and rectum is sigmoidoscopy. Barium enema is not as accurate as sigmoidoscopy in determining depth of injury and carries grave risks of contamination by barium and feces if perforation occurs. CT, MRI, and aortography are not useful in evaluating the colon for early ischemia.

417. The answer is b. (*Townsend, pp 2022-2023.*) This patient's underlying problem is unilateral primary lymphedema. Lymphedema is classified as primary when the etiology is unknown. Hypoplasia of the lymphatic system of the lower extremity accounts for more than 90% of cases of primary lymphedema. If edema is present at birth, it is referred to as congenital; if it starts early in life (as in this woman), it is called praecox; if it appears after the age of 35 years, it is tarda. The inadequacy of the lymphatic system accounts for the repeated episodes of cellulitis that these patients experience. Swelling is not seen with acute arterial insufficiency. Deep venous thrombophlebitis will result in tenderness and is generally not a predisposing factor for cellulitis of the foot. Venous insufficiency is usually accompanied by varicose veins, brawny skin discoloration in the distal leg and ankle, and skin ulcers.

418. The answer is d. (*Greenfield, pp 1728-1729.*) The patient's presentation of acute onset, persistent back pain, and hypotension is classic for ruptured abdominal aortic aneurysm. The CT scan reveals a fractured ring of calcification in the abdominal aorta with significant density (blood) in the para-aortic area. The incidence of ischemic colitis following abdominal aortic repair is about 2%. The incidence dramatically increases following a ruptured aneurysm repair. The sigmoid colon is affected most frequently. Blood flow to the left colon is normally derived from the IMA with collateral flow from the middle and inferior hemorrhoidal vessels. The SMA may also contribute via the marginal artery of Drummond. If the SMA is stenotic or occluded, flow to the left colon will be primarily dependent on an intact IMA. The IMA is usually ligated at the time of aneurysm repair. Patients at highest risk for diminished flow through collateral vessels are those with a history of visceral angina, those found to have a patent IMA at the time of operation, those who have suffered an episode of hypotension following rupture of an aneurysm, those in whom preoperative angiograms reveal occlusion of the SMA, and those in whom Doppler flow signals along the mesenteric border cease following occlusion of the IMA. Bowel ischemia recognized at the time of operation should be treated by reimplantation of the IMA into the graft to restore flow.

419. The answer is c. (*Greenfield, pp 1711-1719.*) The patient has an asymptomatic abdominal aortic aneurysm (AAA). An aneurysm is defined as a focal dilation of an artery exceeding 1.5 times the normal diameter. The diameter of a normal abdominal aorta in a man is approximately 2 cm. This patient's arteriogram demonstrates an aneurysm diameter close to three times the size of his normal aorta. This would make the patient's aneurysm 5 cm to 6 cm in diameter. All symptomatic AAAs should be repaired, regardless of size. In asymptomatic patients, the minimum size for repair is controversial. For good surgical candidates (young, low operative risks), repair is advocated for aneurysms larger than 4 cm in diameter. Smaller AAAs may warrant repair only if rapidly enlarging owing to the increased risk for rupture. The patient's age is not a contraindication to surgery, because several studies have demonstrated a low mortality rate (<5%) and satisfactory long-term survival and quality of life in elderly, even octogenarian, patients.

420. The answer is b. (*Greenfield, pp 1545-1548.*) Doppler ultrasonography (duplex) is the best initial test for screening patients with carotid disease. It has become a highly accurate test, often obviating the need for carotid arteriography prior to carotid endarterectomy. Carotid arteriography remains the gold standard when quantifying the degree of carotid stenosis, but it is usually performed after noninvasive testing suggests significant stenosis. Spiral CT angiography is a noninvasive modality that has been used to evaluate many segments of the vascular tree, but as yet its accuracy does not approach that of standard arteriography and it would certainly not be used in the initial evaluation of a patient with an asymptomatic bruit. MRA is also a modality that has enjoyed success in the investigation of carotid disease. Although not quite as accurate as standard arteriography, it has been used in conjunction with the duplex as a complementary study. Once again, because of its cost, MRA would not be used as the primary screening modality. Transcranial Doppler studies are used to assess the intracranial vasculature.

421. The answer is d. (*Executive Committee for the Asymptomatic Carotid Atherosclerosis Study, pp 1421-1428.*) In a prospective, randomized, multicenter trial involving 1662 patients in a study known as the Asymptomatic Carotid Atherosclerosis Study, patients with asymptomatic carotid artery stenosis causing 60% or greater reduction in diameter and whose general health made them good candidates for elective surgery were found to have a significant reduction in the 5-year risk for ipsilateral stroke with surgery compared with medically treated cohorts (5.1% vs 11.0%). Medically treated patients were treated with aspirin on a daily basis. Warfarin has not been shown to be effective in the management of patients with carotid disease. Angioplasty of carotid stenoses is being performed in some institutions but to date has not replaced surgery as the treatment for high-grade carotid stenoses.

422. The answer is d. (*Townsend, pp 545-547.*) This patient should undergo four compartment fasciotomy (anterior, lateral, superficial posterior, and deep posterior) since he satisfies two conditions that lead to a compartment syndrome of the leg: acute arterial occlusion without collateral inflow and rapid reperfusion of ischemic muscle. Another common cause of compartment syndrome is orthopedic trauma to the leg. The need for fasciotomy is based on clinical judgment. If a fasciotomy is indicated, all four compartments should always be opened. Electromyographic studies and compartment pressure measurements would probably be abnormal, but are unnecessary in view of the known findings and would delay treatment. Application of a splint has no role in the acute management of this problem.

423. The answer is e. (*Brunicardi, pp 767-770.*) The major threat to patients with arterial occlusive disease is limb loss. Rest pain and gangrene represent advanced stages of arterial insufficiency and warrant arterial reconstructive surgery whenever clinically feasible. This patient does not have rest pain which is defined as persistent pain in the extremity. Claudication, in most cases, reflects mild ischemia; the majority of affected patients are successfully managed without surgery. Most will stabilize or improve with development of increased collateral blood flow following institution of a program of daily exercise, cessation of smoking, and weight loss. Ankle-brachial index is a useful preoperative tool but does not by itself determine whether someone is a candidate for revascularization. Palpable pulses are usually absent in patients with claudication. Vasodilator drugs have been shown to have little benefit in the conservative management of intermittent claudication.

424. The answer is a. (*Willerson, pp 12A-18A.*) Antiplatelet agents are generally used to prevent thrombotic and embolic events in the arterial circulation. The Canadian Cooperative Study demonstrated antiplatelet therapy to be effective in preventing strokes in men with carotid artery disease. Antiplatelet therapy has also been shown to increase graft patency rates following coronary artery bypass grafting if the medication is started preoperatively and continued postoperatively. Aspirin exerts an antiplatelet effect that will last for the life of the platelet (approximately 7-10 days). Patients who take aspirin will experience its effect for 7 to 10 days after stopping the medication. Aspirin interferes with platelet function by inhibiting the synthesis of thromboxane A2 and the subsequent production of prostaglandins. The platelet does not have a nucleus and thus cannot remanufacture the prostaglandins necessary for its functioning. Antiplatelet therapy has no role in treatment of thrombophlebitis in the deep venous system.

425. The answer is e. (*Brunicardi, pp 796-797.*) Atherosclerotic occlusion of the subclavian artery proximal to the vertebral artery is the anatomic situation that results in the subclavian steal syndrome. On being subjected to exercise, the involved extremity (usually the left, which is more prone to atherosclerosis because of anatomic differences) develops relative ischemia, which gives rise to reversal of flow through the vertebral artery with consequent diminished flow to the brain. The upper extremity symptom is intermittent claudication. Venous occlusive disease is not a feature of the syndrome. The operative procedure for treating the subclavian steal syndrome consists of delivering blood to the extremity by creating either a carotid-subclavian bypass or a subclavian-carotid transposition. Dilatation and stenting of the artery by endovascular techniques is effective as well.

426. The answer is a. (*Greenfield, pp 1634-1639.*) Patients with aortoiliac atherosclerotic disease, or Leriche syndrome, often present with claudication of the hips, buttocks, and thighs; absent femoral pulses; and impotence. The slow progression of aortoiliac atherosclerotic occlusive disease leads to enlargement of a network of collateral channels around the diseased segments. Important collateral arterial pathways around the aortic bifurcation and common iliac segments are the intercostal and lumbar arteries to circumflex iliac and iliolumbar arteries, the superior to inferior epigastric arteries, and the superior and inferior mesenteric arteries to rectal and internal pudendal arteries. Collateral pathways bypassing occlusive lesions of the external iliac arteries include the hypogastric to circumflex femoral channels. This network of collateral vessels provides sufficient blood flow to meet the metabolic needs of the lower extremities, but do not have the capacity to increase blood flow to the levels necessary during exercise. Erectile dysfunction is another common complaint in men secondary to the reduced hypogastric perfusion. Retrograde ejaculation usually occurs with disruption of the sympathetic chain overlying the distal aorta and left iliac after dissection around these vessels during vascular reconstructions. Gangrene of the feet or toes is rarely seen unless distal embolization of atherosclerotic material from the aorta occludes the pedal or digital arteries. Dependent rubor is usually a sign of significant ischemia resulting from lower extremity occlusive and not aortoiliac disease. Causalgia or reflex sympathetic dystrophy is a disorder of the sympathetic nervous system that can affect the upper or lower extremities.

427. The answer is d. *(Boucher, pp 389-394. Pasternack, pp 13-17.)* When gated blood pool scans (eg, MUGA or multiple gated acquisition scan) demonstrate ejection fractions of 35% or less and reversible perfusion defects on dipyridamole-thallium imaging they are predictive of perioperative ischemic cardiac events among patients undergoing peripheral vascular reconstruction. Ischemic rest pain or early onset of claudication after minimal exercise limits the effectiveness of stress testing as a screening procedure for occult coronary artery disease in this group of patients. Screening coronary angiography, followed by angioplasty or bypass of asymptomatic lesions, had an adverse effect on patient survival in a large prospective study of patients who had peripheral vascular surgery. Transesophageal echocardiography has no role in the preoperative screening of peripheral vascular patients.

428. The answer is c. *(Belkin, pp 769-773. Eisbud, pp 160-165.)* Management of acute graft occlusion must include both reestablishment of peripheral perfusion and correction of any underlying hemodynamic problem. Urokinase is associated with fewer allergic reactions than streptokinase and is the preferred thrombolytic agent. Treatment results in total clot lysis in 75% of patients. However, high reocclusion rates are observed (20% within 1 year) even if angioplasty or anastomotic revision is performed after successful lysis. Without surgical revision following clot lysis, a 50% reocclusion rate is expected within 3 months. Urokinase has proved equally successful in opening both vein and prosthetic graft thromboses.

429. The answer is a. *(Greenfield, pp 1637-1643.)* Immediate surgical intervention is the appropriate management for patients presenting with acute arterial insufficiency with neurologic compromise of the lower extremities from thromboembolic disease. The heart is the most common source of arterial emboli and accounts for 90% of cases. Sources include diseased valves, endocarditis, the left atrium in patients with unstable atrial arrhythmias, and mural thrombus on the wall of the left ventricle in patients with myocardial infarction. The diagnosis in this patient is clear, and therefore neither noninvasive testing nor arteriography is indicated. In the absence of neurologic symptoms arteriography with directed thombolysis of the clot is an acceptable alternative to surgery. However, if neurologic symptoms are present, arteriography may delay treatment and lead to limb loss. Embolectomy of the femoral artery can be performed under local anesthesia with minimal risk to the patient. Emboli typically lodge in one femoral artery; contralateral exploration is not indicated in the absence of signs or symptoms. The contralateral groin should always be prepared in case flow is not restored via simple thrombectomy, and femoral-femoral bypass is needed to provide inflow to the affected limb.

430. The answer is b. (*Brunicardi, pp 750-751.*) Popliteal artery aneurysms are the most common peripheral arterial aneurysms. They are bilateral up to 70% of the time and are associated with extrapopliteal aneurysms 55% of the time (aortic, femoral). Many patients are asymptomatic when diagnosed (40%), but can develop embolization (25%) or thrombosis (40%) with resultant gangrene. Rupture of the aneurysm (less than 5%) can occur but is an uncommon presentation compared with distal emboli. All symptomatic popliteal aneurysms should undergo surgical repair with exclusion of the aneurysm (which is ligated and left in situ) combined with a surgical bypass. Because of the risk of complications, asymptomatic popliteal aneurysms greater than 2 cm, should be repaired as well.

431. The answer is b. (*Greenfield, pp 1649-1654.*) This patient has occlusion of the right superficial femoral artery caused by atherosclerosis. This is confirmed by both the physical examination and the flow study findings which indicate a sharp decrease in the blood pressure below the level of the common femoral artery. Fewer than 10% of patients with claudication progress to gangrene and the need for amputation. Operative therapy would not be suggested at this time because it is quite likely that, with cessation of cigarette smoking and adherence to an exercise program, the patient could markedly improve his walking radius as collateral vessels enlarge to deliver more blood to the affected tissues. Operative therapy (femoropopliteal bypass) would be indicated at this time in this patient only if symptoms of rest pain or ischemic ulceration were present. Physical examination and flow studies indicate disease distal to the aortoiliac distribution.

432. The answer is a. *(Brunicardi, p 346)* The Greenfield filter pictured on the x-ray is used to interrupt migration of emboli to the lungs from the veins below the level of the filter. It is indicated in patients who sustain a recurrent pulmonary embolus despite adequate anticoagulant therapy or in patients with pulmonary emboli who cannot receive anticoagulants because of a contraindication (eg, bleeding ulcer, intracranial hemorrhage). The filter is not used in patients who sustain a single pulmonary embolus. It is placed in the inferior vena cava just below the renal veins and therefore would not be effective for emboli that arise cephalad to its position. Despite the hypercoagulable state seen in some patients with metastatic pancreatic cancer, anticoagulation can still be used as a first-line defense.

433. The answer is b. *(Greenfield, pp 1614-1618.)* Abdominal pain out of proportion to findings on physical examination is characteristic of intestinal ischemia. The etiology of ischemia may be embolic or thrombotic occlusion of the mesenteric vessels or nonocclusive ischemia due to a low cardiac index or mesenteric vasospasm. Differentiation among these etiologies is best made by mesenteric angiography. While not without serious risks, angiography also offers the possibility of direct infusion of vasodilators into the mesenteric vasculature in the setting of nonocclusive ischemia. This patient, with a recent myocardial infarction and a low cardiac index, is at risk for embolism of clot from a left ventricle mural thrombus as well as low-flow mesenteric ischemia. If embolism or thrombosis is found angiographically (usually involving the superior mesenteric artery), thrombolytic therapy can be attempted in the absence of suspicion of ischemic bowel. Otherwise, operative embolectomy or vascular bypass is indicated to restore flow. If occlusive disease cannot be demonstrated, efforts should be made to simultaneously increase cardiac output with inotropic agents and dilate the mesenteric vascular bed by angiographic instillation of papaverine, nitrates, or calcium-channel blockers. Computed tomography is not helpful in delineating the cause of intestinal ischemia because it does not provide a sufficiently detailed image of the mesenteric vessels. Laparoscopy and/or laparotomy would be useful if ischemic bowel were suspected, although laparoscopy would not allow for adequate assessment of the visceral vessels. Flexible sigmoidoscopy, while useful in patients with ischemic colitis, has no role in the workup of mesenteric ischemia, which involves primarily the small intestine and right colon. Serum lactate is helpful in raising the suspicion of intestinal ischemia, but no absolute level should be used to decide whether or not to explore a patient.

434. The answer is b. (*Greenfield, pp 1781-1783.*) The sensitivity, specificity, and positive and negative predictive values of duplex scanning (Doppler analysis and B-mode ultrasonography) are more than 95% in *symptomatic* patients with acute DVT. A high negative predictive value means that if the patient tests negative, there is a high probability of *not* having the disease. Therefore, a negative duplex scan is sufficient to withhold anticoagulation. Duplex scanning is less sensitive in detecting calf thrombi in asymptomatic patients. Duplex scanning can differentiate between acute and chronic venous thromboses. Acute DVTs are characterized by an enlarged noncompressable vein without collateral vessels whereas chronic DVTs have normal-sized veins with significant collaterals. The duplex scanning device is portable, and therefore the study is easily performed at the bedside, in a vascular laboratory, or in a radiology suite. It is completely noninvasive, painless, and safe.

435. The answer is a. (*Brunicardi, pp 742-744.*) The patient has a mycotic aortic aneurysm, which is a sequela of infection, most commonly with either *Staphylococcus* or *Salmonella*. Treatment for infrarenal mycotic aortic aneurysms has traditionally been that an axillofemoral bypass is performed and then the involved intra-abdominal aorta is excised. If the aorta is debrided and replaced, autogenous graft material is used (eg, superficial femoral vein). Antibiotic therapy is also administered for 3 to 6 months.

436. The answer is b. (*Greenfield, pp 1640-1648.*) Given her comorbidities, the patient should undergo axillofemoral bypass grafting. In a patient with severe symptoms of claudication that are interfering with his or her lifestyle, intervention is indicated. In a young, healthy patient with unilateral iliac artery occlusive disease, when angioplasty is not a treatment option, an aortofemoral bypass offers excellent long-term relief. Aortobifemoral bypass, while clearly the most risky of the treatment options offered, provides the best long-term patency. In elderly patients with severe comorbidities who are considered at high risk for complications, extra-anatomic bypasses (femoro-femoral or axillofemoral bypasses) offer fair long-term patencies while not subjecting the patient to the risks of general anesthesia. Femorofemoral bypass offers the additional benefit of not disturbing sexual function; however, femorofemoral bypass is not an option in a patient with bilateral iliac artery disease. Axillofemoral bypass grafts are an alternative to aortofemoral procedures, but have a lower 5-year patency rate and should be reserved for high-risk patients with bilateral iliac disease or an infected aortic aneurysm or graft.

Urology

Questions

437. A 65-year-old woman complains of urinary incontinence and desires a surgical consultation regarding treatment options. Which of the following statements about incontinence is correct?

a. Pelvic floor exercises improve symptoms in patients with mild urge incontinence.
b. Continuous urinary incontinence suggests the presence of a vesicovaginal or vesicocutaneous fistula.
c. Anticholinergic medications may improve symptoms in patients with mild stress incontinence.
d. Spinal cord injuries at the level of the cauda equina can result in urge incontinence.
e. Urge incontinence never improves after a urethral sling procedure.

438. A 26-year-old man is seen in the emergency ward because of symptoms of urinary burning, frequency, and urgency. Urinalysis shows bacteriuria. His meatus is inferiorly displaced on the glans. Which of the following statements regarding hypospadias is correct?

a. It is often associated with chordee (ventral curvature of the penis).
b. It is associated with undescended testes in more than 50% of cases.
c. It is a rare fusion defect of the posterior male urethra.
d. It occurs sporadically, without evidence of familial inheritance.
e. The most common location is penoscrotal.

439. A 60-year-old man sees a urologist for what he describes as bloody urine. A urine sample is positive for cytologic evidence of malignancy. Cystoscopy confirms the presence of superficial transitional cell carcinoma. Which of the following is the recommended treatment for stage A (superficial and submucosal) transitional cell carcinoma of the bladder?

a. Local excision
b. Radical cystectomy
c. Radiation therapy
d. Topical (intravesicular) chemotherapy
e. Systemic chemotherapy

440. A 36-year-old man presents to the emergency room with renal colic. A radiograph reveals a 1.5-cm stone. Which of the following statements regarding this disorder is correct?

a. Conservative treatment including hydration and analgesics will not result in a satisfactory outcome.
b. Serial kidney-ureter-bladder (KUB) radiographs should be used to follow this patient.
c. Urinalysis will nearly always reveal microhematuria.
d. When the acute event is correctly treated, this disease seldom recurs.
e. Elevated blood urea nitrogen (BUN) and creatinine are expected.

441. An 8-month-old boy is seen by a pediatrician for the first time. The physician notes that there are no testes in the scrotum. Which of the following is the optimal management of bilateral undescended testicles in an infant?

a. Immediate surgical placement into the scrotum.
b. Chorionic gonadotropin therapy for 1 month; operative placement into the scrotum before age one if descent has not occurred.
c. Observation until the child is 2 years old because delayed descent is common.
d. Observation until age 5; if no descent by then, plastic surgical scrotal prostheses before the child enters school.
e. No therapy; reassurance of the parent that full masculinization and normal spermatogenesis are likely even if the testicle does not fully descend.

442. A 32-year-old medical student notes an asymptomatic mass in his right testicle. On examination, the mass cannot be transilluminated. The urologist suspects seminoma. Seminoma is accurately described by which of the following statements?

a. It is the most common type of testicular cancer.
b. Metastases to liver and bone are frequently found.
c. It does not respond to radiation.
d. The 5-year survival rate approaches 50%.
e. Common presentation is that of a painful lump that transilluminates.

443. A 10-year-old boy presents to the emergency room with acute onset of pain in the left testicle. On physical examination, he is noted to have a high-riding, indurated, and markedly tender left testis. Urinalysis is unremarkable. Which of the following statements regarding the patient's diagnosis and treatment is true?

a. There is a strong likelihood that this patient's father or brother has had or will have a similar event.
b. Operation should be delayed until a technetium scan clarifies the diagnosis.
c. The majority of testicles that have undergone torsion can be salvaged if surgery is performed within 24 hours.
d. If torsion is found, both testes should undergo orchiopexy.
e. The differential diagnosis includes spermatocele.

444. A patient is noted incidentally on an ultrasound to have a right renal mass. Which of the following statements is true regarding further workup and treatment of a renal mass?

a. Presence of a simple cyst requires follow-up imaging in a year.
b. Diagnosis of an angiomyolipoma of the kidney requires surgical resection.
c. Presence of a 3-cm lesion suspicious for renal cell carcinoma can be treated with a partial nephrectomy.
d. Computed tomographic (CT) scanning is diagnostic for oncocytomas.
e. Presence of a solid, enhancing lesion in the right kidney should always be biopsied percutaneously.

445. A 48-year-old African-American man is found to have a mass in the prostate on a digital rectal examination. His prostate-specific antigen (PSA) is high and a biopsy of the prostate confirms carcinoma. Which of the following statements regarding carcinoma of the prostate is true?

a. It has a higher incidence among African Americans than among other American ethnic group.
b. A single microscopic focus of prostate cancer discovered on transurethral resection of the prostate (TURP) is an indication for radical prostatectomy.
c. It arises initially in the gland's central portion.
d. It commonly produces osteoclastic bony metastases.
e. Screening for elevated PSA offers no advantage over simple rectal examination in the detection of the disease.

446. A 60-year-old man seeks medical attention because of increasing difficulty in urination (decreased flow, straining, hesitancy). A prostate biopsy proves benign. Which of the following statements regarding benign prostatic hyperplasia (BPH) is true?

a. Initial management of BPH is transurethral resection of the prostate.
b. Low bladder pressures and low flow rates are suggestive of outflow obstruction.
c. All patients with BPH should be treated to prevent renal failure due to outflow obstruction.
d. Indications for surgery include urinary retention refractory to medical therapy and recurrent urinary tract infections (UTIs).
e. Hypernatremia is a complication of transurethral resection of the prostate for BPH.

447. The left ureter is partially transected (50% of circumference) during the course of a difficult operation on an unstable, critically ill patient. Which of the following would be the most appropriate management of this injury given the patient's unstable condition?

a. Placement of an external stent through the proximal ureteral stump with delayed reconstruction
b. Ipsilateral nephrectomy
c. Placement of a catheter from the distal ureter through an abdominal wall stab wound
d. Placement of a closed suction drain adjacent to the injury
e. Bringing the proximal ureter up to the skin as a ureterostomy

448. A pedestrian is hit by a speeding car. Radiologic studies obtained in the emergency room, including a retrograde urethrogram (RUG), are consistent with a pelvic fracture with a rupture of the urethra superior to the urogenital diaphragm. Which of the following is the most appropriate next step in this patient's management?

a. Immediate percutaneous nephrostomy
b. Immediate placement of a Foley catheter through the urethra into the bladder to align and stent the injured portions
c. Immediate reconstruction of the ruptured urethra after initial stabilization of the patient
d. Immediate exploration of the pelvis for control of hemorrhage from pelvic fracture and drainage of pelvic hematoma
e. Immediate placement of a suprapubic cystostomy tube

449. A 25-year-old man presents with a painful, fully erect penis lasting several hours. Which of the following statements regarding the patient's diagnosis and treatment is true?

a. It can be associated with sickle disease.
b. It can cause systemic hypoxia and acidosis.
c. The peak incidence is seen from ages 10 to 30 years.
d. It is not recommended to give treatment through the intracorporal route.
e. Treatment is primarily surgery with corporosaphenous, corporoglandular, or corporospongiosal shunts.

450. A 55-year-old man presents with fever and pain in the perineal region. Upon further questioning he also complains of frequency, urgency, dysuria, and a decreased urinary stream. On physical examination his abdomen is soft, nondistended, and nontender. Digital rectal examination demonstrates exquisite tenderness on the anterior aspect. Laboratory examination reveals leukocytosis and findings on urinalysis consistent with a bacterial infection. Which of the following is the most likely diagnosis?

a. Urinary tract infection
b. Benign prostatic hyperplasia
c. Prostatitis
d. Pyelonephritis
e. Nephrolithiasis

Urology

Answers

437. The answer is b. *(Brunicardi, pp 1543-1544.)* There are several types of urinary incontinence: stress, urge, overflow, and total. Stress incontinence in women is associated with previous birth trauma, aging, and neurologic injuries. Nonoperative treatment includes estrogen therapy, pelvic floor exercises, and timed voiding. Surgical therapy in women consists of a urethral sling procedure. Urge incontinence can be treated symptomatically with anticholinergic medications, biofeedback, and timed voiding. If there is a contributory component from stress incontinence, urge incontinence may improve with a urethral sling procedure. A spinal cord injury above the level of the sacrum results in a hyperreflexic bladder and urges incontinence. Overflow incontinence may result from bladder outlet obstruction. Total incontinence, or continuous leakage of urine, suggests the presence of a fistula and typically requires surgical intervention.

438. The answer is a. *(Brunicardi, pp 1555-1556.)* Hypospadias is a common congenital anomaly of the penis resulting from incomplete development of the anterior urethra. It occurs in about 1 in 300 live births and is believed to have a multifactorial genetic mode of inheritance. Of those with hypospadias, about 7% have a father with the disorder, 14% a brother, and 20% a second family member. Hypospadias occurs in the corona in about 75% of cases, where it is often accompanied by chordee. Undescended testes occur in about 10% of cases of hypospadias, as do inguinal hernias. Hypospadias in the scrotal area is associated with bilateral undescended testes and infertility and must be differentiated from pseudohermaphroditism and adrenogenital syndrome.

439. The answer is d. *(Greenfield, pp 2084-2086.)* Bladder cancer represents 2% of all cancers, and 90% of bladder cancers are of transitional cell origin. It is most prevalent among men with a history of heavy smoking and is usually multifocal and superficial, even when recurrent. When the disease is still superficial, transurethral resection of visible lesions and intravesicular chemotherapy are most often recommended. More radical surgical resection is reserved for advanced stages of the disease.

440. The answer is a. (*Greenfield, pp 2078-2081.*) Initial management of kidney stones should include hydration and analgesics. However, as this patient's stone is larger than 1 cm, it is unlikely to pass spontaneously, though stones smaller than 0.5 cm usually do pass spontaneously. The size of the stone also makes a high-grade obstruction more likely; therefore, an intravenous pyelogram (IVP) must be urgently performed. A high-grade obstruction will require nephrostomy or a ureteral stent. If the stone is completely occluding the lumen of the ureter, urinalysis may not show microhematuria and thus may be misleading. Approximately 50% of patients may have a recurrence within 5 to 10 years. If both kidneys are functioning, then obstruction of one ureter will not result in an elevation in BUN and creatinine; such findings are expected only in the setting of an obstructed single functioning kidney.

441. The answer is b. (*Greenfield, p 1953.*) Surgical intervention consisting of inguinal orchiopexy, should be performed before 1 year of age. By the second year, a testicle not in the cooler environment of the scrotal sac will begin to undergo histologic changes characterized by reduced spermatogonia. Testicles left longer in the undescended state not only have a higher incidence of malignant degeneration, but are inaccessible for examination. If a malignancy should occur, diagnosis will be delayed. There is also a substantial psychological burden when children reach school age or are otherwise subjected to exposure of their deformed genitalia. Gel-filled prostheses are generally inserted when a testicle cannot be placed in the scrotum. Close follow-up by a physician until the late teens is indicated in all patients who have had an undescended testicle. Since these patients may be at increased risk for malignancy throughout life, careful training should be given in self-examination.

442. The answer is a. (*Greenfield, pp 2091-2093.*) Seminomas tend to grow slowly and metastasize late. They usually present as a nonpainful lump that does not transilluminate. They represent about 40% of malignant testicular tumors; embryonal cell carcinoma and teratocarcinoma each represent about 25%. Because most tumors have mixed elements, they are usually classified according to the most malignant cell type encountered, whatever the predominant cell type. When metastases occur, they are usually along the regional lymphatic drainage pathways to the iliac, aortic, and renal lymph nodes. Because of their slow growth and radiosensitivity, seminomas are associated with a 90% 5-year survival rate. Therapy generally consists of removing the affected testis and sampling the lymph nodes (usually external iliac) for evidence of metastasis. If metastases are present, radiation therapy is given locally to areas of known involvement. Radiation therapy is highly effective in seminoma, and metastatic disease may be palliated for extended periods.

443. The answer is d. (*Townsend, p 2266.*) Testicular torsion is a surgical emergency that requires rapid diagnosis and intervention to maintain testicular viability. If left untreated testicular torsion leads to strangulation of the blood supply to the testicle. Testicular torsion usually occurs in adolescent boys 12 to 18 years of age. The underlying pathology is secondary to an abnormally narrowed testicular mesentery with tunica vaginalis surrounding the testis and epididymis in a bell clapper deformity. As the testis twists, it comes to lie in a higher position within the scrotum. Presentation is acute onset of testicular pain and/or swelling. Diagnosis of testicular torsion is mainly made with clinical presentation and examination. A technetium 99m (^{99m}Tc) pertechnetate scan or Doppler ultrasound may be helpful in making the diagnosis if clinical suspicion of torsion is low; however, operation should not be delayed in order to maximize testicular salvage. This patient's presentation warrants immediate operation. If treated within the first 4 to 6 hours of onset of symptoms, the chance of saving the testicle is high. During surgery the affected testicle is rotated to its normal position. If it is viable, orchiopexy is performed on both the affected and the unaffected testes. If the affected testicle is nonviable, orchiectomy is performed with orchiopexy of the nonaffected testicle. Both epididymitis and testicular torsion presents with pain and swelling of the testicle, and it is sometimes difficult to differentiate between the two conditions. In the case of epididymitis Doppler ultrasound would demonstrate increased blood flow to the testicle, while there would be no blood flow to the testicle in torsion. A spermatocele presents as a painless fluid-filled sac located above and posterior to the testicle.

444. The answer is c. (*Brunicardi, pp 1531-1532.*) Lesions that are solid and enhancing on CT scan should raise the suspicion for a renal cell carcinoma. Because of a high false-negative rate, suspicious lesions should not routinely be biopsied. For renal cell cancers less than 4 cm, a partial nephrectomy can be performed, but for larger lesions, a radical nephrectomy (which includes the kidney, ipsilateral adrenal gland, and perirenal fat) is indicated. Benign kidney lesions include simple cysts, angiomyolipomas, and oncocytomas. Simple cysts do not require further follow-up, but multiple septations or calcifications should increase suspicion for malignancy. Angiomyolipomas can be diagnosed based on appearance on CT scan and do not require removal; larger lesions are at increased risk for hemorrhagic complications. Oncocytomas can be diagnosed only on pathology.

445. The answer is a. *(Brunicardi, pp 1535-1538; Greenfield, pp 2088-2091.)* Prostate cancer is the most common cancer in men affecting one in every six men in the United States during their lifetime. Family history, African American race, and diet have all been implicated as risk factors. Prostate cancer (adenocarcinoma) arises initially in the periphery of the gland. Therefore, one of the best screening tests is careful digital rectal examination (DRE). Screening for prostate cancer with PSA has resulted in an improvement in the diagnosis of early-stage disease. However, routine PSA screening is controversial because of the low positive predictive value. Spread of prostate cancer is by direct local extension and via lymphatic and vascular channels. The most common locations of distant metastases are in the axial skeleton with osteoblastic bony lesions. A single focus of disease discovered on TURP or simple prostatectomy is considered stage T1 by the TNM classification system and management of these lesions is dependent on the patient's life expectancy. For example, patients older than 65 years of age are treated with expectant management. More locally advanced disease is treated with radiation or surgical prostatectomy.

446. The answer is d. *(Brunicardi, pp 1528-1531.)* Indications for surgery in patients with BPH include urinary retention refractory to medical therapy, upper tract dilation, renal insufficiency secondary to outflow obstruction, and bladder stones. Recurrent urinary tract infections are also an indication for surgical intervention. BPH increases in incidence with age, and is almost universal in men in their 90s. Treatment should be directed at alleviating symptoms; initial management consists of α-blockade. Outflow obstruction is characterized by high bladder pressures and low flow rates. Low bladder pressures and low flow rates are present when the bladder muscles are poorly contractile because of overdistention and persistent obstruction. Although persistent outflow obstruction can ultimately lead to renal failure, BPH does not always progress to this stage. Surgical treatment for BPH consists of transurethral resection of the prostate. Because of the use of large volumes of hypotonic fluid during TURP, patients should be monitored postoperatively for hyponatremia secondary to absorption of the irrigation solution resulting in hemodilution.

447. The answer is a. (*Greenfield, pp 442-444; Moore, pp 811-814.*) If the patient is too unstable to perform a definitive repair, placement of a catheter into the proximal ureter is an acceptable alternative that will allow reconstruction to be performed later. Suction drainage adjacent to the injured segment alone is inadequate. If time and the patient's condition permit, primary ureteral reconstruction should be carried out. In the middle third of the ureter, this will usually consist of ureteroureterostomy (primary anastamosis) using absorbable sutures over a stent. If the injury involves the upper third, ureteropyeloplasty may be necessary. In the lower third, ureteral implantation into the bladder using a tunneling technique is preferred. The creation of a watertight seal is difficult and nephrectomy may be required if the injury occurs during a procedure in which a vascular prosthesis is being implanted (eg, an aortic reconstructive procedure) and contamination of the foreign body by urine must be avoided.

448. The answer is e. (*Brunicardi, pp 1545-1546.*) If a rupture of the urethra is suspected, a retrograde urethrogram should be obtained before any attempts are made to place a Foley catheter, as efforts to do so may result in the creation of multiple false passages or conversion of a partial laceration into complete rupture. If there is incomplete disruption of the urethra, a transurethral Foley catheter can be cautiously placed across the injury. However, if there is complete disruption, a suprapubic catheter is placed temporarily and definitive repair is delayed four to six months, at which time the hematoma will have resolved and the prostate will have descended into the proximity of the urogenital diaphragm. Percutaneous nephrostomy has no role in the management of this problem.

449. The answer is a. (*Townsend, pp 2266-2267.*) The patient has priapism, a pathologic condition of a penile erection that lasts beyond or is unrelated to sexual stimulation. In the younger age group, priapism is most often associated with sickle cell disease or neoplasm. In the older group it is most often caused by pharmacologic agents. It can occur in all age groups, but the peak incidence is from ages 5 to 10 and 20 to 50 years. There is decreased venous outflow and increased intracavernosal pressure causing local hypoxia and acidosis. In patients with sickle cell disease (or trait) treatment is intravenous (IV) hydration, alkalinization with bicarbonate in the IV fluids, analgesia, and supplemental oxygen to help reduce the veno-occlusive state in the corporal bodies. If the priapism persists then sickle cell patients are given red blood cell transfusions to reduce the hemoglobin S below 30% of total hemoglobin. In non-sickle cell patients, α-adrenergic intracorporal injections are given while monitoring blood pressure and pulse. When the intracorporal α-adrenergic treatment fails, surgical procedures with shunts (corporosaphenous, corporoglandular, or corporospongiosal) are needed to divert the occluded corporal blood.

450. The answer is c. *(Brunicardi, p 1542.)* The patient has signs and symptoms classic for acute prostatitis. Occasionally, patients may present in shock with hypotension and tachycardia. On rectal examination the prostate is extremely tender to palpation and it should be performed gently to prevent releasing bacteria into the blood stream. The treatment is broad-spectrum IV antibiotics until the patient is afebrile and hemodynamically normal. Then the treatment is continued for a total of 3 weeks with oral antibiotics. A urinary tract infection also presents with the same complaints of frequency, urgency, dysuria, and decreased urinary stream but it is not associated with perineal pain or pain on rectal exam. Benign prostatic hyperplasia does not present with pain or fever. Pyelonephritis and nephrolithiasis are not associated with pain in the perineum.

Orthopedics

Questions

451. An 18-year-old football player is seen in the emergency ward with severe knee pain incurred after being hit by a tackler while running. Physical examination is consistent with tearing of a meniscus. Meniscal tears usually result from which of the following circumstances?

a. Hyperextension
b. Flexion and rotation
c. Simple hyperflexion
d. Compression
e. Femoral condylar fracture

452. A 34-year-old man is extracted from an automobile after a motor vehicle collision. The patient has an obvious deformity of his right thigh consistent with a femur fracture. Upon closer examination of the right thigh there is bone visible through an open wound. Which of the following is the most appropriate initial management of his open femur fracture?

a. Intravenous (IV) antibiotics and cast or splint placement
b. IV antibiotics and internal or external fixation
c. Early irrigation and debridement, IV antibiotics, and cast or splint placement
d. Early irrigation and debridement, IV antibiotics, and internal or external fixation
e. Early irrigation and debridement, IV antibiotics, compartment decompression, and internal or external fixation

453. A 6-year-old boy is brought into the emergency room by his mother for walking with a limp for several weeks. On examination, the patient has tenderness over his right thigh without evidence of external trauma. An x-ray of the pelvis shows a right femoral head that is small and denser than normal. Which of the following is the correct diagnosis?

a. Slipped capital femoral epiphysis (SCFE)
b. Legg-Calve-Perthes (LCP) disease
c. Dysplasia of the hip
d. Talipes equinovarus
e. Blount disease

454. A 65-year-old man presents with acute onset of pain, swelling, and erythema of the left knee. He denies previous episodes or trauma to the knee. The differential diagnosis includes septic arthritis and gout. Which of the following is the best study to differentiate between gout and septic arthritis?

a. White blood cell count
b. X-ray of the knee
c. Magnetic resonance imaging (MRI) of the knee
d. Bone scan
e. Evaluation of synovial fluid aspirate

455. While playing with his children, a 44-year-old man falls and lands on his right shoulder. There is immediate pain and deformity. In an uncomplicated dislocation of the glenohumeral joint, the humeral head usually dislocates primarily in which of the following directions?

a. Anteriorly
b. Superiorly
c. Posteriorly
d. Laterally
e. Medially

456. A 10-year-old girl falls and fractures her femur. You try to explain what, if any, growth disturbances might be expected in the future because of the location of the fracture. The most severe epiphyseal growth disturbance is likely to result from which of the following types of fracture?

a. Fracture dislocation of a joint adjacent to an epiphysis
b. Fracture through the articular cartilage extending into the epiphysis
c. Transverse fracture of the bone shaft on the metaphyseal side of the epiphysis
d. Separation of the epiphysis at the diaphyseal side of the growth plate
e. Crushing injury compressing the growth plate

457. A 29-year-old construction worker fell 15 ft from a roof and broke his right humerus, as depicted in the accompanying radiograph. Given his injury, which of the following nerves is most at risk?

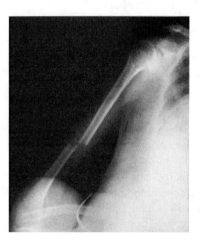

a. Median nerve
b. Radial nerve
c. Posterior interosseous nerve
d. Ulnar nerve
e. Ascending circumflex brachial nerve

458. In a failed suicide gesture, a depressed student severs her radial nerve at the wrist. Which of the following is her expected disability?

a. Loss of ability to extend the wrist
b. Loss of ability to flex the wrist
c. Wasting of the intrinsic muscles of the hand
d. Sensory loss over the thenar pad and the thumb web
e. Palmar insensitivity

459. After being injured by a bull on his mother's farm, a young man is placed in a cast for a supracondylar fracture of his humerus. He begins to experience intense pain and weakness in the ipsilateral hand. Compartment pressures are measured and are markedly elevated. Which of the following statements regarding compartment syndromes following orthopedic injuries is true?

a. The first sign is usually loss of pulse in the extremity.
b. Passive flexion of the extremity proximal to the involved compartment will aggravate the pain.
c. Surgical decompression (fasciotomy) is necessary only as a last resort.
d. These syndromes are most commonly associated with supracondylar fractures of the humerus and tibial shaft.
e. The syndrome is often painless.

460. Your son falls and breaks his tibia while ice skating. The orthopedic surgeon suggests an operation to reduce and fixate the fracture. You recall from your medical school reading that there is controversy regarding open versus closed treatment of fractures. In contrast to closed reduction, which of the following is true regarding the open reduction of a fracture?

a. Produces a shorter healing time
b. Decreases trauma to the fracture site
c. Produces a higher incidence of nonunion
d. Reduces the risk of infection
e. Requires longer periods of immobilization

Questions 461 to 464

For each description, select the type of fracture or dislocation with which it is most likely to be associated. Each lettered option may be used once, more than once, or not at all.

a. Navicular (scaphoid) fracture
b. Monteggia deformity
c. Greenstick fracture
d. Spiral fracture
e. Posterior shoulder dislocation

461. A patient has a seizure with gross tonic-clonic movements.

462. A patient experiences prolonged pain and radiologic evidence of non-healing after an injury.

463. A 30-year-old cyclist falls and injures her forearm. The radial head is dislocated and the proximal third of the ulna is fractured.

464. A patient has tenderness in the anatomical snuffbox.

Questions 465 to 468

For each description, select the type of bone disease with which it is most likely to be associated. Each lettered option may be used once, more than once, or not at all.

a. Osteogenesis imperfecta
b. Osteopetrosis
c. Osteitis fibrosa cystica
d. Osteomalacia
e. Osteitis deformans (synonym for Paget disease)

465. Your patient has renal stones and needs an operation in the neck. Parathyroid hormone levels are elevated.

466. Your patient is taking high doses of vitamin D to supplement a defect in the mineralization of adult bone due to abnormalities in vitamin D metabolism.

467. A genetically determined disorder in the structure or processing of type I collagen may require your patient to wear various orthoses to protect himself.

468. A patient has bossing of his frontal bones and an abnormal skull radiograph.

Questions 469 to 471

For each description, select the type of bone lesion with which it is most likely to be associated. Each lettered option may be used once, more than once, or not at all.

a. Osteoma
b. Osteoid osteoma
c. Osteoblastoma
d. Osteosarcoma
e. Paget disease
f. Ewing sarcoma

469. An 11-year-old boy presents with pain in his right leg. A radiograph shows a sunburst appearance with bone destruction, soft tissue mass, new bone formation, and sclerosis limited to the metaphysis of the lower femur.

470. A 25-year-old man presents with severe pain in the left femur. The pain is relieved by aspirin. On plain film, a 0.5-cm lucent lesion, which is surrounded by marked reactive sclerosis, is seen.

471. A 12-year-old boy complains of pain in his left leg that is worse at night. He has been experiencing fevers and also has a 9-lb weight loss. X-ray demonstrates an aggressive lesion with a permeative pattern of bone lysis and periosteal reaction. There is an associated large soft tissue mass as well. Pathology demonstrates the tumor to be of the round cell type.

Orthopedics

Answers

451. The answer is b. *(Brunicardi, p 1711.)* Most meniscal tears are produced by flexion and rapid rotation. A classic example (football knee) involves a player who is hit while running. The knee, supporting the entire player's weight, usually is slightly flexed, and the foot is anchored to the ground by cleats. Impact from an opposing player usually causes rotation almost entirely restricted to the knee. The injury involves rapid rotation of the flexed femoral condyles about the tibial plateau, which most frequently tears the medial meniscus. (Less frequently, the lateral meniscus is torn.) A tear in the inner free border of the cartilage is also common whenever excessive rotation without flexion or extension occurs. Early surgical removal of the displaced menisci is usually recommended to prevent further damage to the cartilage or ligaments.

452. The answer is e. *(Townsend, pp 547-551.)* Early irrigation and debridement are the mainstays in management of an open fracture. Debridement requires meticulous removal of all foreign material and resection of all nonviable tissue from the wound to reduce the bacterial count. IV antibiotics do not penetrate nonviable tissue. The wound is aggressively explored because the area of injury is always larger than expected from merely observing the wound. Irrigation with copious amounts of saline is performed with repeat debridements 48 to 72 hours later to assess for further necrosis. Given the significant amount of muscle damage in open fractures, fasciotomies are liberally performed during debridement. Skeletal stabilization is crucial for soft tissue healing in an open fracture. Compared to cast and splints, internal or external fixation allows greater access to wound care and is the preferred method of stabilization. Wound coverage is usually accomplished within 1 week of injury.

453. The answer is b. *(Brunicardi, pp 1716-1719.)* The patient's presentation and x-ray findings are most consistent with LCP. LCP can occur between the ages of 2 and 12, is 3 to 5 times more common in boys, and is bilateral in 10% to 20% of cases. The pathogenesis is thought to involve a period of ischemia in the proximal femoral epiphysis followed by revascularization. Patients with LCP present with a limp and pain in the groin, thigh, or knee. Plain radiographs show a small and denser than normal femoral head on the affected side. Slipped capital femoral epiphysis is a disorder involving dissociation between the epiphysis and metaphysis of the proximal femur. SCFE usually occurs during the adolescent growth spurt and is bilateral in one-third of cases. Patients with SCFE also present with a limp and pain in the thigh or knee. The physical examination is most remarkable for limitation of internal rotation of the hip. Plain films of the pelvis in SCFE show displacement of the metaphysis of the proximal femur. Developmental dysplasia of the hip involves a spectrum of disorders with differing degrees of instability of the hip and underdevelopment of the acetabulum. Talipes equinovarus is "clubfoot". Blount disease involves infants born with physiologic genu varum (bow legs).

454. The answer is e. *(Brunicardi, p 1680.)* The patient's presentation is consistent with both septic arthritis and gout. The most definitive study to differentiate between the two diagnoses is synovial fluid aspiration. In gout, urate crystals are seen on analysis of the joint fluid. In septic arthritis, synovial fluid aspirate demonstrates bacteria and white blood cells with high neutrophils on differential count. White blood cell count can be elevated with both processes. X-ray and MRI would show tissue swelling around the joint consistent with both conditions. A bone scan would target the area of inflammation but not give any information as to the source of the inflammation.

455. The answer is a. *(Brunicardi, pp 1694-1696.)* The glenohumeral joint is bounded posteriorly by the teres minor and infraspinatus muscles and partially by the long head of the triceps. It is bounded laterally by the powerful deltoid muscle; superiorly, the acromion process precludes upward dislocation. However, anteriorly and inferiorly the pectoralis major and the long head of the biceps do not completely stabilize the glenohumeral joint; in this region the articular ligaments and joint capsule provide the major structural support. Thus, the joint is not strongly supported in its anteroinferior aspect and consequently anterior (or anteroinferior) dislocations are the most common glenohumeral dislocations. The humeral head is driven anteriorly, which tears the shoulder capsule, detaches the labrum from the glenoid, and produces a compression fracture of the humeral head. Most glenohumeral dislocations result from a posteriorly directed force on an arm that is partially abducted. Posterior dislocation is much rarer and should raise the possibility of a seizure as the precipitating cause. Clinical suspicion and physical examination are important in diagnosis of glenohumeral joint dislocations; diagnosis can be confirmed by radiologic plain films (antero-posterior, scapular lateral, and axillary views).

456. The answer is e. *(Brunicardi, pp 1654-1655.)* Longitudinal growth of bone follows ossification of cartilage that forms at the epiphyseal plate. Fractures that involve separation of the growth plate (type I; almost always on the diaphyseal side) may be realigned; normal growth usually follows epiphyseal separation because the proliferative cells are still attached to their blood supply in the bone epiphysis. Fractures that extend perpendicular to and through the epiphysis (types II, III, IV) may result in the formation of bony bridges across the epiphysis that can disrupt later growth. Though all the fractures listed place the epiphyseal growth plate in some jeopardy, crushing injuries to the epiphysis (type V) have the worst prognosis; numerous bony bridges may form and prevent longitudinal growth.

457. The answer is b. *(Brunicardi, p 1696.)* The radiograph demonstrates a transverse fracture of the distal half of the humeral shaft. The radial nerve runs in a groove on the posterior aspect of the humerus as it courses into the forearm compartment and is therefore at high risk of injury. If the nerve injury is apparent before any manipulation has been done, the fracture should be reduced; the nerve injury should be observed, since the nerve function will likely improve with time. If the nerve injury is present only after reduction, immediate surgical exploration is warranted because the nerve might be trapped in the fracture site. At this level of the arm, the ulnar and median nerves are well protected by muscle. The posterior interosseous nerve is a distal branch of the radial nerve and may be injured in fractures near the radial head, but it is in no danger from injuries at the level seen in this radiograph. There is no ascending circumflex brachial nerve.

458. The answer is d. *(Brunicardi, p 1771.)* An injury to the radial nerve at the wrist would cause primarily sensory abnormalities. The dorsum of the hand from the radial aspect of the fourth digit over the thumb, including the thenar pad and thumb web, becomes insensate after severance of the radial nerve at the wrist. Radial injuries more proximally would impair extension of the wrist and digits as well as forearm supination.

459. The answer is d. *(Brunicardi, p 349.)* Compartment syndromes result from increasing pressures in the fascial compartments of the arm or leg.

Capillary blood flow is compromised first resulting in loss of oxygen delivery to tissues and increased extremity edema because of increased capillary permeability. Next, venous and lymphatic flow are compromised resulting in further edema. Arterial flow is the last to be compromised, which is why pulselessness is an unreliable sign. Extreme pain (out of proportion to the injury), pain on passive extension of the fingers or toes, pallor of the extremity, motor paralysis, and paresthesias are all components of the syndrome. The patient will usually hold the injured part in a position of flexion to maximally relax the fascia and reduce the pain; passive extension will usually produce severe pain. The diagnosis can be confirmed by measuring intracompartmental pressures, but whenever physical findings or symptoms are suspicious, immediate surgical decompression by fasciectomy is indicated, since delay is likely to lead to irreversible damage.

460. The answer is c. *(Brunicardi, pp 1681-1682.)* Open reduction of a fracture involves the restoration of normal bone alignment under direct observation at surgery. In effect, open reduction converts a simple fracture into a compound (or open) fracture and thereby increases the risk of infection. Operative manipulation also increases trauma at the fracture site and may consequently add to the probability of infection. Hematomas at the site of fracture may be important for early healing; open reduction, which usually involves removing the clots in the field, could contribute to a delay in bone healing and to nonunion. The major advantage of open reduction is the shorter period of immobilization it allows, an advantage that often outweighs all the disadvantages previously mentioned, as in the open reduction of femoral neck fractures in the elderly. This allows these patients to get out of bed much sooner than if they were treated with several weeks of traction.

461 to 464. The answers are 461-e, 462-a, 463-b, 464-a. *(Brunicardi, pp 1694-1696, 1730-1736.)* Fractures of the navicular bone of the wrist should be suspected in anyone, particularly a young person, who falls on an outstretched hand. Although x-rays are mandatory, it is important to realize that the fracture may not be seen on the initial x-ray and that a presumptive diagnosis can and should be made on clinical grounds alone. Typically, there will be tenderness to palpation over the navicular tuberosity and limitation of wrist flexion and extension. Immobilization of the wrist for about 16 weeks and sometimes up to 6 months is required.

Nonunion or avascular necrosis is not uncommon and may require bone grafting for correction. Dislocation of the radial head with a fracture of the proximal third of the ulna is known as Monteggia deformity. Usually, the radial head is dislocated anteriorly. The injury is usually caused by forced pronation. The injury can be treated by reduction and stabilization of the ulna followed by reduction of the radial head via supination and direct pressure.

Greenstick fractures are common in children. The bones of young children are able to bend to a greater degree than those of adults; the fracture may occur only at the site of maximal cortical stress but not at the opposite cortex, the site of maximal longitudinal compression. A spiral fracture, frequently seen in the tibia in skiers, results from the application of torque to a long bone. Anterior shoulder dislocations occur more frequently than posterior dislocations. However, posterior dislocations are seen in special situations, such as during an epileptiform convulsion and during electroshock therapy. Closed reduction followed by immobilization is usually sufficient therapy.

465 to 468. The answers are 465-c, 466-d, 467-a, 468-e. *(Brunicardi, pp 231, 1655.)* Osteitis fibrosa cystica is commonly associated with hyperparathyroidism. Hemorrhagic cystic lesions (brown tumors) usually occur in the long bones. Treatment is parathyroidectomy. Osteomalacia is defined as a defect in mineralization of adult bone that results from abnormalities in vitamin D metabolism. Treatment generally involves vitamin D supplementation. Osteogenesis imperfecta is a genetically determined disorder in the structure or processing of type I collagen. Treatment is surgical and involves orthoses to prevent fractures and correction of deformities by multiple osteotomies. Osteitis deformans is also known as Paget disease.

Osteopetrosis is a rare skeletal deformity associated with increased density of the bones.

469 to 471. The answers are 469-d, 470-b, 471-f. *(Brunicardi, pp 1664-1673.)* Osteosarcoma, or osteogenic sarcoma, usually is seen in patients between the ages of 10 and 25 years. The distal femur is the site most frequently involved. The radiograph has a blastic, or sunburst, appearance. The tumor is not sensitive to radiation but does respond well to combination chemotherapy followed by surgical resection or amputation.

An osteoid osteoma typically presents with severe pain that is characteristically relieved by aspirin. On radiograph, the lesion appears as a small lucency (usually <1.0 cm) within the bone that is surrounded by reactive sclerosis. These lesions gradually regress over 5 to 10 years, but most are excised to relieve symptoms. Surgical extirpation is usually curative.

Ewing's sarcoma is a round cell–type tumor. This is a highly malignant tumor that affects children (age range 5-15 years) and tends to occur in the diaphyses of long bones. The spine and pelvis can also be primary sites.

There is a permeative pattern of bone lysis and periosteal reaction often associated with a large soft tissue mass. Fever and weight loss are common. The pain is often more pronounced at night. Treatment usually involves a combination of radiation and systemic chemotherapy, with 5-year survivals around 50%. Adjuvant surgery in combination with radiation and chemotherapy improves the 5-year survival rate to about 75%.

Neurosurgery

Questions

472. A severely traumatized woman is seen in the emergency room (ER) with a Glasgow coma scale of 5T. Her family asks what the significance of this measurement is. Which of the following statements regarding the Glasgow coma scale is true?

a. It serves to assess the long-term sequelae of head trauma.
b. A high score correlates with a high mortality rate.
c. It includes measurement of intracranial pressure (ICP).
d. It includes measurement of pupillary reflexes.
e. It includes measurement of verbal response.

473. A 25-year-old unhelmeted man involved in a motorcycle collision has multiple cerebral contusions on head computed tomographic (CT) scan. He is agitated but hemodynamically stable, with a heart rate of 80 beats per minute and a mean arterial pressure (MAP) of 90 mm Hg. An intracranial pressure monitor is placed, and the initial ICP reading is 30 mm Hg. Which of the following is the most appropriate in the management of his traumatic brain injury (TBI) over the next few days?

a. Hyperventilation to maintain a cerebral P_{CO_2} of 25 to 30 mm Hg
b. Administration of neosynephrine to increase his MAP and, consequently, his cerebral perfusion pressure (CPP)
c. Administration of mannitol (1 g/kg) to reduce his ICP
d. Placement of the patient in Trendelenburg position to increase cerebral perfusion
e. Avoidance of all sedating drugs in the first 24 to 48 hours in order to accurately assess his neurologic status

474. A 50-year-old woman complains of headaches and lateralizing weakness. A CT scan of the brain reveals an irregular mass in the right cerebral hemisphere. A biopsy documents that this is a glioblastoma. Which of the following statements regarding glioblastoma multiforme is true?

a. It is a neuronal cell tumor.
b. It arises from the malignant degeneration of an astrocytoma.
c. With aggressive treatment, most patients can live up to 10 years with this disease.
d. It is the most common childhood intracranial neoplasm.
e. With combined surgery, chemotherapy, and radiation therapy, cure rates now approach 50%.

475. A 60-year-old otherwise healthy woman presents to her physician with a 3-week history of severe headaches. A contrast CT scan reveals a small, circular, hypodense lesion with ringlike contrast enhancement. Which of the following is the most likely diagnosis?

a. Brain abscess
b. High-grade astrocytoma
c. Parenchymal hemorrhage
d. Metastatic lesion
e. Toxoplasmosis

476. During the secondary survey of a trauma patient, it becomes apparent that there is a depressed skull fracture. You must decide if this changes the management plan for this patient in any way. Which of the following statements regarding skull fractures is true?

a. Depressed fractures are those in which the patient's level of consciousness is diminished or absent.
b. Compound fractures are those in which the skull is fractured and the underlying brain is lacerated.
c. Any bone fragment displaced more than 1 cm inward should be elevated surgically.
d. Drainage of cerebrospinal fluid via the ear or nose requires prompt surgical treatment.
e. Most skull fractures require surgical treatment.

477. A 39-year-old man presents to his physician with the complaint of loss of peripheral vision. Which of the following findings are demonstrated by the subsequent magnetic resonance imaging (MRI) scan, shown here?

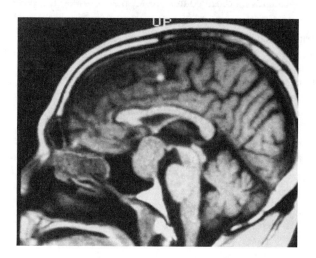

a. Cerebral atrophy
b. Pituitary adenoma
c. Optic glioma
d. Pontine hemorrhage
e. Multiple sclerosis plaque

478. An 18-year-old male is admitted to the ER following a motorcycle accident. He is alert and fully oriented, but witnesses to the accident report an interval of unresponsiveness following the injury. Skull films disclose a fracture of the left temporal bone. Following x-ray, the patient suddenly loses consciousness and dilation of the left pupil is noted. Which of the following is the most likely diagnosis?

a. A ruptured berry aneurysm
b. An acute subdural hematoma
c. An epidural hematoma
d. An intra-abdominal hemorrhage
e. A ruptured arteriovenous malformation

479. A 42-year-old woman presents to the ER with the worst headache of her life. A noncontrast CT scan of the head is negative for lesions or hemorrhage. She then undergoes a lumbar puncture, which appears bloody. All four tubes collected have red blood cell counts greater than 100,000/mL. Which of the following steps is the most appropriate management of this patient?

a. Repeat the head CT scan with intravenous contrast.
b. Perform an angiogram of the aorta and lumbar branches for immediate embolization of the injured vessel.
c. Perform a four-vessel cerebral angiogram.
d. Administer a dose of mannitol.
e. Consult neurosurgery for immediate ventriculostomy.

480. A trauma patient with a closed head injury is being monitored in the neurosurgical intensive care unit (ICU). His ICP measurement is seen to rise precipitously. An acute increase in ICP is characterized by which of the following clinical findings?

a. Respiratory irregularities
b. Decreased blood pressure
c. Tachycardia
d. Papilledema
e. Compression of the fifth cranial nerve

481. A 32-year-old nonsmoking housewife has a chest x-ray, which shows a posterior mass in the right upper chest. Computed tomography documents a pleural-based rounded mass in the posterior mediastinum. The clinical diagnosis is schwannoma of the intercostal nerve. Which of the following statements about schwannomas is true?

a. They represent central nerve tumors.
b. Treatment is via excision.
c. They arise most frequently in motor nerves.
d. They often degenerate to malignancy.
e. The most common presentation is a painful mass.

482. An 18-year-old high school senior develops peripheral vision abnormalities. A CT scan of the brain reveals a cystic suprasellar mass with some calcification noted. Clinically, this is compatible with a craniopharyngioma. Which of the following statements about craniopharyngiomas is true?

a. The tumors are uniformly solid.
b. The tumors are usually malignant.
c. Children with these tumors often develop signs and symptoms of acromegaly.
d. The tumors may cause compression of the optic tracts and visual symptoms.
e. The primary mode of treatment is radiation therapy.

483. Following significant head trauma, a 34-year-old woman receives a CT scan that demonstrates bilateral frontal lobe contusions of the brain. There is no midline shift. Which of the following statements regarding cerebral contusions is true?

a. They occur most frequently in the occipital lobes.
b. They may occur opposite the point of skull impact.
c. They are rarely accompanied by parenchymal bleeding.
d. They may occur spontaneously in patients receiving anticoagulants.
e. Anticonvulsants have no role in the early management of this disorder.

484. A 45-year-old woman presents with left-sided weakness. A CT scan of the head demonstrates a well-circumscribed mass abutting the skull in the right hemisphere. Work up of the mass reveals a meningioma. Which of the following statements is true regarding meningiomas?

a. They are malignant in 50% of cases.
b. They occur predominantly in men.
c. They are treated primarily by surgical excision.
d. They are cured, when properly treated, in nearly 95% of cases.
e. They arise from the dura.

485. A middle-aged homeless man is brought to the ER by EMS for altered mental status, seizures, and vomiting. On physical examination he has no fever, neck stiffness, nor evidence of head trauma. He does, however, have multiple dental caries and a focal neurologic deficit. Which of the following is the best next step in the patient's workup?

a. Lumbar puncture
b. Noncontrast head CT
c. Contrast-enhanced head CT
d. Placement of ICP monitor
e. Placement of ventriculoperitoneal shunt

Questions 486 to 487

For each description, select the type of vascular event with which it is most likely to be associated. Each lettered option may be used once, more than once, or not at all.

a. Subdural hematoma
b. Epidural hematoma
c. Carotid dissection
d. Brain contusion
e. Ruptured intracranial aneurysm

486. While watching a golf tournament, a 37-year-old man is struck on the side of the head by a golf ball. He is conscious and talkative after the injury, but several days later he is noted to be increasingly lethargic, somewhat confused, and unable to move his right side.

487. A 42-year-old woman complains of the sudden onset of a severe headache, stiff neck, and photophobia. She loses consciousness. She is later noted to have a dilated pupil.

Neurosurgery

Answers

472. The answer is e. *(Townsend, pp 485-486.)* The Glasgow coma scale was developed to enable an initial assessment of the severity of head trauma. It is now also used to standardize serial neurologic examinations in the early postinjury period. It measures the level of consciousness using three parameters: verbal response (5 points), motor response (6 points), and eye opening (4 points); a "T" is used in lieu of a verbal score when the patient is intubated. The score is the sum of the highest number achieved in each category and ranges from 3 for a completely unresponsive patient to 15 for a fully oriented and alert patient. A score of 13 to 15 is considered a mild traumatic brain injury (TBI), 9 to 12 a moderate TBI, and 8 or less a severe TBI. The GCS score can be used to prognosticate outcome and likelihood of neurosurgical intervention.

473. The answer is c. *(Townsend, pp 2090-2094.)* The cerebral perfusion pressure is calculated as the difference between the MAP and the ICP; optimally the CPP should be maintained at greater than 70 mm Hg and the ICP at less than 20 mm Hg. Methods for reducing ICP include elevation of the head of the bed (reverse Trendelenburg), administration of mannitol or other diuretics to improve cerebral blood flow, use of short-acting sedatives to decrease patient agitation (the drugs should be intermittently held to perform neurological examinations), prevention of hypovolemia and treatment of hypotension, and prevention of hypoventilation and hypercapnia. Hypoventilation and hypercapnia cause vasodilation of the cerebral vessels, which increases the intracranial volume and pressure. Hyperventilation may still be used in cases of herniation or impending herniation to acutely lower ICP. However, prolonged hyperventilation is not recommended because of decreased perfusion (secondary to vasoconstriction) to an already ischemic brain. Furthermore, the brain resets to the new target P_{CO_2} within 48 to 72 hours, limiting the beneficial effects of hyperventilation and resulting in increased ICP when the P_{CO_2} is later normalized. Therefore, hypercarbia should be avoided but hypocapnia below 30 mm Hg cannot be recommended except in extreme circumstances. Use of pressors to maintain a CPP above 70 mm Hg is controversial.

474. The answer is b. (*Townsend, p 2106.*) Glioblastoma multiforme is the most common form of primary intracranial neuroepithelial tumor. It is a heterogeneous glial cell tumor derived from the malignant degeneration of an astrocytoma or anaplastic astrocytoma. These tumors are most commonly found in the cerebral hemispheres during the fifth decade of life. CT and MRI scans typically reveal an irregular lesion with hypodense central necrosis, peripheral ring enhancement of the highly cellular tumor tissue, and surrounding edema and mass effect. Curative resections are rare. Therapy consists of surgical resection followed by external beam radiation. The course of the disease progresses rapidly after presentation, with median survival being 1 year.

475. The answer is d. (*Townsend, p 2110.*) The CT findings are consistent with any of the suggested lesions. However, the most likely diagnosis in an immunocompetent patient is metastatic disease, which has an incidence of approximately 150,000 to 250,000 cases per year as compared to primary intracranial tumors, which have an incidence of 35,000 per year. Roughly 15% to 30% of cancer patients develop intracranial metastases during the course of their disease. The cancers that most frequently metastasize to the brain parenchyma include those of the lung, breast, kidney, gastrointestinal (GI) tract, and melanomas. Leukemia shows a predilection for the leptomeninges. A large majority of these lesions become symptomatic owing to mass effect from white matter edema. Treatment is dependent on the number and size of the lesions and the physical condition of the patient, but may include a combination of surgery, radiosurgery, and whole-brain radiation therapy. Immunocompromised patients are at increased risk for toxoplasmosis and central nervous system lymphomas. Both immunocompetent and immunocompromised hosts can develop pyogenic brain abscesses, which typically occur in the setting of known infection (which can spread either locally or hematogenously).

476. The answer is c. (*Brunicardi, pp 1615-1617.*) Most skull fractures do not require surgical treatment unless they are depressed or compound. A general rule is that all depressed skull fractures—defined as fractures in which the cranial vault is displaced inward—should be surgically elevated, especially if they are depressed more than 1 cm, if a fragment is over the motor strip, or if small, sharp fragments are seen on x-ray (as they may tear the underlying dura). Compound fractures, defined as fractures in which the bone and the overlying skin are broken, must be cleansed and debrided and the wound must be closed. When a skull fracture occurs in the area of the paranasal sinuses, the mastoid air cells, or the middle ear, a tear in the meninges may result in cerebrospinal fluid drainage from the ear or nose. The presence of rhinorrhea or otorrhea requires observation; although meningitis is a serious sequela, the role of pro-phylactic antibiotics is controversial. Otorrhea usually heals within a few days. Persistent cerebrospinal fluid from the nose or ear for more than 14 days requires surgical repair of the torn dura.

477. The answer is b. *(Brunicardi, p 1636.)* This T1-weighted sagittal MRI scan reveals a dumbbell-shaped homogeneous mass involving the sella turcica and the suprasellar region. This lesion is most consistent with a pituitary adenoma, a benign tumor arising from the adenohypophysis. Pituitary ade-nomas are the most common sellar lesion and constitute 10% to 15% of all intracranial neoplasms. Macroadenomas are greater than 1 cm in size and microadenomas less than 1 cm. Pituitary adenomas may be functional, resulting in endocrinopathies from excessive hormone secretion, such as prolactin (amenorrhea or galactorrhea), growth hormone (gigantism or acromegaly), or adrenocorticotrophic hormone (ACTH) (Cushing syndrome). The tumor pictured is a macroadenoma; these larger tumors may cause symptoms sec-ondary to mass effect; for example, a bitemporal visual field defect can result from compression of the optic chiasm. This tumor's dumbbell shape results from impingement on the adenoma by the diaphragm of the sella turcica. The suprasellar extension seen here makes a frontal craniotomy rather than the more commonly utilized transsphenoidal approach more appropriate.

478. The answer is c. *(Brunicardi, p 1619.)* Epidural hematomas are typ-ically caused by a tear of the middle meningeal artery, and they may be associated with linear skull fractures, usually in the temporal region. The lesion appears as a hyperdense biconvex mass between the skull and the brain on CT scan. Clinical presentation is highly variable, and outcome depends largely on promptness of diagnosis and surgical evacuation. The typical history is one of head trauma followed by a momentary alteration in consciousness and then a lucid interval lasting for up to a few hours. This is followed by a loss of consciousness, dilation of the pupil on the side of the epidural hematoma, and then hemiparesis of the contralateral side. If treated promptly, outcome is favorable in 85% to 90% of cases. Treatment consists of temporal craniectomy, evaluation of the hemorrhage, and control of the bleeding vessel.

479. The answer is c. *(Townsend, pp 2098-2102.)* The patient's history of the "worst headache of her life" and initial examination findings are highly suggestive of a subarachnoid hemorrhage. A CT scan without contrast will show a localized clot, diffusely distributed hemorrhage, intraventricular hemorrhage, or intraparenchymal hemorrhage 80% to 90% of the time.

If the CT scan is negative, and the history and physical examination strongly support a subarachnoid hemorrhage, then a lumbar puncture is obtained. As opposed to traumatic lumbar taps, the red blood cell count does not diminish between the first and last tubes collected when a subarachnoid hemorrhage is present. Xanthochromia is the yellow appearance of cerebrospinal fluid caused by the degradation of heme to bilirubin in the red blood cells entering the CSF during the bleeding. Workup should then proceed to a four-vessel cerebral angiogram to assess for a cerebral aneurysm. Given that only about 85% of cerebral aneurysms are identified on the initial study, a second angiogram should be performed within 7 to 10 days after the first study to completely rule out an aneurysm. Initial management consists of medical therapy to counteract vasospasm, blood pressure control, and anticonvulsant therapy. Although hydrocephalus can result from blockage of the arachnoidal channels, ventriculostomy is not the surgical management of choice. Surgical treatment should be initiated early and consists of craniotomy with clipping of the aneurysm.

480. The answer is a. *(Brunicardi, pp 1613-1614.)* The onset of irregular respirations, bradycardia, and, finally, increased blood pressure with acutely increasing ICP is termed the Cushing response or triad. Irregular respirations are due to hypoperfusion of the brainstem. The hypertension and bradycardia are due to decreased cerebral perfusion and the compensatory response. Cerebral perfusion pressure is the difference between the MAP and ICP. When the blood pressure is inadequate for cerebral perfusion, vasoconstriction and an increase in cardiac output occur to increase blood pressure and therefore CPP. The resultant hypertension stimulates the baroreceptors in the carotid bodies resulting in bradycardia. Focal mass lesions can result in herniation. Depending upon the direction of the mass effect, the herniation can cause compression of different areas of the brain. Herniation of brain parenchyma through the tentorial incisura or foramen magnum causes brainstem compression. Herniation usually causes compression of the third cranial nerve and thus leads to a fixed and dilated pupil on that side. Papilledema is a finding with chronic increases in ICP.

481. The answer is b. *(Townsend, p 2108.)* Benign schwannomas, or peripheral nerve sheath tumors that arise from perineural fibroblasts (Schwann cells), are treated with surgical excision. Because schwannomas do not involve the motor roots, sacrifice of the involved nerve and affected nerve root are of no significant consequence. Malignant schwannomas, which are rare, are treated with radiation therapy if curative resection is not possible. Intracranial schwannomas most frequently originate in the vestibular branch of the eighth cranial nerve and represent 10% of all intracranial neoplasms. Symptoms include hearing loss, tinnitus, and vertigo. Bilateral vestibular schwannomas are associated with neurofibromatosis-2; patients with this disease also present with meningiomas and ependymomas. Neurofibromas are also Schwann cell tumors but are histologically distinguishable from schwannomas; patients with multiple neurofibromas typically have neurofibromatosis-1 or von Recklinghausen disease. Other peripheral nerve tumors include ganglioneuromas, neuroblastomas, chemodectomas, and pheochromocytomas.

482. The answer is d. *(Brunicardi, p 1637.)* Craniopharyngiomas are cystic tumors with areas of calcification and originate in the epithelial remnants of Rathke pouch. These usually benign tumors are found in the sellar and suprasellar region and lead to compression of the pituitary, optic tracts, and third ventricle. As a result, they show up on radiographic imaging as an area of sellar erosion with calcification within or above the sella. Craniopharyngiomas are most commonly found in children but may also present in adulthood. In children, they can cause growth retardation because of hypothalamic-pituitary dysfunction. Treatment consists of subfrontal or transsphenoidal excision with adjuvant radiotherapy if total removal is not possible.

483. The answer is b. *(Brunicardi, p 1618.)* Cerebral contusions are bruises of neural parenchyma that most commonly involve the convex surface of a gyrus. The most frequent sites of cerebral contusion are the orbital surfaces of the frontal lobes and the anterior portion of the temporal lobes. The etiology of the contusion is always traumatic. Injuries may be seen both at the site of impact (coup) and in parenchyma opposite the site (contrecoup). Patients deemed to have a substantial contusion should receive anti-convulsive medication to prevent seizures in the early posttraumatic period.

484. The answer is c. *(Townsend, pp 2107-2108.)* Meningiomas are slow-growing, relatively benign tumors that arise from the arachnoid layer of the meninges. They occur predominantly in women, with a peak incidence at age of 45 years. They are treated primarily by surgical excision. Even after gross total resection, recurrence occurs in 11% to 15% of cases.

485. The answer is c. *(Townsend, p 2128.)* The patient's presentation is most consistent with a brain abscess, which is diagnosed by contrast-enhanced CT or MRI. In this condition, fever, elevated white blood cell count, and signs of meningeal irritation are often absent. Brain abscesses develop by either contiguous spread from adjacent structures or hematogenous spread from a distant site. Common sites of infection include paranasal sinus infection, dental caries, and ear infection. Contrast-enhanced CT and MRI reveal a ring-enhancing lesion usually at the gray-white interface with surrounding edema. Treatment involves accurate identification of the causative organism and appropriate antibiotic therapy, relief of mass effect with aspiration versus surgical excision, and treatment of the underlying cause. A lumbar puncture, ICP monitor, or ventriculoperitoneal shunt would not be helpful in the workup of a brain abscess. A noncontrast head CT is valuable in the work-up of an intracranial hemorrhage. It does not provide the images needed to diagnose a brain abscess.

486 to 487. The answers are 486-a, 487-e. *(Townsend, pp 2112-2116.)* Subdural hematomas usually arise from tears in the veins bridging from the cerebral cortex to the dura or venous sinuses, often after only minor head injuries. They can become apparent several days after the initial injury. Treatment is drainage of the hematoma through a burr hole; a formal craniotomy may be required if the fluid reaccumulates. Significant brain contusions from blunt trauma are usually associated with at least transient loss of consciousness; similarly, epidural hematomas results in a period of unconsciousness, although a lucid interval may follow, during which neurologic findings are minimal.

Subarachnoid hemorrhage (SAH) in the absence of antecedent trauma most commonly arises from a ruptured intracranial aneurysm, which typically is found at the bifurcation of the major branches of the circle of Willis. Other, less frequent causes of SAH include hypertensive hemorrhage, trauma, and bleeding from an arteriovenous malformation. Patients typically present with the sudden onset of an excruciating headache. Complaints of a stiff neck and photophobia are common. Loss of consciousness may be transient or may evolve into frank coma. Cranial nerve palsies are seen as a consequence both of increased ICP because of hemorrhage and pressure of the aneurysm on adjacent cranial nerves. CT scans followed by cerebral arteriography help to confirm the diagnosis as well as to identify the location of the aneurysm. Treatment consists of surgical ligation of the aneurysm by placing a clip across its neck. Early surgical intervention (within 72 hours of SAH) may prevent aneurysmal rebleeding and allow aggressive management of posthemorrhage vasospasm.

Otolaryngology

Questions

488. A 14-year-old boy is brought to medical attention because of nasal full-ness and bleeding. Inspection and biopsy confirm nasopharyngeal carci-noma. Which of the following statements concerning nasopharyngeal cancer is true?

a. A strong correlation exists between nasopharyngeal cancer and the presence of Epstein-Barr virus infections.
b. It occurs primarily after the sixth decade of life.
c. It undergoes early metastasis to the lungs.
d. The treatment of choice is wide surgical excision of the primary tumor.
e. Radiation therapy has little role in the treatment of nasopharyngeal cancer.

489. A young motorcycle driver is thrown against a concrete bridge abut-ment and sustains severe trauma about the face, with marked deformity and bleeding. Regarding these injuries, which of the following statements is true?

a. Evaluation of the cervical spine should precede that of the facial injuries.
b. Severe hemorrhage from the nasopharynx rarely occurs with LeFort fractures.
c. Direct oral or nasotracheal intubation should be performed promptly to prevent airway obstruction.
d. Standard facial x-ray series are preferable to computed tomography (CT) to assess facial fractures because they may be obtained in the emergency depart-ment, are performed faster, and are equally accurate.
e. Definitive management of fractures of facial bones should not be delayed.

490. A 48-year-old man with a strong history of cigarette use and heavy alcohol intake presents with an intraoral mass. Biopsy shows squamous cell cancer. Which of the following statements regarding squamous cell carcinoma of the head and neck is true?

a. Squamous cancers of the head and neck are caused by smoking tobacco rather than chewing tobacco.
b. Chemotherapy rarely produces a response with pharyngeal carcinoma and is not employed.
c. Squamous cancers of the nasopharynx are best treated by radiotherapy; surgery is reserved for lymph node metastases that have not responded to radiation.
d. Squamous cancers of the oropharynx are best treated by radiotherapy; surgery is not recommended.
e. For squamous cancers of the hypopharynx, radical neck dissection is performed only if lymph nodes are enlarged.

491. Your patient presents with a complaint of small masses inside her lips, which have been slowly enlarging. Biopsy shows a pleomorphic adenoma. You must discuss this tumor with your patient in preparation for surgery. Pleomorphic adenomas (mixed tumors) of the salivary glands are characterized by which of the following?

a. They occur most commonly on the lips, tongue, and palate.
b. They grow rapidly.
c. They rarely recur if simply enucleated.
d. They present as rock-hard masses.
e. They have no malignant potential.

492. A 5-year-old child presents with a small mass near the anterior border of the sternocleidomastoid muscle. Which of the following statements about branchial cleft anomalies is true?

a. A fistula that lies between the external auditory canal and the submandibular region originates from the second branchial cleft.
b. The course of the first branchial cleft fistula is through the bifurcation of the carotid artery.
c. Injury to the hypoglossal nerve may occur during excision of a second branchial cleft fistula.
d. The internal opening of the second branchial cleft fistula is usually found in the maxillary sinus.
e. The internal opening of the first branchial cleft cyst is just underneath the base of the tongue.

493. A 21-year-old woman asks you to evaluate a small painless lump in the midline of her neck that moves with swallowing. You make the clinical diagnosis of thyroglossal duct cyst. Which of the following statements regarding symptomatic thyroglossal duct cysts is true?

a. More than 90% manifest themselves before the age of 12 years.
b. Treatment includes resection of the hyoid bone.
c. They usually present as a painful swelling in the lateral neck.
d. Approximately 10% to 15% contain malignant elements.
e. They can contain ectopic thyroid tissue.

494. A 60-year-old smoker is seen because of an ulcerating mass on his tongue. Biopsy establishes that this is cancer. He declines surgical intervention. Which of the following statements regarding cancer of the tongue is true?

a. Carcinomas of the tongue are best treated by irradiation alone rather than surgery.
b. Metastases to the preauricular lymph nodes is common.
c. Cancer of the tongue most commonly occurs near the frenulum.
d. Local invasion may result in hypoglossal or lingual nerve dysfunction.
e. Elective neck dissection is not indicated in early-stage tumors.

495. A dentist notices a shaggy white mass in the gingivobuccal recess of a 68-year-old man. Biopsy of the mass reveals carcinoma of the buccal mucosa. Which of the following is characteristic of this cancer?

a. It is not associated with tobacco chewing.
b. Stage I and II tumors are best treated initially with chemotherapy.
c. Surgery followed by radiation therapy is the treatment of choice for advanced buccal carcinomas.
d. Involvement beyond the cheek mucosa at presentation is rare.
e. Lymphatic drainage is primarily to the submental lymph nodes.

496. A 4-year-old boy is brought into the emergency room by his parents for difficulty in breathing and swallowing. On physical examination the child is febrile, tachycardic, and tachypneic. He is anxious, drooling, and becomes increasingly exhausted while struggling to breath. Which of the following is the most appropriate management of this patient?

a. Examine the larynx at bedside
b. IV antibiotics and admission to the floor
c. Immediate endotracheal intubation in the emergency room
d. Immediate endotracheal intubation in the operating room
e. Immediate tracheostomy in the operating room

497. A 58-year-old man is found to have a small mass in the right neck on a yearly physical examination. The patient reports the mass has been slowly growing for the last few months and is not associated with pain or drainage. He has an otherwise negative review of systems. On examination there is a hard, mobile 2-cm mass along the mid-portion of the right sternocleido-mastoid muscle. Which of the following is the most appropriate initial step in the workup of the neck mass?

a. No further workup needed. Reevaluate the mass after a course of antibiotics for 2 weeks.
b. Fine-needle aspiration (FNA).
c. Core needle biopsy.
d. Incisional biopsy.
e. Excisional biopsy.

498. A 62-year-old man presents with a 3-month history of an enlarged lymph node in the left neck. He is a longtime smoker of cigarettes and denies fevers, night sweats, fatigue, or cough. On physical examination there is a 1.5 cm hard, fixed mass below the angle of the mandible in the left neck. Which of the following is the most likely cause of an enlarged lymph node in the neck?

a. Thyroglossal duct cyst
b. Dermoid tumor
c. Carotid body tumor
d. Branchial cleft cyst
e. Metastatic squamous cell carcinoma

Otolaryngology

Answers

488. The answer is a. *(Brunicardi, pp 532-533.)* Risk factors for nasopharyngeal carcinoma include environment, ethnicity, and tobacco. There is an unusually high incidence of nasopharyngeal cancer in southern China, Africa, Alaska, and in Greenland Eskimos. A strong association exists with Epstein-Barr virus (EBV) infections, such that EBV titers may be used as to follow a patient's response to treatment. The incidence of nasopharyngeal carcinoma has a bimodal distribution in the teen years and between ages 45 and 55. Most patients present with a neck mass, and up to 20% of patients may already have bilateral cervical nodal involvement at that time. Less than 5% of patients have distant metastases on presentation. Diagnosis of nasopharyngeal cancer, which tends to arise in relatively young people, should be made by biopsy of the primary tumor. Radiation therapy is the initial treatment of choice for the primary nasopharyngeal cancer.

489. The answer is a. *(Greenfield, pp 389-395.)* In patients with severe facial or mandibular trauma, airway difficulties may develop secondary to the effects of massive hemorrhage, tissue swelling, or associated laryngeal trauma. If oral or nasotracheal intubation cannot be performed easily, cricothyroidotomy or emergency tracheostomy should be performed. Evaluation of the cervical spine is a top priority and should be performed in any patient with head trauma prior to further facial studies. Although most facial fractures can be diagnosed easily with a standard radiographic facial series, computed tomography (CT) is more accurate and allows assessment of areas (eg, intracerebral contents) that cannot be evaluated by conventional techniques. CT is the preferred method of evaluation for patients with severe maxillofacial trauma. Maxillary fractures are categorized by the LeFort classification, and, unlike other facial fractures, are frequently associated with severe nasal and nasopharyngeal hemorrhage. This may be treated with head elevation and ice compresses. Nasal packing also affords good control of hemorrhage, and in extreme cases ligation or embolization of the internal maxillary artery may be necessary. Definitive reduction and fixation of fractures may be delayed while other injuries and medical problems are addressed. In addition to control of hemorrhage, initial management of facial fractures may include temporary stabilization and wound closure.

490. The answer is c. *(Brunicardi, pp 515-536.)* Squamous cell cancers of the head and neck appear to arise as a response to tobacco in general (including chewing tobacco), rather than just to cigarette smoking, especially when used in combination with alcohol ingestion. Chemotherapy for squamous cell pharyngeal cancer has been used very successfully in childhood and adolescence, although its role in adult pharyngeal cancer is uncertain. Treatment of nasopharyngeal squamous cell carcinoma is by radiation, followed by radical neck dissection if lymph node metastases have not been controlled. Oropharyngeal cancers have responded equally well to surgery and radiation, and both treatments are routinely employed. In the hypopharynx, surgery is the optimal treatment, often supplemented by postoperative radiation therapy. Surgery for hypopharyngeal cancers includes radical neck dissection because lymph node metastases occur frequently and are not well controlled by radiation alone.

491. The answer is a. *(Brunicardi, pp 538-540.)* Pleomorphic adenomas (mixed tumors) can occur in either the major (submandibular, parotid, and sublingual) or minor salivary glands. These round tumors have a rubbery consistency and are slow-growing; all are potentially malignant. Unless adequately excised, they tend to recur locally in a high percentage of cases. The sites most commonly affected by pleomorphic adenomas of the salivary glands are the lips, tongue, and palate.

492. The answer is c. *(Greenfield, pp 1840-1842.)* Branchial cleft cysts, sinuses, and fistulas are remnants of the first and second branchial pouches. The internal opening of the first branchial pouch is the external auditory canal; for the second, it is the posterolateral pharynx below the tonsillar fossa. The facial nerve may be injured during dissection of the first fistula. The second fistula passes between the carotid bifurcation and adjacent to the hypoglossal nerve. In childhood, most branchial cleft anomalies present as a painless nodule along the lateral border of the sternocleidomastoid muscle. In adults, superinfection of the cyst or fistulous drainage via an orifice in the supraclavicular region may occur. Treatment is surgical excision.

493. The answer is b. *(Greenfield, pp 1842-1845, Brunicardi, p 1475.)* Thyroglossal duct cysts result from retention of an epithelial tract between the thyroid and its embryologic origin in the foramen cecum at the base of the tongue. This tract usually penetrates the hyoid bone. There is no sex predilection, and although these cysts are more frequently detected in children, they may not become symptomatic until adulthood. The most common presentation is a painless swelling in the midline of the neck that moves with protrusion of the tongue or swallowing. They should not be confused with midline ectopic thyroid tissue. The cysts are prone to infection and progressive enlargement. Although rare (< 1%), epidermoid or papillary carcinomas do occur within thyroglossal duct cysts. Surgical resection is the standard therapy. The Sistrunk procedure, which involves local resection of the cyst and the central portion of the hyoid bone, is the operation of choice. Simple excision of the cyst results in an unacceptably high recurrence rate.

494. The answer is d. *(Brunicardi, p 519; Greenfield, p 656.)* Cancers of the tongue commonly present on the lateral or ventral surface of the tongue. Metastases to the submandibular or cervical nodes are common. Local invasion may result in tongue deviation due to involvement of the hypoglossal nerve or decreased sensation due to involvement of the lingual nerve. Treatment is surgical—wide local excision of the tumor and neck dissection as needed. In patients without nodal metastases, elective neck dissection is indicated for more invasive tumors. In contrast to therapeutic nodal dissections which are performed for clinically evident lymph node metastases, elective nodal dissections are performed for staging purposes.

495. The answer is c. *(Townsend, p 822.)* Buccal carcinoma is an uncommon oral cavity cancer. Smoking, chewing tobacco, snuff dipping, alcohol abuse, and lichen planus are all associated with buccal cancer. Approximately 65% of patients have extension beyond the cheek mucosa at presentation. Wide excision is the best initial treatment for this neoplasm. Advanced tumors should be treated with surgery followed by postoperative radiation. Chemotherapy does not have a significant role in the treatment of buccal carcinomas.

496. The answer is d. *(Greenfield, p 1840.)* The patient's history and physical examination is classic for acute epiglottitis. An airway should be emergently secured in the operating room; the surgeon should be prepared to perform a tracheostomy if endotracheal intubation is unsuccessful. Attempts to visualize the patient's larynx, such as at the bedside or in the emergency room, may result in sudden airway occlusion with aspiration and respiratory arrest. Therefore, examination of the patient's airway must be undertaken only in the operating room with personnel prepared to perform endotracheal intubation.

Acute epiglottitis most commonly occurs in children 2 to 4 years of age, and is caused by *Haemophilus influenza* in more than 90% of the cases. It presents as a rapidly progressive illness with symptoms of stridor, airway obstruction, drooling, and difficulty swallowing and signs of systemic toxicity (leukocytosis, fever, tachycardia). If the child's condition permits, lateral neck x-rays can be obtained which show edema of the epiglottis and ballooning of the hypopharynx. In advanced cases, the child is anxious and will sit erect and lean forward.

497. The answer is b. (*Townsend, p 837.*) Neck masses in adults represent malignancy until proven otherwise. One of the initial steps in the workup of neck masses is fine-needle aspiration. FNA has an overall accuracy of 95% for benign neck masses and 87% for malignant masses. It is the least invasive method to biopsy tissue but is more than adequate for identifying benign versus malignant tissue. CT scanning assists in evaluating the masses and potential primary sites, but cannot delineate between benign versus malignant masses.

498. The answer is e. (*Townsend, pp 837-838.*) Most commonly, lymphadenopathy in an adult is indicative of metastatic squamous cell cancer (SCC). Metastatic SCC originates most frequently from the nasopharynx, oropharynx, or hypopharynx. In addition to lymphadenopathy, persistent lateral neck masses in adults may represent neuromas, neurofibromas, carotid body tumors, branchial cleft cysts, lipomas, sebaceous cysts, parathyroid cysts, or a primary soft tissue tumor. Midline neck masses may represent thyroglossal duct cysts, dermoid tumors, thyroid masses, lipomas, or sebaceous cysts.

Pediatric Surgery

Questions

499. A neonate is examined in the nursery and found to have no anal orifice; only a small perineal fistulous opening is visualized. Decision as to the operative approach necessitates determining how high or low the anus has descended. Which of the following statements concerning imperforate anus is true?

a. Imperforate anus affects males more frequently than females.
b. In females, a low imperforate anus often occurs with a persistent cloaca.
c. The rectum usually ends in a blind pouch.
d. The chance for eventual continence is greater when the rectum has descended to below the levator ani muscles
e. Immediate definitive repair of the anatomic defect is required to maximize the chance of eventual continence.

500. A 2-month-old boy is examined because he has been straining while passing stool and has a distended abdomen. He is very low on the growth chart for age. A rectal examination and biopsy is performed. Which of the following statements concerning Hirschsprung disease is true?

a. It is initially treated by colostomy.
b. It is best diagnosed in the newborn period by barium enema.
c. It is characterized by the absence of ganglion cells in the transverse colon.
d. It is associated with a high incidence of genitourinary tract anomalies.
e. It is the congenital disease that most commonly leads to subsequent fecal incontinence.

501. A newborn has a midline defect in the anterior abdominal wall. The parents ask what, if anything, should be done. Spontaneous closure of which of the following congenital abnormalities of the abdominal wall generally occurs by the age of 4?

a. Umbilical hernia
b. Patent urachus
c. Patent omphalomesenteric duct
d. Omphalocele
e. Gastroschisis

502. A neonate is found to have an imperforate anus. As the pediatric surgeon you recommend studies to search for other anomalies because infants with anorectal anomalies tend to have other congenital anomalies. Associated abnormalities include which of the following?

a. Abnormalities of the cervical spine
b. Hydrocephalus
c. Duodenal atresia
d. Heart disease
e. Corneal opacities

503. A 36-hour-old infant presents with bilious vomiting and an increasingly distended abdomen. At exploration, the segment pictured here is found as the point of obstruction. Which of the following statements regarding this finding is true?

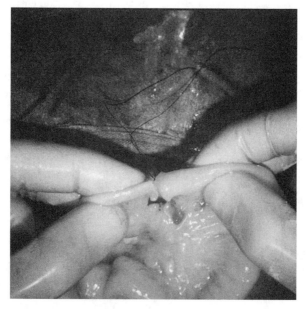

a. Resection with primary anastomosis should not be performed.
b. Gentle, persistent traction on the specimen usually corrects the defect and removes the need for a resection.
c. The lesion is much more common in the jejunum than in the ileum in this age group.
d. This problem is probably related to mesenteric vascular insufficiency.
e. A properly monitored barium enema might have corrected this defect and removed the need for an operation.

504. A 1-year-old child has repeated episodes of vomiting and abdominal distention. An x-ray shows obstruction at the second portion of the duodenum. Laparotomy is performed and an annular pancreas is discovered. For a symptomatic partial duodenal obstruction secondary to an annular pancreas, which of the following is the operative treatment of choice?

a. A Whipple procedure
b. Gastrojejunostomy
c. Vagotomy and gastrojejunostomy
d. Partial resection of the annular pancreas
e. Duodenoduodenostomy

505. Approximately 2 weeks after a viral respiratory illness, an 18-month-old child complains of abdominal pain and passes some bloody mucus per rectum. A long, thin mass is palpable in the right upper quadrant of the abdomen. Intussusception is suspected. Correct statements concerning intussusception in infants include which of the following?

a. Recurrence rates following treatment are high.
b. It is frequently preceded by a gastrointestinal viral illness.
c. A 1- to 2-week period of parenteral alimentation should precede surgical reduction when surgery is required.
d. Hydrostatic reduction without surgery rarely provides successful treatment.
e. The most common type occurs at the junction of the descending colon and the sigmoid colon.

506. An 18-year-old female presents with abdominal pain, fever, and leukocytosis. With the presumptive diagnosis of appendicitis, a right lower quadrant (McBurney) incision is made and a lesion 60 cm proximal to the ileocecal valve is identified (see photo). Which of the following statements regarding this lesion is true?

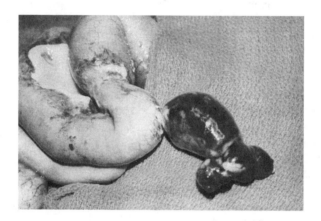

a. Can best be diagnosed by preoperative angiogram, which should be done whenever the diagnosis is suspected.
b. Should routinely be removed when incidentally discovered during celiotomy.
c. Is embryologically derived from a persistent vitelline duct (omphalomesenteric duct).
d. Often contains ectopic adrenal tissue.
e. Is frequently associated with cutaneous flushing and episodic tachycardia.

507. A newborn infant born from a mother with polyhydramnios presents with excessive salivation along with coughing and choking with the first oral feeding. An x-ray of the abdomen shows gas in stomach and a nasogastric tube coiled in the esophagus. Which of the following is the most likely diagnosis?

a. Esophageal atresia
b. Tracheoesophageal fistula
c. Esophageal atresia and tracheoesophageal fistula (TEF)
d. Omphalocele
e. Gastroschisis

508. An infant is born with a defect in the anterior abdominal cavity. Upon examination there are abdominal contents (small bowel and liver) protruding directly through the umbilical ring. Which of the following is true regarding this condition?

a. The abdominal contents are covered with a membrane composed of the peritoneum on the outside and amnion on the inside.
b. There is no sac covering the abdominal contents.
c. Karyotype abnormalities are present in roughly 30% of infants.
d. The intestine is often thickened, edematous, matted together, and foreshortened.
e. A silastic silo allows for immediate reduction of the viscera into the abdominal cavity.

509. A 2-week-old infant presents with sudden onset of bilious emesis. Plain films of the abdomen show evidence of an intestinal obstruction. An upper gastrointestinal (UGI) contrast series reveals a midgut volvulus with the site of obstruction at the third portion of the duodenum. Which of the following is the most likely diagnosis?

a. Necrotizing enterocolitis (NEC)
b. Intussusception
c. Hirschsprung disease
d. Anomalies of intestinal rotation and fixation
e. Hypertrophic pyloric stenosis

510. A 29-week-old previously healthy male infant presents with fevers, abdominal distention, feeding intolerance and bloody stools at 3 weeks of age. An abdominal x-ray reveals pneumatosis intestinalis. Which of the following is true regarding this condition?

a. Prematurity is the single most important risk factor.
b. It only affects the distal ileum and ascending colon.
c. Operative management is initiated immediately after the diagnosis is made.
d. It is the second leading cause of short gut syndrome in children.
e. Intestinal strictures may develop after the acute episode in roughly 50% of infants.

511. A newborn presents with signs and symptoms of distal intestinal obstruction. Abdominal x-rays reveal dilated loops of small bowel, absence of air-fluid levels, and a mass of meconium within the right side of the abdomen mixed with gas to give a ground-glass appearance. Which of the following is true regarding this condition?

a. It represents the earliest clinical manifestation of sickle cell disease.
b. Initial treatment is bowel rest with nasogastric tube decompression and IV antibiotics.
c. Initial treatment is a contrast enema.
d. Initial treatment is surgical evacuation of the luminal meconium.
e. Initial treatment is resection of the dilated terminal ileum.

512. A 4-week-old male infant presents with projectile, nonbilious emesis. Ultrasound of the abdomen reveals a pyloric muscle thickness of 8 mm (normal 3-4 mm). Which of the following is true regarding this condition?

a. Gastric outlet obstruction leads to hyperchloremic, metabolic alkalosis.
b. The highest incidence is found among African Americans and Chinese.
c. Males and females are equally affected.
d. Underlying metabolic alkalosis needs to be corrected prior to surgery.
e. Treatment is pyloroplasty.

513. A 1-month-old female infant presents with persistent jaundice. A serum direct bilirubin is 4.0 mg/dL and an ultrasound of the abdomen shows a shrunken gallbladder and inability to visualize the extrahepatic bile ducts. Which of the following is the most appropriate initial management of this patient?

a. NPO and total parenteral nutrition
b. Oral choleretic bile salts
c. Methylprednisolone
d. IV antibiotics
e. Exploratory laparotomy

514. A full-term male newborn experiences respiratory distress immediately after birth. A prenatal sonogram was read as normal. An emergency radiograph is shown here. The patient is intubated and placed on 100% O_2. Arterial blood gases reveal pH 7.24, P_{O_2} 60 kPa, and P_{CO_2} 52 kPa. The baby has sternal retractions and a scaphoid abdomen. Which of the following statements correctly refers to this condition?

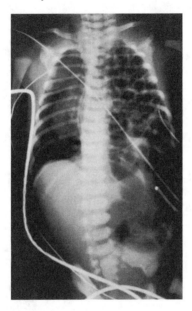

a. The most likely cause of this problem is in utero traumatic rupture of the diaphragm.
b. The most important aspect in management is immediate exploration and repair of the defect.
c. The size of the defect directly correlates with severity of the disease.
d. The defect is usually anteromedial in location.
e. Any abdominal organ can be involved.

515. A 2-year-old asymptomatic child is noted to have a systolic murmur, hypertension, and diminished femoral pulses. Which of the following is true about this child's disorder?

a. Atrial septal defects (ASDs) are frequently associated.
b. The child is unlikely to become normotensive even with surgical intervention.
c. Rib notching is often seen on x-ray.
d. Claudication is frequently noted.
e. Older children with this disorder almost always have symptoms of heart failure.

516. A 35-week term infant presents with cyanosis shortly after birth. His arterial oxygen saturation is only 30%. Which of the following is the most likely diagnosis?

a. Patent ductus arteriosus
b. Coarctation of the aorta
c. Atrial septal defect
d. Ventricular septal defect
e. Transposition of the great vessels

Questions 517 to 518

For each patient, select the most likely congenital cardiac anomaly. Each lettered option may be used once, more than once, or not at all.

a. Tetralogy of Fallot
b. Ventricular septal defect
c. Tricuspid atresia
d. Transposition of the great vessels
e. Patent ductus arteriosus

517. A noncyanotic 2-day-old child has a systolic murmur along the left sternal border; examination is otherwise normal. Chest x-ray and electrocardiogram are normal.

518. A 3-year-old child has congenital cyanosis.

Pediatric Surgery

Answers

499. The answer is d. *(Brunicardi, pp 1497-1499.)* Imperforate anus affects males and females with equal frequency, occurring in 1 in 5000 live births. It is due to failure of descent of the urorectal septum. Imperforate anus may be broadly classified into high or low, depending on whether the rectum ends above or below the level of the levator ani complex. The rectal fistula may end in the prostatic urethra or vagina in the high cases, while the low cases terminate in a perineal fistula. In females, high imperforate anus often occurs with a persistent cloaca (where the rectum, vagina, and urethra share a single perineal orifice). For the low cases, only a perineal operation may be required, and these children will be expected to be continent. A pull-through procedure will be required for the high imperforate anus, and the likelihood of continence is smaller. If there is doubt about the level or location of the termination of the rectum, it is better to perform a temporary colostomy than to compromise the ultimate chances of continence by an injudicious perineal approach.

500. The answer is a. *(Brunicardi, pp 1496-1497.)* Hirschsprung disease, which is the congenital absence of ganglion cells in the rectum or rectosigmoid colon, is definitively diagnosed by rectal biopsy. The typical findings on barium enema—a distal narrow segment of bowel with markedly distended colon proximally—may not be seen early in life. Symptoms may go unrecognized in the newborn period, with consequent development of malnutrition or enterocolitis. Initial treatment is colostomy decompression. Definitive repair is best delayed until nutritional status is adequate and the chronically distended bowel has returned to normal size. Unlike the situation with imperforate anus, which is associated with a high incidence of genitourinary tract anomalies and risk of long-term fecal incontinence, in Hirschsprung disease repair leads to satisfactory bowel function in most affected patients.

501. The answer is a. *(Brunicardi, pp 1501-1504.)* In most children, umbilical hernias close spontaneously by the age of 4 and need not be repaired unless incarcerated or symptomatic. Omphalocele and gastroschisis result in evisceration of bowel and require emergency surgical treatment to effect immediate or staged reduction and abdominal wall closure. Patent urachal or omphalomesenteric ducts result from incomplete closure of embryonic connections from the bladder and ileum, respectively, to the abdominal wall. They are appropriately treated by excision of the tracts and closure of the bladder or ileum.

502. The answer is d. (*Brunicardi, p 1498.*) Congenital anorectal anomalies are frequently associated with other congenital anomalies including heart disease, esophageal atresia (EA), abnormalities of the lumbosacral spine, double urinary collecting systems, hydronephrosis, and communication between the rectum and the urinary tract, vagina, or perineum. Patients may present with a number of anomalies collectively known as the VACTERL syndrome: **V**ertebral anomalies, **A**nal atresia, **C**ardiac defect (eg, ventricular septal defect [VSD]), **T**racheo**E**sophageal fistula, **R**enal anomalies, and **L**imb defects (eg, radial dysplasia). They occur in approximately 1 in 5000 live births. A variety of surgical procedures have been devised to treat the problem, depending on the type of anomaly (whether the rectum ends above or below the level of the levator ani complex). However, even when anatomic integrity is established, the prognosis for effective toilet training is poor. In 50% of cases, continence is never achieved. Cervical spine abnormalities, hydrocephalus, duodenal atresia, and corneal opacities have no significant association with congenital anorectal anomalies.

503. The answer is d. (*Brunicardi, p 1488.*) This is an example of an ileal atresia. Whether the atresia is jejunal or ileal does not affect treatment, and there is no predilection for one site over the other. The basis of jejunoileal atresia is probably a mesenteric vascular accident during intrauterine growth. Resection and primary anastomosis should be performed if possible, but the bowel should be exteriorized if there is a question of viability or a large size discrepancy between two segments. Plain films will reveal a small-bowel obstruction with no gas beyond the lesion. A carefully administered Gastrografin enema can help in the differential diagnosis. Midgut volvulus and meconium ileus can be apparent on an enema, which is important, as meconium ileus should be managed nonoperatively.

504. The answer is e. (*Brunicardi, pp 1487-1488.*) A bypass procedure is the operation of choice for obstruction secondary to an annular pancreas.

A Whipple procedure (pancreaticoduodenectomy) is too radical a therapy for this benign condition, and a partial resection of the annular pancreas often is complicated by fistula. Duodenoduodenostomy is much more physiologic than gastrojejunostomy and does not require a vagotomy to prevent marginal ulceration; it is therefore the procedure of choice.

505. The answer is b. *(Brunicardi, pp 1493-1494.)* Intussusception is the result of invagination of a segment of bowel into distal bowel lumen. The most common type is ileocolic, which typically appears as a coiled spring on barium enema. Ileoileal and colocolic intussusceptions occur less commonly and are not easily diagnosed on barium enema. If bloody mucus, peritonitis, or systemic toxicity have not developed, hydrostatic reduction by barium enema is the appropriate initial treatment. Most patients are successfully managed this way and do not require surgical intervention. Immediate treatment should be instituted to avert the danger of bowel infarction. Recurrence is surprisingly uncommon after either surgical or nonsurgical treatment.

506. The answer is c. *(Brunicardi, pp 1495-1496.)* This is an inflamed Meckel diverticulum. This common lesion is often clinically indistinguishable from acute appendicitis. It is the remnant of the vitelline duct. Meckel diverticula are usually located 60 cm proximal to the ileocecal valve, are antimesenteric, and may contain either gastric and pancreatic or only pancreatic tissue. Hemorrhage or obstruction is a more common presentation than inflammation. Technetium 99m (^{99m}Tc) pertechnetate has affinity for gastric mucosa, and a scan with this isotope can aid in the diagnosis of this anomaly as a cause of lower gastrointestinal hemorrhage in a child. Angiography is more useful when looking for arteriovenous malformations. Since complications are relatively rare, most surgeons do not recommend removing asymptomatic diverticula when they are incidentally discovered during abdominal procedures. Those diverticula with a narrow neck, palpable heterotopic tissue, or nodularity are prone to obstruction and should be excised. In addition, patients explored for abdominal pain of unknown etiology should also undergo diverticulectomy, as should those operated on for appendicitis who are to be left with a scar of the right lower quadrant.

507. The answer is c. *(Townsend, pp 2055-2056.)* The diagnosis of EA should be entertained in an infant who presents with excessive salivation along with coughing and choking during the first oral feeding. A maternal history of polyhydramnios is often present. The inability to pass a nasogastric tube into the stomach is seen with EA. If gas is present in the gastrointestinal tract, then an associated tracheoesophageal fistula (TEF) is confirmed. In an infant with EA and TEF the air is introduced into the stomach via the fistula between the distal esophagus and the trachea with each inspired breath. Reflux of gastric contents into the trachea through the TEF may result in cough, tachypnea, apnea, or cyanosis. After evaluating for VACTERL abnormalities, surgical repair of the EA and TEF is performed.

508. The answer is c. *(Townsend, pp 2067-2069.)* The infant has an omphalocele. During normal development of the embryo, the midgut herniates outward through the umbilical ring and continues to grow. It returns back into the abdominal cavity by the eleventh week of gestation and undergoes normal rotation and fixation. If the intestines fail to return the infant is born with abdominal contents protruding through the umbilical ring, termed an omphalocele. A sac composed of the peritoneum on the inside and amnion on the outside covers the bowel protecting it from the surrounding amniotic fluid. Sometimes the sac is torn in utero and the bowel is exposed to the amniotic fluid. This abdominal wall defect is called a gastroschisis and the defect is always seen on the right side of the umbilical ring with an intact umbilical cord. The risk for associated anomalies with gastroschisis is low. In contrast, more than half of infants with an omphalocele have other major or minor malformations, and karyotype abnormalities are present in roughly 30% of infants (including trisomies 13, 18, and 21). In giant omphaloceles a Silastic silo allows for gradual reduction of the viscera into the abdominal cavity over several days. In patients with gastroschisis, the intestine is often thickened, edematous, matted together and foreshortened leading to impaired motility, digestion and absorption. Both conditions are repaired surgically.

509. The answer is d. *(Townsend, pp 2060-2061.)* The patient's presentation and radiologic findings are most consistent with anomalies of intestinal rotation and fixation (aka malrotation). Rotational anomalies may present as a volvulus, duodenal obstruction, or intermittent or chronic abdominal pain. When the midgut returns to the abdominal cavity by the tenth week of gestation it rotates around the axis of the superior mesenteric artery for 270° in a counterclockwise direction placing the final position of the ligament of Treitz in the left upper quadrant and the cecum in the right lower quadrant of the abdomen. Interruption or reversal of any of these coordinated movements leads to the range of anomalies seen. The most frequently encountered anomaly is complete nonrotation of the midgut, in which the proximal jejunum and ascending colon are fused together as one pedicle. The midgut volvulus occurs on this pedicle leading to ischemic necrosis of the entire midgut. Necrotizing enterocolitis (NEC), Hirschsprung disease, hypertrophic pyloric stenosis, and intussusception are not associated with a midgut volvulus.

510. The answer is a. (*Townsend, pp 2061-2062.*)The patient's presentation and radiologic findings are classic for NEC. NEC is the most common gastrointestinal emergency in the neonatal period. Prematurity is the single most important risk factor. Other significant risk factors include ischemia, bacteria, cytokines, and enteral feeding. About 80% of cases occur within the first month of life. The radiologic hallmark of NEC is pneumatosis intestinalis (air within the walls of the bowel). The distal ileum and ascending colon are usually affected, but the entire gastrointestinal tract may be involved (NEC totalis). Initial management consists of bowel rest with nasogastric tube decompression, fluid resuscitation, and broad-spectrum antibiotics. Medical management is successful in half of cases and surgery is reserved for patients with overall clinical deterioration, abdominal wall cellulitis, falling white blood cell count or platelet count, palpable abdominal mass, persistent fixed loop on abdominal films, or intestinal perforation. NEC is the single most common cause of short gut syndrome in children. Intestinal strictures may develop after either medical or surgical management of NEC in roughly 10% of infants.

511. The answer is c. (*Townsend, pp 2062-2063.*) The patient has a meconium ileus. In meconium ileus, the terminal ileum is dilated and filled with thick, tarlike, inspissated meconium. Meconium ileus in the newborn represents the earliest clinical manifestation of cystic fibrosis. The initial treatment is a water-soluble contrast enema. This is successful in relieving the obstruction in up to 75% of cases with a bowel perforation rate of less than 3%. Operative management is required when the contrast enema fails to relieve the obstruction. A small enterotomy is made in the dilated terminal ileum and a red rubber catheter is used to irrigate the proximal and distal bowel with either warm saline or 4% N-acetylcysteine. The meconium is either manipulated into the distal colon or removed through the enterotomy. The enterotomy is closed in two layers at the end of the case.

512. The answer is d. (*Townsend, pp 2058-2059.*) The patient's symptoms and findings on ultrasound are consistent with hypertrophic pyloric stenosis. The highest incidence is found among whites of Scandinavian decent and males outnumber females by a ratio of 4:1. Loss of hydrochloric acid with repeated episodes of emesis leads to development of hypochloremic, metabolic alkalosis. Before surgery, it is important to hydrate the infant and slowly correct the metabolic alkalosis with normal saline. If the underlying metabolic alkalosis is not corrected the infant will compensate with respiratory acidosis and postoperative apnea may occur. Treatment of hypertrophic pyloric stenosis is a pyloromyotomy. This involves cutting of the thickened pyloric musculature while preserving the mucosal layer.

513. The answer is e. *(Townsend, pp 2077-2078.)*An infant with persistent jaundice after the first few weeks of life needs to be evaluated with laboratory studies and an abdominal ultrasound. This infant has findings consistent with biliary atresia. Biliary atresia is characterized by progressive obliteration of the extrahepatic and intrahepatic bile ducts. Delay in the diagnosis of biliary atresia leads to irreversible hepatic fibrosis. Success with surgical correction is much improved if undertaken before 60 days of life. If an abdominal ultrasound or liver-needle biopsy is consistent with biliary atresia, exploratory laparotomy is performed expeditiously. The initial goal at surgery is to confirm the diagnosis with demonstration of fibrotic biliary remnants and absent proximal and distal bile duct patency. Surgical correction of biliary atresia is with the Kasai hepatoportoenterostomy.

514. The answer is e. *(Brunicardi, pp 1476-1478.)* This radiograph of a child with a scaphoid abdomen and respiratory disease is characteristic of a congenital diaphragmatic hernia. These defects are posterolateral and occur due to failure of the embryologic diaphragm to fuse between the eighth and twelfth weeks of intrauterine life. The size of the defect does not correlate with the symptoms. Even a large diaphragmatic hernia can be missed on prenatal sonogram if the abdominal contents have slipped back into the abdomen at the time of the study. Hernias of Morgagni are anteromedial and do not present as emergencies at birth. Any abdominal organ—pancreas, kidney, small and large intestine, stomach, liver, or spleen—can herniate into the chest. The abdominal organ acts as a space-occupying lesion and retards growth of the lung, which results in pulmonary hypoplasia. Respiratory problems at birth stem from primary pulmonary hypertension, the consequence of hypoplasia, rather than from compression of the lung by abdominal contents. Most experts recommend stabilizing the pulmonary hypertensive crisis medically or with extracorporeal membrane oxygenation (ECMO) prior to attempting repair.

515. The answer is c. (*Greenfield, pp 1448-1449.*) Coarctation of the aorta is a congenital anomaly that usually causes narrowing of the aorta just distal to the left subclavian artery in the area of the ligamentum arteriosum. Collateral circulation develops around the obstruction by way of intercostal vessels and accounts for the classic x-ray appearance of rib notching. Without surgery, complications in adults arise with eventual death from cardiac failure, rupture of aortic aneurysms or of a cerebral artery, and bacterial endocarditis. Coarctation is often associated with VSDs and aortic stenosis. Patients who are operated on earlier in life have a better chance of becoming normotensive. Claudication is not a common feature of this disorder.

516. The answer is e. (*Greenfield, pp 1432-1452.*) With the exception of coarctation, in which no shunt (or cyanosis) exists, the anomalies listed cause a shunting of blood between the systemic and lower-pressure pulmonary circulation. Transposition of the great vessels is a right-to-left shunt that leads to cyanosis. Except where there is persistent congenital pulmonary hypertension, patent ductus arteriosus and atrial septal defects cause a shunting of oxygenated blood from the aorta and left atrium, respectively, back into the pulmonary artery and right atrium. These anomalies cause recirculation of oxygenated blood within the cardiopulmonary circuit but not cyanosis. When a VSD is combined with pulmonary artery atresia (tetralogy of Fallot), the resulting undercirculation in the pulmonary system joins transposition as a cause of cyanosis. Other, less common congenital lesions in which the pulmonary arterial blood flow is relatively decreased include tricuspid atresia, Ebstein anomaly, and hypoplastic right ventricle.

517 to 518. The answers are 517-b, 518-a. (*Greenfield, pp 1432-1452.*) VSD accounts for 20% to 30% of all congenital cardiac anomalies. It may lead to cardiac failure and pulmonary hypertension if the defect is larger than 1 cm, or it may be asymptomatic if the defect is small. Surgery is not indicated for the asymptomatic patient with a small defect since a substantial number of these anomalies close spontaneously during the first few years of life. Operation is indicated in infants with congestive heart failure or rising pulmonary vascular resistance (owing to the left-to-right shunt). Additionally, operation is indicated if the VSD has not closed by age of 5. Tetralogy of Fallot, transposition, and tricuspid atresia are cyanotic lesions. Congenital cyanosis that persists beyond the age of 2 years is associated, in the vast majority of cases, with tetralogy of Fallot. Patent ductus arteriosus is associated with the characteristic continuous machinery murmur.

Bibliography

Belkin M, Belkin B, Buchman CA, et al. Intra-arterial fibrinolytic therapy. Efficacy of streptokinase vs urokinase. *Arch Surg.* 1986;121:769-773.

Blumgart LH, Fong Y. *Surgery of the Liver and Biliary Tract.* 3rd ed. New York, NY: W.B. Saunders; 2000.

Boucher CA, Brewster DC, Darling RC, et al. Determination of cardiac risk by dipyridamole-thallium imaging before peripheral vascular surgery. *N Engl J Med.* 1985;312:389-394.

Brunicardi FC, Andersen DK, Billiar TR, et al, eds. *Schwartz's Principles of Surgery.* 8th ed. New York, NY: McGraw-Hill; 2005.

Bunt TJ, Malone JM, Moody M, et al. Frequency of vascular injury with blunt trauma–induced extremity injury. *Am J Surg.* 1990;160:226-228.

Charlson ME, MacKenzie CR, Gold JP, et al. The preoperative and intraoperative hemodynamic predictors of postoperative myocardial infarction or ischemia in patients undergoing noncardiac surgery. *Ann Surg.* 1989;210:637-648.

Cosentino CM, Luck SR, Raffensperger JG, et al. Choledochal duct cyst: Resection with physiologic reconstruction. *Surgery.* 1992;112:740-748.

Cummings RA, Wesly RL, Adams DH, et al. Pneumopericardium resulting in cardiac tamponade. *Ann Thorac Surg.* 1984;37:511-518.

Dutky PA, Stevens SL, Maull KI, Factors affecting rapid fluid resuscitation with large-bore introducer catheters. *J Trauma.* 1989;29:856-860.

Eisenbud DE, Brener BJ, Shoenfeld R, et al. Treatment of acute vascular occlusions with intraarterial urokinase. *Am J Surg.* 1990;160:160-165.

Executive Committee for the Asymptomatic Carotid Atherosclerosis Study, Endarterectomy for asymptomatic carotid artery stenosis. *JAMA.* 1995;273:1421-1428.

Flint L, Babikian G, Anders M, et al. Definitive control of mortality from severe pelvic fracture. *Ann Surg.* 1990;211:703-707.

Gobbi PG, Dionigi P, Barbier F, et al. The role of surgery in the multimodal treatment of primary gastric non-Hodgkin's lymphomas. *Cancer.* 1990;65(11):2528-2536.

Goodnough LT, Shuck JM. Risks, options, and informed consent for blood transfusion in elective surgery. *Am J Surg.* 1990;159:602-609.

Greenfield LJ, Lillemoe KD, Mulholland MW, et al, eds. *Surgery: Scientific Principles and Practice.* 4th ed. Philadelphia, PA: Lippincott-Raven; 2005.

Heys SD, Park KG, Garlick PJ, et al. Nutrition and malignant disease: Implications for surgical practice. *Br J Surg.* 1992;79:614-623.

Landercasper J, Merz BJ, Cogbill TH, et al. Perioperative stroke risk in 173 consecutive patients with a past history of stroke. *Arch Surg.* 1990;125: 986-989.

Mahmoodian S. Appendicitis complicating pregnancy. *South Med J.* 1992;85:19-24.

McQuaid KR, Isenberg JI. Medical therapy of peptic ulcer disease. *Surg Clin North Am.* 1992;72:285-316.

Merrell SW, Schneider PD. Hemobilia: Evolution of current diagnosis and treatment. *West J Med.* 1991;155:621-625.

Moore EE, KL Mattox, DV Feliciano, et al, eds. *Trauma.* 6th ed. New York, NY: McGraw-Hill; 2007.

Pasternack PF, Imparato AM, Bear G, et al. The value of the radionuclide angiogram in the prediction of perioperative myocardial infarction in patients undergoing lower extremity revascularization procedures. *Circulation.* 1985;72:13-17.

Podolosky DK. Inflammatory bowel disease. *N Engl J Med.* 1991;325:928-937. *N Engl J Med.* 1991;114:593-597.

Reilly HF, al-Kawas FH. Dieulafoy's lesion. Diagnosis and management. *Dig Dis Sci.* 1991;36:1702-1707.

Rhame FS. Preventing HIV transmission. Strategies to protect clinicians and patients. *Postgrad Med.* 1992;91:141-152.

Robinson T, Birrer R, Mandava N,et al. Body smuggling of illicit drugs: Two cases requiring surgical intervention. *Surgery.* 1993;113:709-711.

Schwesinger WH. Is *Helicobacter pylori* a myth or the missing link? *Am J Surg.* 1996;172:411-416.

Thoren T, Wattwil M. Effects on gastric emptying of thoracic epidural analgesia with morphine or bupivacaine. *Anesth Analg.* 1988;67:687-694.

Tondini C, Giardini R, Bozzetti F, et al. Combined modality treatment for primary gastrointestinal non-Hodgkin's lymphoma in the Milan Cancer Institute experience. *Ann Oncol.* 1993;4:831-837.

Townsend CM Jr, Beauchamp RD, Evers BM, et al, eds. *Sabiston Textbook of Surgery.* 18th ed. Philadelphia, PA: Saunders; 2007.

Trunkey DD. Shock-trauma. *Can J Surg.* 1984;27:479-486.

Way LW, Doherty GM. *Current Surgical Diagnosis & Treatment,* 11th ed. New York, NY: McGraw-Hill; 2003.

Weissman C. The metabolic response to stress: An overview and update. *Anesthesiology.* 1990;73:308-327.

Willerson JT, Golino P, McNatt J,et al. Role of new antiplatelet agents as adjunctive therapies in thrombolysis. *Am J Cardiol.* 1991;67:12A-18A.

Wilson SE, Williams RA, Robinson G. Operating on HIV-positive patients. What are the risks to healthcare workers? To patients? *Postgrad Med.* 1990;88:193-194,199-201.

Index

A

Abdomen, free fluid in, 111, 133–134
Abdominal decompression, 213, 241
Abdominal injuries
 diagnosis and treatment, 91–93,
  113–114, 116
 duodenal hematoma, 95, 117–118
 fluid resuscitation, 104, 127–128
 gunshot wounds, 98, 122
 repair of, 106, 130
Abdominal-perineal resection,
  225, 250
Achalasia, 198, 227, 264, 277–278
Acidosis
 metabolic, 4, 16, 21–22, 34
 non-anion-gap, 13, 16, 32, 34
 oxygen dissociation curve, 57
 respiratory, 21, 39, 57
Addison disease, 50, 68, 169, 183
Adenomas
 adrenal, 171, 185–186
 liver, 207, 237
 pleomorphic, 340, 344
 thyroid gland, 169, 183, 191
Adrenal adenomas, 171, 185–186
Adrenal insufficiency, 8, 27, 169, 183
Adrenocortical insufficiency,
  50, 67–68
Adrenocortical tumors, 174, 188–189
Adriamycin (doxorubicin), 149, 165
Airway management, 50, 68–69
Airway obstructions, 109, 112, 134
Albumin, serum levels of, 47, 64
Alcohol use, 158
Alkalosis
 metabolic, 3, 21, 47, 64
 respiratory, 4, 21–22
Alveolar ventilation, 46, 63
Amino acids, 124
Anaerobic infections, 79, 88
Analgesia, epidural, 42, 59
Anaphylactoid reactions, 45, 63

Anesthetics (*See also specific types*)
 local, 44, 61
 types of, 52, 70–71
Angina, 274
Angiography, 5, 23
Angiomyolipomas, 311
Antibiotic therapy
 perioperative, 79, 88
 as prophylactic treatment, 2, 20, 79,
  82, 88
Antiplatelet agents, 285, 296
Antrectomy, 200, 229
Anus
 carcinomas of, 211, 225, 240, 250–251
 imperforate, 347–348, 355–356
Aortic aneurysm
 abdominal
  cardiac function assessment, 53
  cecal volvulus, 213, 241
  colitis, ischemic, 282, 293–294
  diagnosis and repair, 283, 294
  fluid management, 41, 58, 281, 292
  mycotic, 290, 300
  thoracic, 259, 265, 274, 278
Aortic coarctation, 265, 279, 353–354, 361
Aortic dissection, 255, 270
Aortic injury, thoracic, 108, 131
Aortic regurgitation, 265, 278
Aortic stenosis, 253, 268
Aortoiliac atherosclerosis, 285
Appendectomy, 208, 238, 248
Appendiceal adenocarcinomas,
  198, 226–227
Appendiceal carcinoid tumors, 181–182,
  195, 218, 222, 245, 247
Appendicitis, 214, 241–242
Argyll Robertson pupil, 265, 278
Arterial embolus, 286, 298
Arterial injuries, 93, 102, 105, 115, 125, 130
Arterial insufficiency, 285, 295
Aspiration of gastric contents, 48, 66,
  68–69

Aspiration cytology, 142, 159
Aspirin intoxication, 4, 21–22
Aspirin prophylaxis, 285, 296
Atrial septal defect, 361
Axillofemoral bypass, 291, 300–301

B

Bacteroides fragilis, 79, 88
Basal cell carcinoma, 75, 80, 83, 89
Beck triad, 43, 60–61
Bile ducts
    obstruction of, 206
    repair of, 94, 116–117, 209, 238
    vanishing bile duct syndrome, 153
Biliary atresia, 352, 360
Biopsies, 144, 161
Bladder cancer, 303, 308
Bleeding time, 10, 28, 53–54, 71–72
Blood gases
    alveolar ventilation, 46, 63
    oxygen dissociation curve, 39, 56–57
Blood transfusions
    hypocalcemia, 19, 29–30
    reactions to, 4, 6, 9, 16, 22, 25, 28,
        34–35, 38, 46, 56, 63
    timing of, 8, 27
    viral illness risks, 40, 57–58
Boerhaave syndrome, 257, 272
Bone marrow transplantation, 140, 157
Bowel (*see* Intestines)
Brachial cleft anomalies, 340, 344
Brain abscess, 331, 337–338
BRCA mutations, 149, 165
Breast(s)
    cystosarcoma phyllodes of, 178, 192
    cysts in, 172, 186
    fat necrosis in, 174, 188
    fibroadenomas of, 173, 187
    and nipple discharge, 179, 193
    Paget disease and, 175, 189–190
Breast cancer, 148–149, 164–165, 170,
        172, 175, 184, 187–188
    conservation therapy for, 170, 184
        risks for, 179, 194
        staging system for, 180, 194–195
        treatments for, 182, 195–196
    lumpectomy for, 146, 163, 195
        mastectomy versus, 170, 184

Bronchial carcinoid tumors, 262, 276
Bronchogenic carcinoma, 254, 269
Buccal carcinomas, 341, 345
Burn(s)
    chemical, 74, 82
    energy requirements, 17, 35
    thermal burns, 121
    treatment of, 76, 84

C

Calcium gluconate, 12, 15, 30, 33
Cancer (*see specific types*)
Carbon dioxide, 47
Carbon monoxide poisoning, 97, 120
Carcinoembryonic antigen (CEA), 150,
        166, 223, 249
Carcinoid syndrome, 195, 247, 276
Carcinoid tumors, 181, 195, 218, 222,
        245, 247–248, 262, 276
Carcinomas
    acinar cell, 144, 161
    basal cell, 75, 80, 83, 89
    BRCA mutations, 149, 165
    buccal, 341, 345
    of colon (*see* Colon, carcinomas of)
    of esophagus, 210, 238–239
    lung, 253, 268–269
    medullary, 143, 160
    metastatic disease, 328, 334
    nasopharyngeal, 339–340, 343–344
    nutrition and, 147, 163
    oropharyngeal, 344
    parotid, 144, 161
    pharyngeal, 344
    squamous cell, 75–77, 84–85, 87, 89,
        340, 342, 344, 346
    tumor grading and staging, 142, 159
Cardiac allografts (*see* Heart, transplantation)
Cardiac events, ischemic, 286, 297
Cardiac injuries, 101, 123–124
Cardiac myxoma, 258, 273
Cardiac output, 42–43, 58–59
Cardiac risks, surgery, 44, 61
Cardiac tamponade, 43, 60–61, 104, 110,
        128–129, 132, 258, 272–273
Cardiomyopathy, 149, 165
Carotid artery disease, 283, 294
Carotid artery stenosis, 284, 295

Carotid endarterectomy, 53, 71
Carpal tunnel syndrome, 76, 85, 275
CEA (carcinoembryonic antigen), 150, 166, 223, 249
Cecal volvulus, 213, 241
Cellulitis, 293
Central venous pressure, 50, 67
Cerebral contusions, 331, 337
Cerebral perfusion pressure, 109, 327, 333
Cervical lymph nodes, 142, 159
Charcot triad, 220, 246
Chemical burn, 74, 82
Chemotherapy, 145, 149, 161–162, 166, 175, 189
Chest injuries, 96, 101, 109, 112, 119, 123–124, 134–135, 257, 272
Cholangitis, 220, 224, 246, 250
Cholecystectomy, 75, 83, 203, 234
Cholecystitis, 42, 59–60, 220, 246
Cholecystostomy, 220, 246
Choledochal cysts, 219, 245
Choledochojejunostomy, 94, 116, 209, 238
Choledocholithiasis, 224, 250
Cholelithiasis, 224, 249–250
Cholesterol atheroembolism, 50, 67
Chorionic gonadotropin, human, 141, 159
Chromium deficiency, 31
Chylothorax, 258, 262, 273, 276
Claudication, 285, 288, 291, 295–300
Cleft lip and palate, 77, 86
Clostridium difficile, 2, 17, 34–35
Clotting factors, vitamin K dependent, 27
Coagulation
    complications with, 51, 69–70
    factors in measurement of, 53–54, 71–72
    and hemophilia A, 9, 28
    and von Willebrand disease, 6, 24–25, 48, 65
Coin lesions, 263, 276–277
Colectomy, 225, 250–251
Colitis
    Crohn, 216, 243
    ischemic, 206, 236, 281–282, 293–294
    pseudomembranous, 17, 35
    ulcerative, 198, 225, 227–228, 243, 250–251
Collagen, 81–82

Colon
    carcinomas of, 147, 150–151, 163, 166, 203, 207, 233–234, 236–237
    injuries to, 99, 122–123
    polyps in, 209, 238
    postoperative viability, 281, 293
    surgery and antibiotic prophylaxis, 2, 20
Colorectal cancer, 146, 162–163, 202, 229, 231–232
Colorectal tumors, 223, 249
Colostomies, 200, 229
Coma scale, 327, 333
Compartment syndrome, 78, 87–88, 109, 131–132, 284, 295, 318, 322–324
Congenital cyanosis, 354, 361
Contraceptives, oral, 207, 237
Contusion, pulmonary, 110, 133
Coombs test, 46, 63
Coronary artery bypass graft (CABG), 261, 274–275
Coronary artery bypass surgery, 261, 274–275
Coronary artery disease, 5, 23
Corticosteroids, 183
Craniopharyngiomas, 331, 337
Crohn disease, 74, 82, 212, 216, 225, 240, 243, 250–251
Cryoprecipitate, 48, 65
Cryptorchidism, 145, 162
Cushing disease, 179, 193
Cushing response, 336
Cushing syndrome, 179, 186, 192–193
Cyclooxygenase enzyme, 28
Cyclophosphamide, 149, 165–166
Cyclosporine, 138, 152, 154, 156, 167
Cystic teratomas, 265–266, 279
Cytomegalovirus, 40, 57–58, 140, 156–157, 166

D
Deep vein thrombosis (*see* Venous thrombosis)
Dermoid cysts, 265–266, 279
Desmopressin (DDAVP), 6
Diabetes mellitus, 222, 248
Diabetic ulcers, 80, 89
Diaphragmatic hernia, 353, 360
Diaphragmatic injuries, 22, 88, 93, 98, 106–107, 113, 116, 130

Dieulafoy lesion, 221, 247
Diverticulitis, 204, 234
Diverticulosis, 234
Diverticulum
    Meckel, 218, 244–245, 350, 357
    Zenker, 260, 274
Dobutamine, 41, 59
Dopamine, 40, 57, 267, 280
Doxorubicin (Adriamycin), 149, 165
Drug packets, 52, 70
Dukes C tumor, 151
Dumping syndrome, 201, 229–230
Duodenal hematoma, 95, 117–118
Duodenal ulcers, 200
Duodenostomy, 349, 357

E

Echinococcal infections, 214, 241
Electrical injuries, 98, 121
Empyema, 269
Energy requirements, 17, 35
Enflurane, 71
Enteral nutrition, 7, 26
Enteritis, 208, 237–238
Enzyme(s)
    cyclooxygenase, 28
    urokinase, 286, 297
Epiglottitis, 341, 345–346
Epinephrine, 44–45, 61, 63, 266,
    279–280
Epstein-Barr virus, 149, 166, 343
Esophageal atresia, 350, 357–358
Esophageal hernia, 205, 214, 235–236, 242
Esophageal spasm, diffuse, 256, 270–271
Esophagectomy, 254, 270
Esophagogram, 256, 271
Esophagoscopy, 274
Esophagus
    carcinomas of, 210, 238–239
    corrosive injuries to, 256, 271
    hernias, 205, 214, 235–236, 242
    perforation of, 254, 270
    rupture, 257, 272
    varices, 201, 231
Ewing sarcoma, 319, 326
Extracorporeal membrane oxygenation
    (ECMO), 48, 65–66
Extubation, 37, 55

F

Facial injuries, 339, 343–344
Facial nerves, 144, 161
Fasciotomy, 284, 295
Fat embolism syndrome, 50, 68
Femoral arteries, 288, 298–299, 318
Femoral hernia, 206, 318
Femur fracture, open, 315, 321
Fibroblasts, 81, 85–86
Fistulas, 9, 28, 105, 127, 129
Flail chest, 96, 112, 119, 134
Fluid resuscitation, 13, 32, 104, 109,
    127–128, 131–132
Fractures (*See also specific fractures*)
    epiphyseal growth disturbance,
        316, 323
    open versus closed reduction, 318, 324
    types and causes, 318–319, 324–325
Frostbite, 74, 82

G

Gallbladder, 42, 59–60, 204, 222,
    234, 248
Gallstone ileus, 203, 233
Gallstone pancreatitis, 211, 239
Gas gangrene, 51, 69
Gastrectomy, 10, 29
Gastric erosive lesions, 220, 246
Gastric outlet obstruction, 47, 64
Gastric ulcers, 197, 202, 226, 231
Gastrinoma, 210, 239
Gastroschisis, 356
Genitourinary injuries, 103, 127
Glasgow coma scale, 327, 333
Glenohumeral dislocations, 316, 322–323
Glioblastoma multiforme, 328, 334
Glucagonomas, 171, 185
Glutamine, 124
Goiter, 259, 273
Graft-versus-host disease, 140, 157
Greenfield filter (*see* Vena caval filter)
Greenstick fractures, 325

H

Halothane, 71
Hamartoma, 263, 277
Head trauma, 95–96, 99, 118–119, 122,
    339, 343

Heart
   arterial embolus of, 286, 298
   congenital defects, 354, 361
   graft occlusion, 286, 297
Heart failure, congestive, 5, 23
Herat transplantation, 140, 147,
      156–157, 164
Helicobacter pylori infection, 202, 232
Hemangiomas, 223, 248–249
Hematemesis, 249
Hematomas
   epidural, 329, 335, 338
   subdural, 332, 338
   retroperitoneal, 51
   wound, 170, 184
Hemianopsia, 170, 184–185
Hemobilia, 215, 243
Hemodialysis, 138, 145, 154–155, 162
Hemolysis, 56
Hemophilia A, 9, 28
Hemorrhage
   esophageal varices, 201, 231
   heparin reversal, 7, 26
   retroperitoneal, 69
   subarachnoid, 330, 332, 335–336, 338
Hemothorax, 110, 132
Heparin, 4, 7, 22, 24, 26, 51, 69
Hepatitis, 40, 58
Hernias
   diaphragmatic, 353, 360
   esophageal, 205, 214, 235–236, 242
   femoral, 206, 318
   inguinal, 202, 219, 232–233, 245
   paraesophageal, 217, 244
   types and causes, 232–233
   umbilical, 347, 355–356
Hirschsprung disease, 347, 355
HIV (human immunodeficiency virus),
      148, 164
Hodgkin disease, 265–266, 279
Hormonal response to injuries, 94, 101,
      116, 124
Horner syndrome, 262, 276
Hyoid bone, 341, 345
Hyperaldosteronism, 178, 191–192
Hypercalcemia, 171, 174, 185, 187–188
Hyperkalemia, 15, 33, 102, 126
Hypermagnesemia, 1, 18

Hyperoxaluria, 1, 19
Hyperparathyroidism, 150, 166, 171, 174,
      176–177, 185, 187–188, 190–191
Hyperthermia, malignant, 13, 31–32, 49,
      66–67
Hypocalcemia, 11, 29–30
Hypomagnesemia, 2, 19–20
Hyponatremial, 18–19, 50, 67
Hypophosphatemia, 7, 26–27
Hypospadias, 308
Hypotension, 3, 99, 122
Hypovolemia, 2, 19, 21
Hypoxemia, 57, 64
Hypoxia, 38, 56–57

I
Ileal atresia, 348, 356
Ileostomy, 225, 250
Inappropriate ADH secretion syndrome,
      14, 33
Incontinence, 303, 308
Infections
   anaerobic, 79, 88
   echinococcal, 214, 241
   necrotizing skin and soft tissue, 51, 69
   nosocomial, 8, 27, 79, 88
   postoperative, prevention of, 12, 30–31
Inflammatory bowel disease, 74, 82
Inguinal hernia, 202, 219, 232–233, 245
Injuries (*see also specific injuries*)
   body's response to, 94, 101, 116, 124
   hormonal response to, 94, 101, 116, 124
Insulin, 94, 116
Insulinomas, 179, 194, 239–240
Interleukin 2, 138, 154
Intestines
   carcinoid tumors of, 181, 195
   injuries to, 105, 129
   ischemia, 290, 299–300
   obstructions in, 38, 56, 95, 118, 203,
      212, 233–234, 240
   surgery and enteral nutrition, 7, 26
Intracranial metastases, 328, 334
Intracranial pressure, 53, 71, 95–96, 119,
      132, 327, 330, 333, 336
Intravenous catheters, 104, 127–128
Intubation, 51, 68–69
Intussusception, 349, 357

Ischemia, intestinal, 281, 293
Ischemic ulcers, 80, 89

J
Jejunoileal bypass, 1, 19
Joint dislocation, 98, 121–122

K
Kidney
  cancer of, 310–311
  dialysis, 138, 154–155
    versus transplantation, 145, 162
  failure of, 50, 67
  injuries to, 103, 126–127
  lesions, 305, 310–311
Kidney stones, 304, 309
Kidney transplantation, 137–138, 141, 147,
    150–151, 153–156, 158, 164, 166
Knees
  dislocation of, 98, 121–122
  vascular injury to, 98

L
Laparotomy, 52, 70, 91, 113, 130–131
Laryngeal obstructions, 112, 134
Legg-Calve-Perthes (LCP) disease, 315,
    321–322
Leukoplakia, 77, 86
Lidocaine, 44, 61
Li-Fraumeni syndrome, 148, 165
Lips
  cleft, and palate, 77, 86
  squamous cell carcinoma of, 76, 84–85
Liver
  abscesses, 205, 235
  adenomas, 207, 237
  cysts, 214, 241
  hemangiomas, 223, 248–249
  lesions, 207, 237
  metastases, 202, 232
Liver transplantation, 137, 141, 153,
    157–158
Lobectomy, 253, 268
Lungs
  abscesses, 255, 270
  coin lesions, 263, 276–277
  metastases, 147, 164
  tumor types, 263, 277

Lymph nodes, 142, 159
Lymphadenopathy, 342, 346
Lymphedema, 282, 293
Lymphomas, 144, 159, 161

M
Malignant hyperthermia, 13, 31–32, 49,
    66–67
Mallory-Weiss syndrome, 249
Malrotation, intestinal, 351, 358–359
Mannitol, 327, 333
Marjolin ulcer, 78, 87, 89
Maxillary fractures, 343–344
Meckel diverticulum, 218, 244–245, 350, 357
Meconium ileus, 352, 359
Median nerve, 97, 119–120
Mediastinal hematoma, 258, 273
Mediastinum, 108, 131, 259, 273
Melanomas, 73, 78, 81, 87
MELD (model for end-stage liver disease)
    score, 139
Meningiomas, 331, 337
Meniscal tears, 315, 321
Mesenteric arteries, 5, 23–24, 290,
    293–294, 299–300, 348, 356
Metastatic disease, 328, 334
Methemoglobinemia, 76, 84
Methoxyflurane, 71
Mohs surgery, 75, 83
Molybdenum deficiency, 31
Monoclonal antibody drug, 141, 158
Monocytes, 73, 81
Monteggia deformity, 318–319, 325
Morphine, 52–53, 71
Multiple endocrine neoplasia (MEN),
    160, 162
Myocardial contusion, 257, 272
Myocardial infarction, 5, 23
Myocarditis, 265, 278
Myotomy, 256, 271

N
Nasogastric decompression, 48, 66
Nasopharyngeal carcinoma, 339–340,
    343–344
Navicular fracture, 318–319, 324
Neck mass, 342, 346
Neck wounds, 94, 117

Necrotizing enterocolitis, 351, 359
Necrotizing fasciitis, 100, 123
Nephrectomy, 305, 310
Nephroblastomas, 143, 159–160
Neurofibromas, 337
Neurofibromatosis, 146, 162
Nitroprusside, 266, 280
Nitrous oxide, 38, 52–53, 56, 71
Non-Hodgkin lymphoma, 144, 161
Nonsteroidal anti-inflammatory drugs,
    10, 28–29
Norepinephrine, 280
Nosocomial infections, 8, 27, 79, 88
Nutrition
    cancers and, 147, 163
    enteral, 7, 26
    parenteral total, 7, 26–27, 105, 129
    protein, adequacy of, 47, 64
    resting energy expenditures, 17, 35

O

Octreotide, 171, 185, 201, 230
Ogilvie syndrome, 215, 242
OKT3, 141, 158
Oliguria, 2, 19, 281, 292
Omeprazole (Prilosec), 197, 226
Omphalocele, 351, 356, 358
Opiate antagonists, 42, 59
Orbital fractures, 103, 126
Orchiopexy, 304–305, 309–310
Organ transplantation, 150, 166 (See also
    specific organs)
Oropharyngeal carcinoma, 344
Osteitis deformans, 319, 325
Osteitis fibrosa cystica, 10, 29, 190,
    319, 325
Osteogenesis imperfecta, 319, 325
Osteogenic sarcoma, 320, 325
Osteoid osteoma, 320, 325
Osteomalacia, 319, 325
Osteopetrosis, 325
Osteosarcoma, 148, 165, 320, 325
Oxygen dissociation curve, 39, 56–57

P

p53 tumor suppressor gene, 148, 165
Paget disease, 319, 325
    of breast, 175, 189–190

Palate, cleft, 77, 86
Pancoast tumors, 262, 276
Pancreas
    annular, 349, 356–357
    carcinomas, 218, 244, 248
    cystadenocarcinomas, 199, 228
    injuries, 104, 127
    pseudocysts, 199, 221, 228, 246–247
    tumors, 175, 179, 190, 194, 200, 211,
        229, 239–240
Pancreatic transplantation, 141, 158
Pancreatectomy, 248
Pancreaticoduodenectomy, 200, 229, 248
Pancreatitis, 208, 211, 237, 239
Paraesophageal hernia, 217, 244
Parathyroid adenomas, 177, 191,
    265–266, 279
Parathyroid hormone (PTH), 185
Parathyroidectomy, 166, 319, 325
Parenteral nutrition, total, 7, 26–27,
    105, 129
Parotid carcinoma, 144, 161
Patent ductus arteriosus, 361
Pelvic fractures, 104, 127–128
Peptic ulcer disease, 261, 275
Pericardial tamponade, 112, 134–135
Perirectal abscesses, 145, 161–162
Peritoneal lavage, 108
Peutz-Jeghers syndrome, 203, 234
Pharyngeal carcinoma, 344
Pheochromocytomas, 146, 162, 189,
    265–266, 279
Physiologic monitoring, 53, 71
Pilonidal cyst, 206, 236
Pituitary tumors, 170, 184–185, 329, 335
Platelet-derived growth factor (PDGF), 81
Platelet dysfunction, 6, 9, 24–25, 28–29
Pneumatic antishock garment, 104, 128
Pneumonia, aspiration, 48, 66
Pneumopericardium, 261, 275–276
Pneumothorax, 93–94, 102, 112, 115,
    117, 125, 135, 256, 271
Poiseuille law, 127
Popliteal aneurysms, 287, 298
Positive-pressure ventilation, 43, 45, 60, 62
Postoperative complications, 4, 22–23
Postoperative energy requirements, 17, 35
Potassium, 12, 15, 30, 33

Pregnancy
    appendicitis during, 214, 241–242
    carpal tunnel syndrome, 76, 85
    chemotherapy during, 175, 189
    venous thrombosis during, 5, 24
Preoperative testing, 3, 20–21
Priapism, 307, 312
Prilosec (omeprazole), 197, 226
Proctocolectomy, 225, 250
Prostate cancer, 305, 311
Prostatic hyperplasia, benign, 306, 311
Prostatitis, 307, 313
Protamine sulfate, 51, 69
Protein nutrition, adequacy of, 47, 64
Prothrombin time, 54, 71
PTH (parathyroid hormone), 185
Pulmonary artery atresia, 361
Pulmonary artery catheter, 53, 71
Pulmonary capillary wedge pressure, 45, 62
Pulmonary embolus, 51, 69, 289, 299
Pulsus paradoxus, 61
Pupillary dilation, 96, 119
Purpura, idiopathic thrombocytopenic,
    197, 226
Pyelogram, 10, 29, 103
Pyoderma gangrenosum, 74, 82, 89

Q
Quincke pulse, 265, 278

R
Radial nerve, 95, 118, 317, 323
Radiation therapy, 146, 163, 189
Rectal abscesses, 206, 236
Rectal carcinoid tumors, 222, 247–248
Rectal injuries, 101, 124–125
Rectus sheath hematoma, 205, 235
Reiter syndrome, 265, 278
Renal failure, 50, 67
Renal transplantation (*see* Kidney
    transplantation
Respiratory distress syndrome
    acute, 43, 60–61
    adult, 38, 56
Resting energy expenditures, 17, 35
Rib fractures, 92, 113–114
Ringer lactate solution, 11, 14, 30, 32–33,
    79, 103, 126

S
Salicylate intoxication, 4, 21–22
Salivary gland tumors, 340, 344
Sarcomas, soft tissue, 142, 144,
    160–161
Schwannomas, 330, 336–337
Seatbelt sign, 91, 113
Selenium deficiency, 31
Seminomas, 304, 309–310
Sepsis
    body's response to, 101, 124
    central venous pressure, 50, 67
    energy requirements, 35
    signs and symptoms, 15, 34
    tumor necrosis factor and, 137, 153
Shivering, 47, 65
Shock
    biochemical changes, 102, 126
    cardiogenic, 41, 59, 97, 120
    hypovolemic, 41, 58, 103, 126
    neurogenic, 44, 61–62, 109, 131
    septic, 43, 60
Shoulder dislocations, 318–319, 325
Sigmoid volvulus, 213, 241
Silver nitrate, 76, 84
Skin abnormalities, 75, 83–84
Skull fractures, 328, 334–335
Smoke inhalation injuries, 52, 70
Spinal cord injuries, 109, 131
Spiral fracture, 325
Spleen, 92, 108, 114, 130–131
Splenectomy, 208, 237
Squamous cell carcinomas, 75–77, 84–85,
    87, 89, 340, 342, 344, 346
Staphylococcus infections, 79, 88
Stenosis
    aortic, 253, 268
    hypertrophic pyloric, 352, 359–360
Stomach, non-Hodgkin lymphoma, 144,
    161
Stress tests, 3, 20–21
Stress ulceration, 220, 246
Strokes, 45, 62
Subarachnoid hemorrhage, 330, 332,
    335–336, 338
Subclavian steal syndrome, 285, 296
Superior vena cava syndrome, 254,
    269–270

Surgery, cardiac risks and, 44, 61
Surgical wounds (*see* Wounds)

T
T cells, 138, 141, 154, 158
Tendon injuries, 74, 82–83
Testicles, undescended, 304, 309
Testicular cancer, 141, 145, 159, 162, 304,
    309–310
Testicular torsion, 305, 310
Tetany, 2, 19–20
Tetralogy of Fallot, 354, 361
Thermal burns, 121
Thiamine deficiency, 31
Thoracic duct injury, 258, 273–274
Thoracic outlet syndrome, 261, 275
Thoracotomy, 105, 110, 128–129, 132,
    254, 256, 262, 269, 271, 276
Thrombin time, 54, 72
Thrombocytopenia, 4, 6, 22, 25, 197, 226
Thromboplastin time, 72
Thymomas, 265–266
Thyroglossal duct cyst, 341,
    344–345, 358
Thyroid gland
    adenomas, 169, 183, 191
    carcinomas, 172, 178, 186, 192–193
    embryologic origination, 358
    nodules, 178, 192–193
Thyroid hormones, 116
Thyroid storm, 176–177, 190–191
Thyroidectomy, 11, 30
Tongue cancer, 341, 345
Tracheobronchial injury, 111, 133
Tracheoesophageal fistula, 350, 356
Tracheoinnominate artery fistula (TIAF),
    55, 64
Tracheostomy, 48, 66, 68
Transposition of great vessels, 354, 361
Trauma victims, 35
Tricuspid regurgitation, 265, 278
Tumor grading and staging, 142, 159
Tumor lysis syndrome, 138, 154
Tumor necrosis factor (TNF), 81,
    137, 153
Turner syndrome, 265, 278–279

U
Ulnar nerve, 73, 81
Umbilical hernia, 347, 355–356
Ureteral injury, 10, 29, 306, 312
Urethral injuries, 103, 111, 127, 134,
    306, 312
Urinary incontinence, 303, 308
Urinary tract infections, 9, 27
Urokinase, 286, 297

V
VACTERL syndrome, 348, 356
Vagotomy, 201–202, 229–231
Vascular injuries, 92–93, 98, 114–115,
    121–122
Vasopressin, 116
Vena caval filter, 7, 24, 26, 289, 299
Venous statis ulcers, 80, 89
Venous thrombosis
    diagnosis and treatment, 5, 24, 290, 300
    portal, 137, 153, 208, 237
    splenic, 208, 237
    treatment of, 281, 292
Ventricular septal defect, 354, 361
Vitamin K, 27
Vitelline duct, 350, 357
Vocal cord dysfunction, 184
von Hippel-Lindau disease, 164
von Willebrand disease, 24–25, 65

W
Warfarin, 24
Wilms tumor, 143, 159–160
Wounds (*See also* Infections)
    bacterial contamination classifications,
    75, 83
    contraction, 77, 85–86
    healing, 74, 81–82
    management of, 76, 84
    treatment of, 78, 88

Z
Zenker diverticulum, 260, 274
Zinc, deficiency of, 13, 31
Zollinger-Ellison syndrome, 175, 190,
    210, 239

Notes